MON BIO-MEDICAL SCIENCES SERIES

Editor: Roger Maickel
Indiana University
Bloomington

Environmental Health and Safety
PBMSS-1

Environmental
Health and Safety

Herman Koren
Indiana State University
Terre Haute, Indiana

PERGAMON PRESS INC.

New York · Toronto
Oxford · Sydney
Braunschweig

PERGAMON PRESS INC.
Maxwell House, Fairview Park, Elmsford, N.Y. 10523

PERGAMON OF CANADA LTD.
207 Queen's Quay West, Toronto 117, Ontario

PERGAMON PRESS LTD.
Headington Hill Hall, Oxford

PERGAMON PRESS (AUST.) PTY. LTD.
Rushcutters Bay, Sydney, N.S.W.

VIEWEG & SOHN GmbH
Burgplatz l, Braunschweig

Library of Congress Cataloging in Publication Data

Koren, Herman.
    Environmental health and safety.

    (Pergamon bio-medical sciences series, 1)
    1. Hospitals--Hygiene.   2.   Hospitals--Safety
measures.   I.   Title.   II.   Series.
[DNLM: 1.   Accident prevention.   2.   Environmental
health.   3.   Sanitation.   WA670 K84e 1973]
RA969.K67   1973   614.7'93   72-11634
ISBN 0-08-017077-3
ISBN 0-08-017623-2 (pbk.)

Printed in the United States of America

*To my darling wife Donna, whose
love and support inspire me to
improve the environment of man.*

The Author

Herman Koren, H.S.D., Indiana University and M.P.H., University of Michigan, is currently Associate Professor of Health and Safety specializing in Environmental Health, Department of Health and Safety, Indiana State University, Terre Haute.

Dr. Koren has been an Environmental and Public Health practitioner, applied researcher consultant to hospitals, federal, state and local agencies, and a teacher for more than twenty years.

He has been Chief of Environmental Health and Safety, Philadelphia General Hospital; Associate, Department of Preventive Medicine, University of Pennsylvania Medical School; and Chairman, Committee on Hospital Sanitation, National Environmental Health Association. He is also a Founder Diplomate, American Academy for Certification of Sanitarians, a Registered Professional Sanitarian, as well as a Member of the Editorial Board of the *Journal of Environmental Health* and the *Journal of Milk and Food Technology.*

Contents

Foreword

The successful design and practice of an environmental health and safety program in an institutional setting is a considerable undertaking requiring the integration of a broad range of diverse and complementary resources and skills. The present volume makes available for the first time a complete source where the student or the instructor can find a detailed overview of this emerging public health specialty; and a source where the practicing environmental health and safety specialist can find accurate, comprehensive, practical and concise guidelines for effective action.

This volume also has much of interest and value for the institutional administrator or superintendent who wishes the latest information on the mechanics of environmental health and safety. Likewise, it contains much material of relevance for physicians, nurses, and paramedical personnel affiliated with institutions. The environmental health specialists draw heavily on their experience and judgment in designing and developing many of the programs necessary to achieve the common aim of maximum well-being for residents and staff.

Many of the procedures formerly used in environmental health practice were principally designed to quantitate problems, e.g., the use of culture plates to estimate levels of bacterial contamination. Factual as such precise information is, this type of methodology has, in general, tended to compartmentalize and obscure the larger view of environmental health as it is evolving within the scheme of present-day comprehensive medical care programming.

As an institutional concern and responsibility, the practice of environmental health and safety has developed as a kind of eclectic function. In the past, for example, the dietary department, the engineering department, the nursing division, and other discrete units of the institution were each concerned with segments of the problem of health maintenance and safety requirements for the resident population and staff. Below the level of institutional director, there was usually no designated administrative official to coordinate their individual activities. Obviously, there was duplication in certain areas, complete voids of activity in others, and generally little or no quality control. Furthermore, there was no clear-cut line of authority permitting a follow-through of recommendations and policies when their origin or execution involved members of more than one department. This fault was particularly evident in problem solving requiring the participation of both professional and nonprofessional personnel, such as food handling and preparation or aspects of infection control as determined by the engineering of the ventilation and heating system.

Those of us in the health-related professions realize the many dangers inherent when improper or incomplete provisions exist for the safety and general health of institutional residents. Such populations are frequently compromised by physical and/or mental disability and are particularly prone to suffer from omission of protective controls or lack of sufficiently high standards of sanitation and disease prevention.

Within the past few years, the science of environmental health has progressed sufficiently so that it is now a unified discipline. In the exercise of his profession, the specialist is involved primarily in para-medical and preventive care activities. He not only leans heavily on management practices, statistical techniques, and various psychosocial concepts, but he must also keep current with much basic and applied biomedical information.

Each of the contributors to this volume is a specialist in his own right. Each has oriented his contribution towards giving the reader a more comprehensive view of practical workable programs to achieve maximum effectiveness in his exercise of institutional environmental infection control and safety measures.

Vice President for Medical Affairs   LUTHER TERRY, M.D.
University of Pennsylvania

Acknowledgments

To my teachers F. Carlyle Roberts, Dr. P. Walton Purdom, Russel B. Franklin, William Gibson (deceased), Dr. John Hall, and Dr. John E. Emich, who provided me with an education which never could have been gained in a textbook, a work experience or a university; to Dr. Henry W. Kolbe, an enlightened hospital administrator who guided me, encouraged me, and gave me the opportunity to develop many new programs in Hospital Environmental Health, Infection Control and Safety; to Dr. Johannes Ipsen and the University of Pennsylvania Medical School, who provided a grant for secretarial services at the inception of the manuscript; to the University of Pennsylvania Medical Library who obtained over 800 articles on infections which were listed in Indexus Medicus from 1960–June 1967; to Austin Pryor, friend and colleague, who gave valuable counsel on the Environmental Health chapter; to Mrs. Marlyn Jones, who typed many of the Environmental Health programs and portions of the textbook voluntarily; to Mrs. Ora Lou Leisure for typing portions of this manuscript. A special thank you to my very competent secretary Jeanette Hauer for final typing of the manuscript.

My contributing authors whose extensive experience and training in the fields of hospital administration, medicine, nursing, engineering, environmental health, and hospital safety made this comprehensive text possible.

A special acknowledgment to Dr. Donald Ludwig, Professor of Health and Safety, for final proofreading of the manuscript.

H. K.

Contributing Authors

Casswell, H. Taylor, M.D. Professor of Surgery, Temple University Science Center, Philadelphia, Pa.
Author of Section on Infection Control Committee

Cavalli, Ronald B., P.E. Assistant Manager, Insurance and Loss Control, Thomas J. Lipton Tea Co., Engelwood, N.J.; formerly Safety Engineer (Hospital Safety), Continental Casulty Co., New York, N.Y.
Coauthor of Chapter on Patient and Employee Safety

Dvorak, Rodger, M.P.H. (Hospital Adm.) Associate Director of Administration, Presbyterian-University of Pennsylvania Medical Center, Philadelphia, Pa.
Author of Chapter on The Hospital

Fincher, Edward, Ph.D. Associate Professor of Aerobiology, University of North Carolina, Chapel Hill, N.C.
Author of Section on Microbiological Testing, Air and Surface Sampling Techniques

Foster, Virginia L., M.S. Assistant Professor of Nursing, Indiana State University; formerly Director of Nursing, St. Mary's Hospital, East St. Louis, Ill.
Author of Section on Isolation Procedures

Kereluk, Karl, Ph.D. Manager of Research, American Sterilizer Co., Erie, Pa.
Senior Author of Section on Sterilization

Kirkwood, Edna, M.S (Nursing), Consultant in Sterilization Technique, American Sterilizer Co., Erie, Pa.
Coauthor of Section on Sterilization

Lawton, George M., M.D. Diplomate, American Board of Preventive Medicine in Occupational Health; Director, Industrial Environmental Health Division, Bureau of Medicine and Surgery, Navy Department, Washington, D.C.

Author of Chapter on The Hospital Occupational Health Program. Contributor to Sections 1 and 2 of Chapter on Infection Control

Pryor, Austin, M.S. Manager, Marketing Development, Economics Laboratory, New York, N.Y.

Author of Section on Detergents and Disinfectants — Evaluation and Use in Hospital Environmental Sanitation Practice

Shields, Glen, L., P.E. Consultant on Plumbing and former Chief of Detroit Department of Plumbing, Detroit, Mich.

Author of Section on Plumbing and Cross-Connections

Whytock, Donald C., P.E. Director of Safety, Federation of Jewish Philanthropies of New York; New York, N.Y.

Coauthor of Chapter on Fire Safety

PROFESSIONAL READERS

Kolbe, Henry W., M.D., Director, Pondville Hospital, Department of Public Health, Commonwealth of Mass., Walpole, Mass. Formerly Executive Director of Philadelphia General Hospital.

Purdom, Walton, P., Ph.D., Professor of Environmental Engineering and Director of the Institute of Environmental Engineering, Drexel Institute of Technology, Philadelphia, Pa.

FOREWORD

Terry, Luther, M.D., Vice President for Medical Affairs and Professor of Preventive Medicine, University of Pennsylvania, Philadelphia, Pa.; former Surgeon General, United States Public Health Service.

Introduction

There has been an emphasis in the last few years on such environmental health problems as air pollution, water pollution, and solid waste disposal. However, despite the fact that over 31 million people in the United States are patients in hospitals, nursing homes, convalescent homes, and old age homes each year, and over 59 million people spend a good portion of each day in schools and other institutions, inadequate emphasis has been placed on this highly complex portion of our environment.

This book was written to fill the existing need for a complete comprehensive source of information, tools and techniques in the field of institutional environmental health, safety and infection control. The students and instructors in environmental health, nursing, hospital administration dietetics and safety as well as the practitioners in these fields and in medicine can find accurate, comprehensive, practical and concise guidelines for effective action. Many tested practical, workable problems and techniques are described that can aid in the solution of problems of the institutional environment. This book can be of considerable help as a reference to those involved with enforcing or having to comply with the new Occupational Safety and Health Act. Since the problems of institutions of all types are in many cases the same, colleges, universities, prisons, large corporations, etc. can use or adapt material from this text to suit their needs.

The material of the text was developed during the eighteen years the author has worked as a practitioner, supervisor, administrator, consultant and teacher in the field of environmental health and safety. The author has held positions as Chief of Environmental Health and Safety at Philadelphia General Hospital, Teaching Associate, University of Pennsylvania Medical School, Chairman of the National Committee on the Hospital Environment of the National Environmental Health Association, and consultant to various hospitals on environmental health, infection control, safety, and administration. He is currently Associate Professor of Health and Safety, with specialization in the environment, Indiana State University.

Many of the guidelines, programs and techniques were developed and tested during these eighteen years. Frequently the efficacy of the programs was discussed with many of the physicians of the five medical schools in Philadelphia and with many of the author's professional colleagues throughout the United States.

H. K.

1

The
Hospital

1-1 SIGNIFICANCE OF THE HOSPITAL IN OUR SOCIETY

Intensive care units, cobalt therapy, artificial kidneys, home care programs, open heart surgery, inhalation therapy — these are just a few of the hundreds of terms that were virtually unknown in the hospital of 25 years ago. They point out one very significant characteristic of the modern hospital: it has been, and will continue to be, a rapidly changing institution. Not only are the diagnostic and treatment facilities drastically improving, but the staff working in the hospital today are more highly trained than ever before. Even the patient population is changing. The typical patient today is older than his counterpart of 25 years ago and is more likely to have a diagnosis associated with aging.

1-1-1 Functions of the Hospital

Just what are the functions of today's hospital? They include (1) care of the sick and injured, (2) education, (3) research, and (4) promotion of the community health.

Providing *care of the sick and injured* is the primary purpose for which the hospital exists. All aspects of the hospital operation must be developed with the focus centered on the patient and his needs. Each hospital must determine the service and facilities it will provide to patients, based on its potential capabilities and selected needs of the community.

The patterns of care provided by the hospital today are undergoing dramatic changes. A continuum of care has been developed which is centered within the hospital but which extends into the community. At one end of the continuum is highly specialized intensive care, then comes intermediate care, ambulatory care, extended or long term care, and home care. The outpatient and emergency departments are also providing broader and more comprehensive patterns of care.

1

Education is an important function of every hospital. By no means can it be limited to those hospitals which offer internships, residencies, nursing education and other formal training programs. Even the small community hospital has an obligation to provide ongoing educational opportunities for the medical staff and employees. Only through a continuing education program will a hospital be in a position to provide the best care to patients.

Research likewise cannot be limited to the large medical center with extensive research facilities and large patient populations. Again, the small hospital has an obligation to contribute to the advancement of health through medical research. The research efforts of the small hospital may be modest; nevertheless they are an important aspect of the hospital's overall program.

Unless a hospital participates in the *promotion of community health*, it cannot consider that it has met its responsibilities to the community. This must be accomplished through cooperation and coordination with local health authorities and health agencies in the area. Promoting community health goes beyond the proper handling of patients with communicable diseases and must include concern for every aspect of the health of area residents. To meet this responsibility, hospitals must participate in health education programs, as well as disease detection and prevention programs which extend into the community.

1-1-2   Classification of Hospitals

Over 7100 hospitals exist in the United States. Many persons picture the average hospital in this country as the large metropolitan hospital of several hundred beds. In reality, more than one half of the hospitals in this country have less than 100 beds.

In describing the hospitals in the United States, three classifications are commonly used: type of control, service provided, and length of stay of patients. All hospitals fall into a division of each of these classifications.

Type of Control

Three forms of hospital control or ownership are generally recognized: governmental, proprietary, and voluntary nonprofit.

Governmental hospitals may be federally owned, such as those of the Veterans Administration, the Armed Services, or the United States Public Health Service. They may also be owned by a state, county, city, city-county, or hospital district. Governmental hospitals account for close to 60% of the nation's hospital beds.

The voluntary nonprofit hospitals, which account for about 37% of the nations's hospital beds, are brought into existence by community groups, churches or fraternal orders and are structured so that no individuals obtain any financial gain from their operation. When earnings exceed expenses, they are retained and used by the hospital.

Proprietary hospitals are operated for profit and may be controlled either by an individual, a partnership, or a corporation. They contain approximately 3% of the existing hospital beds in the country.

Service Provided

Hospitals are also classified according to the type of service they provide. Special hospitals restrict their service to a particular specialty of medicine, such as psychiatry, pediatrics, maternity, or tuberculosis. Of the specialty hospitals, psychiatric hospitals are the most common and account for over one-third of the hospital beds in the United States.

General hospitals, which do not limit their care to a specialty of medicine, account for about 59% of this country's hospital beds.

Length of Stay

In addition to classification by type of control and service provided, hospitals are also classified according to the length of stay of their patients. The American Hospital Association defines a "short stay hospital" as one in which over 50% of all patients admitted have a stay of less than 30 days. Conversely, a "long stay hospital" is one in which over 50% of all patients admitted have a stay of 30 days or more. Short stay hospitals exceed long stay hospitals over 7–1 but contain only 59% of the hospital beds in the country.

1-2 ORGANIZATION OF THE HOSPITAL

1-2-1 The Governing Board

The governing board is the highest authority of the voluntary nonprofit hospital. The name of the governing board may vary from one institution to another. It may be called the board of trustees, the board of directors, or the board of managers. Regardless of the name, the duty of the board is the same—to determine the direction the institution will move, and to establish policies consistent with its goals.

The board of trustees should represent a cross-section of the community. Businessmen, educators, health leaders, attorneys, and clergymen all might be found on a typical board. Since board members serve without pay and are expected to donate significant portions of time to hospital affairs, it is important that each member has a deep interest in the hospital.

The size of governing boards vary greatly from hospital to hospital. Some are very small—seven or less—while others have 40 or more persons serving on them. Normally, board members are nominated by members of the hospital corporation or sponsoring organization and are elected to serve a certain term as defined in the by-laws of the hospital.

In order to accomplish some of its responsibilities, committees of the board are frequently established. Those most frequently found include the executive committee, finance committee, building committee, and joint conference committee. The executive committee is most commonly found in hospitals with large governing boards. It normally possesses some executive power and handles many of the routine matters which come to the board's attention. The finance committee is charged with overseeing the financial solvency of the hospital. Routinely reviewing the financial operations of the hospital, establishing rates and charges, approving budgets, counseling on investments and fund raising are all included in the responsibilities of the finance committee. The building committee is concerned with the operation of the physical plant and with planning new construction. The joint conference committee, composed of representatives of the governing board, medical staff, and the administrator, provides a communications bridge between the governing board and the medical staff and serves as a medical advisory committee to the board.

How do trustees spend the time which they devote to their hospital? One recent study indicated that board members spend 40% of their time talking about finances, 20% on building improvements and equipment, 10% on nursing and patient care, 15% on medical staff issues, 10% on community relations and fund raising, and 5% on miscellaneous matters, including personnel.

1-2-2 The Chief Executive Officer

The title assigned to the Chief Executive Officer of the hospital by the governing board will vary from one hospital to another. "Administrator," "Director," "Executive Vice-President," and "Executive Director" are commonly used.

The Chief Executive Officer also serves as the day-to-day liaison officer between the governing board and the medical staff. As the board's representative, he interprets to the medical staff the policies and

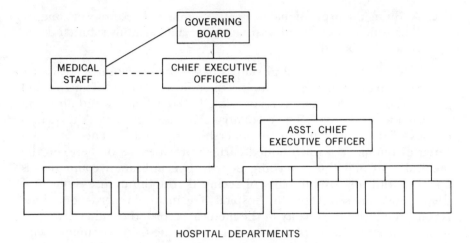

Figure 1-1 Organization chart of a typical voluntary nonprofit hospital.

decisions of the board which are pertinent to the staff. Conversely, he is expected to convey to the board matters of concern to the medical staff which are beyond his administrative authority.

The Chief Executive Officer's responsibility for the day-to-day internal operation of the hospital involves managing, coordinating and directing activities performed by employees. Hospital employees are generally grouped into departments, each of which is supervised by a department head. The department heads report either to the Chief Executive Officer or to a designated member of the administrative staff (*see* Figure 1-1).

Interpreting the hospital to the community and promoting community health are essential aspects of the Chief Executive Officer's position. The hospital exists for the purpose of serving the community, and if it is to fulfill this objective, the Chief Executive Officer must be in close touch with all facets of the community.

1-2-3 Medical Staff

The medical staff of the hospital directs the patient care effort of the hospital. The staff serves the following functions:

a. Providing professional care of the sick and injured in the hospital
b. Maintaining its own efficiency
c. Self government
d. Participating in education

 e. Auditing the professional work

 f. Furnishing advice and assistance to the Administrator and the governing board*

Organization of the medical staff is based on a committee structure. The executive committee, containing the officers of the staff and a small group of other physicians, is responsible for coordinating and directing the activities of the staff. The credential committee evaluates the qualifications of those applying for membership on the staff. The joint conference committee, as mentioned earlier, provides liaison between the medical staff and the governing board. The utilization committee is charged with the responsibility of seeing that optimum use is made of the facilities and services of the hospital. The medical records committee is concerned with the quality of the medical record, the audit committee with the overall quality of care rendered, and the tissue committee with evaluating tissue removed during surgery to insure that operative procedures are justified. Other medical staff committees are developed by each hospital based on needs.

In order to obtain membership on a medical staff, a physician must complete an application form detailing his background. This application is then presented to the credentials committee of the medical staff with appropriate supporting documents and recommendations. If the credentials committee approves the application, it is submitted to the executive committee of the medical staff, then normally to the joint conference committee and finally to the governing board. Only the governing board has the authority and responsibility to make appointments to the medical staff.

Division of the medical staff into departments or services is common in all but the smallest hospitals. The most common of these departments include medicine, surgery, obstetrics-gynecology, pediatrics, pathology, radiology, and anesthesiology. However, in larger hospitals many additional departments may exist as dictated by the specialties represented in the medical staff and the emphasis given them by the hospital.

Each member of the medical staff is not only assigned to a department according to his training and experience, but is further classified according to the degree of his responsibility in contributing to the medical care program of the hospital.

The classification recommended by the Joint Commission on Accreditation of Hospitals, the national hospital accrediting agency, is as follows:

*From MacEachern, M. T. *Hospital Organization and Management.* Berwyn. Ill.: Physician's Record Co., 1957. With permission.

The Honorary Medical Staff:
The honorary medical staff shall consist of physicians and dentists who are not active in the hospital or who are honored by emeritus positions. These may be physicians and dentists who have retired from active hospital practice or who are of outstanding reputation, not necessarily residing in the community. Honorary staff members shall not be eligible to admit patients, to vote, to hold office or to serve on standing medical staff committees.

The Active Medical Staff:
The active medical staff shall consist of physicians and dentists who regularly admit patients to the hospital, who are located closely enough to the hospital to provide continuous care to their patients, and who assume all the functions and responsibilities of membership on the active medical staff, including, where appropriate, emergency service care and consultation assignments. Members of the active medical staff shall be appointed to a specific department, shall be eligible to vote, to hold office and to serve on medical staff committees, and shall be required to attend medical staff meetings.

The Associate Medical Staff:
The associate medical staff shall consist of physicians and dentists who are being considered for advancement to membership on the active staff. They shall be appointed to a specific department and shall be eligible to serve on departmental committees and to vote on matters before such committees. They shall be ineligible to hold office in this medical staff organization. They shall be required to attend medical staff meetings.

The Courtesy Medical Staff:
The courtesy medical staff shall consist of physicians and dentists qualified for staff membership but who only occasionally admit patients to the hospital or who act only as consultants. Courtesy medical staff members shall be appointed to a specific department but shall not be eligible to vote or to hold office in this medical staff organization.

1-2-4 Relationships Between the Governing Board, Chief Executive Officer, and Medical Staff

Liaison between the governing board, its agent the Chief Executive Officer, and the medical staff is essential to maintain smooth and clearly understood hospital-physician relationships. The complexity of these relationships has been well expressed by member Frank M. Stanley, (then president), Board of Directors, South Chicago Community Hospital:

> The great contrast in the positions of the hospital trustee and member of the medical staff is that the trustee carries his tremendous responsibility entirely as a contribution to the community welfare whereas the doctor's membership on the Medical Staff is the greatest single factor in his financial and professional standing. The natural

difference in viewpoint that results from different positions is so great that each must make a constant effort to understand the other's views. In many other situations with contacts of this kind, there are daily inter-relationships, which in turn help to solve differences of opinion and thinking. Unfortunately, the opportunities and avenues with communications between the hospital board and the Medical Staff are relatively limited, and the communication that does exist tends to be formal, rather than an informal day to day give and take, which can most often solve many delicate problems.* (pp. 2–3)

Providing the necessary formal liaison between the governing board, the Chief Executive Officer, and the medical staff can be accomplished in a number of ways. Often times, a Joint Conference Committee is created for this purpose. The committee is composed of members of the governing board, the medical staff, and the Chief Executive Officer.

1-2-5 Departments Within the Hospital

In addition to the division of the medical staff into departments, hospital employees likewise work within a departmental framework. These departments are responsible to the Chief Executive Officer or to a member of the administrative staff. The departments commonly found in the hospital include the following:

Admitting. Responsible for the admission of patients into the hospital in accordance with the policies of the governing board.

Business Office. Handles the management of all accounting activities within the hospital, including patient accounts, accounts payable, payroll, credit and collections, and financial reports.

Central Supply. Prepares, stores and issues sterile supplies and other related items used in the care and treatment of patients.

Chaplain. Coordinates the religious activities program of the hospital.

Data Processing. Deals with the accumulation, processing and presentation of selected information covering the hospital operation.

Development. Cultivates sources of donation income.

Electrocardiography. Responsible for taking electrocardiograms (heart tracings) and preparing them for interpretation by physicians.

Electroencephalography. Responsible for taking electroencephalograms (brain tracings) which are interpreted by physicians.

Emergency Room. Provides screening and emergency treatment to patients.

Engineering Department. Maintains the hospital physical plant including heating, air conditioning, electricity, plumbing, and routine upkeep of the hospital facilities.

*Stanley, Frank M. "The Board, the Staff, the Administrator – Checks and Balances in Hospital Government". Reprinted with permission from the author and *TRUSTEE*, published by The American Hospital Association, February 1965 issue.

Environmental Sanitation. Supervises the environmental health program of the hospital.

Food Service Department. Prepares all of the meals which are served to patients and employees and is responsible for the nutritional education of patients and students.

Housekeeping Department. Keeps the hospital in a clean and sanitary condition in accordance with established standards.

Industrial Engineering. Improves, designs and installs systems and procedures so as to maximize effectiveness at optimum cost.

Inhalation Therapy. Provides treatment concerned with the proper exchange of oxygen and carbon dioxide in the patient's lungs.

Laundry. Launders soiled hospital linens and prepares clean linen for distribution.

Medical Education. Coordinates the educational programs of interns, residents, and medical students.

Medical Library. Maintains medical periodicals and books to assist the hospital staff in keeping aware of recent developments in the field of medicine, and also to assist in medical research.

Medical Records Department. Maintains a file of patient records and handles the release of information from these records in accordance with hospital policy.

Nursing Education. Administers educational programs for nursing students (both professional and licensed practical nurses).

Nursing Service. Provides nursing care to patients in accordance with hospital standards and physician's directives.

Occupational Therapy. Provides therapeutic exercise and training to improve functional ability utilizing techniques and crafts.

Out-Patient Department. Provides diagnosis and treatment to ambulatory patients through scheduled clinics.

Pathology Department. Performs laboratory tests used in the treatment and diagnosis of patients, examines tissue specimens and performs autopsies.

Personnel Department. Handles the recruitment and screening of applicants for vacant positions, and oversees the entire personnel program of the hospital.

Pharmacy. Supplies drugs to both in and out patient areas.

Physical Therapy. Provides treatment to patients using modalities including exercise, electrical stimulation, heat, water, and sound.

Public Relations Department. Interprets the hospital to the community through mass media, published reports and contact with members of the public.

Purchasing Department. Provides a mechanism for the centralized procurement of supplies and equipment.

Radiology Department. Supplies diagnostic as well as therapeutic radiology services to in and out patients.

Security. Coordinates and directs all aspects of the hospital security program.

Social Service Department. Assists the patient, his family, and the patient care team in their understanding of the social, economic, and emotional factors relating to the patient's illness.

Telephone Service. Operates the hospital switchboard and paging system.

Volunteer Service Department. Coordinates the use of volunteer services within the hospital.

1-3 HUMAN RELATIONS

When one considers that between 65% and 70% of the typical voluntary hospital's budget is composed of salaries and wages, the importance of the relationships between people within the organization becomes immediately apparent. The unique nature of these relationships has been noted by Georgopoulos and Mann:

> Work in the hospital is greatly differentiated and specialized, and of a highly international character. It is carried out by a large number of cooperating people whose backgrounds, education, training, skills, and functions are as diverse and heterogeneous as can be found in any part of the most complex organization in existence. Because of this extensive division of labor every person working in the hospital depends upon some other person or persons for the performance of his own organizational role. Specialists and professionals can perform their functions only when a considerable array of supportive personnel and auxiliary services is put at their disposal at all times. Doctors, nurses, and others in the hospital do not, and cannot, function separately or independently of one another. Their work is mutually supplementary, interlocking and interdependent. In turn, such a high interdependence requires that many departments, groups and individuals of the organization be sufficiently coordinated, if the organization is to function effectively and attain its objectives.* (p. 7)

An organizational chart has limitations in indicating how people actually relate to one another within an organization. Its purpose is to define the formal lines of authority, but the extent to which they are followed may be an entirely different matter. The relationships of people within an organization as they seek to accomplish objectives established for them are governed by many things. Included among these factors are past successes and failures in contacts with others, the desire to shortcut complexities, and the intricacies of human personalities with varying motivations, interests, and ideas. The outgrowth of these relationships is the informal organization.

1-3-1 Informal Organization

The informal organization reflects the channels which are utilized to

---

*Reprinted with permission from Georgopoulos, B. S. and Mann, F. C. *The Community General Hospital.* © Macmillan Company, 1962.

accomplish organizational objectives. These channels may be far different from those shown in the organizational chart itself. Examples of the informal organization are found in every hospital. A nurse who stops a plumber as he is walking through her unit and convinces him to repair a leaky faucet in a patient room is a typical example of the informal organization. If she were to follow the organizational lines to accomplish this repair, she would be required to submit a requisition which might be screened at least by her supervisor as well as the plumber's supervisor before the job is accomplished. Another example of the informal organization is the physical therapist who, after finding that patients from one nursing station are constantly arriving late for treatments, resolves the matter by a direct conference with the nurses concerned. If strict organizational channels had been followed, this problem might well have been referred from the physical therapy department to a member of the administrative staff, then to the director of nursing service and finally to the personnel concerned.

1-3-2 Interdepartmental Relations

Departments within the hospital are dependent upon one another. For example, the nursing units are dependent upon the laundry for fresh linen; the operating rooms are dependent upon central supply for sterile supplies; the switchboard depends upon the admitting office for the names of patients who enter the hospital, so that patients will receive phone calls intended for them; the food service department is dependent upon the receiving department for food supplies, and so on and on.

The varying functions of each department added to the backgrounds, skill levels, and motivations of the staff in each department make interdepartmental relations a complex matter. Conflicts and misunderstandings frequently result. For example, it is not unusual for the food service department to have misunderstandings with the nursing department. The nursing department must advise the food service department of varying patient meal needs—the food service department must supply food in the quantity needed and at the designated meal times. Slip-ups, and misunderstandings are inevitable from time to time.

Business office employees, too, may become involved in interdepartmental conflicts. This is due largely to their tasks which are related to financial solvency, although the primary objective of the organization is humanitarian.

Problems between the laundry and the nursing department are

classic. Nursing personnel feel that clean linen should always be available when needed. Unfortunately, the maintaining of realistic inventory levels, and the processing and the delivering of linen to nursing units on a day in, day out basis is highly complicated.

Intricate relationships between departments, such as the examples above, are duplicated all over the hospital. Successful interdepartmental relations are largely dependent upon the spirit of cooperation and understanding which exist and require continued effort on the part of each one concerned.

1-3-3 Intradepartmental Relations

In some departments, a widely varying level of skills exists. Others have personnel with about the same skill levels. Some departments operate within one geographical area, while the activities of others take them into all corners of the hospital.

The pathology department is an example of a department with widely varying skills. The pathologist, a physician with at least three years or more of training beyond his internship, provides the professional direction of the department. Subordinate to him are laboratory technologists, many with college degrees. Further down the line are the laboratory aides and glasswashers whose skill levels may be very basic. A hierarchy exists within such an organizational structure which minimizes the possibility of a warm relationship between all members of the department.

Burling, Lentz, and Wilson in their book *The Give and Take in Hospitals*, have noted:

> The laboratory director is the spokesman for the department to the rest of the hospital. He is responsible for the administration of all the work, but usually delegates the routine aspects to a chief technician. While his reputation is often a source of pride to the technicians, his relationship with them is frequently a somewhat distant one. Each can respect the competence of the others but the tasks of each are sufficiently different that they do not compete with one another. On the other hand, the relationships among the laboratory technicians, including the supervisor, are close and informal, apparently so much so that they satisfy social needs of the workers.* (p. 296)

In contrast to the laboratory, the laundry is composed of a group with about the same skill levels. Working together in the same areas, it is more likely that a feeling of group cohesiveness will develop within such a department. Mr. Thomas R. O'Donovan, Associate Administrator of

*From Burling, T., Lentz, E., and Wilson, R. *The Give and Take in Hospitals*. New York: Putnam's, 1956. With permission.

the Mount Carmel Mercy Hospital, Detroit, has contrasted human relations within the Laundry with those which exist within the House-keeping Department where individuals have the same skill levels but generally do not work together.

> If the nature of the job is such that the workers performing the task do not work together in the same area, this has effect on group cohesiveness in the informal organization. In such cases, their group cohesiveness would be less and morale would tend to be lower among such workers.
>
> In contrast, if the employees work together as a team on projects, there is an opportunity for greater cohesiveness, a strengthening of the morale. In the hospital, we find that housekeeping workers tend to be geographically dispersed through the hospital in their work assignments. Thus, the maids do not have a close-knit informal organization among themselves. However, laundry workers tend to have their working area centralized and therefore their cohesiveness is greater and high ties of acquaintance-ship develop. Thus, we see among female laundry workers a greater homogeneity among the workers, higher morale, lower rate of turnover, and a high average job tenure . . . . It should also be noted that maids in the hospital industry are surrounded by professional personnel as they perform their daily tasks. Thus, they are constantly reminded of their relative status, whereas the laundry employees do not think of status at all while they are performing their work tasks.* (pp. 67–68)

Throughout this discussion on human relations, one thing should have become increasingly apparent. The key to effectiveness within a hospital organization is an understanding of people. The wide variation in backgrounds, skills, and motivations of those who comprise a hospital staff makes this a complex challenge, but if met successfully, one that has many rewards.

1-4 THE HOSPITAL ENVIRONMENTAL HEALTH SPECIALIST

The present and evolving complexities of the modern hospital environment and practices therein support the requirement for a technically trained paramedical or health specialist, whose main concern is the prevention of disease and injury and who can function across the broad but interrelated components forming the modern medical care complex. Experience in recent years has only begun to indicate the significance and interrelationships among these several components. The technical depth and complexity of the problems related to environmental control and medical care which have arisen out of the medical services and support service divisions have indicated the need for tech-

*O'Donovan, T. R. "Human Relations in the Hospital." Reprinted with permission from the quarterly journal of the American College of Hospital Administrators, *Hospital Administration*, Vol. 11, No. 1, Winter 1956, 51–69.

nical direction and consultation that can be provided by a technically trained person with the conceptual competence uniquely applicable to the medical care situation in analyzing and suggesting solutions to the multitudinous problems interpreted in their broadest meaning within the complex.

Such a person is the Hospital Environmental Health Specialist. He has had epidemiological training; exposure to biological, physical and chemical hazards; broad public health and environmental health training and experience; and has participated in many of the activities that are part of the hospital setting. His ultimate function is to promote better patient care by reducing the risk of infection, the opportunity for accidents and by limiting the extent of injuries.

By definition: The Environmental Health Hospital Specialist is "a person whose education and experience in the biological and environmental sciences qualifies him to engage in the promotion of the intramural environment conditions in support of the maintenance and restoration of health." He applies technical knowledge to the analysis and solution of problems of a preventive, medical and environmental nature and develops methods, tools, and utilizes procedures for the control of those factors which effect good patient care.

By education he possesses a master's degree in Public Health, Environmental Health, Environmental Engineering, Environmental Science or Life Science with major course work in Environmental Health and minor course work in epidemiology and statistics.

By training he has had five years of progressive environmental health experience, two years of which should have been in supervision, and one year of which should have been in administration.

His areas of interest would include the development of study techniques, conducting these studies; formulating practical recommendations and issuing reports; and planning and evaluation of environmental health, infection control and safety programs related to good patient care, and satisfactory employee practices.

The logical position for this individual is as a staff assistant to the Chief Executive Officer, for in accomplishing his goals and satisfying the hospital objectives, he must cross all departmental lines. His salary should be commensurate with his position.

Where the state health department is responsible for the hospital program, the chief of the division should have the above qualifications.

The environmental health person who is preparing for this career should have a master's degree as previously mentioned, two years progressive experience, and be given courses and a six month internship in hospitals.

REFERENCES AND SELECTED READINGS

Burling, T., Lentz, Edith, and Wilson, R. *The Give and Take in Hospitals*. New York: G. P. Putnam's Sons, 1956.

Georgopoulos, B. S. and Mann, F. C. *The Community General Hospital*. New York: Mac-Millan, 1962.

Guidelines for the Formulation of Medical Staff By-laws, Rules and Regulations. Departmentalized Hospitals Chicago: Joint Commission on Accreditation of Hospitals, 1971.

MacEachern, M. T. *Hospital Organization & Management*. Berwyn, Ill.: Physicians Record Co., 1967.

O'Donovan, T. R. Human relations in the hospital, *Hospital Administration*, Vol. 11, No. 1, Winter, 1966, pp. 51–69.

Sloan, R. P. *Today's Hospital*. New York: Harper & Row, 1966.

Stanley, F. M. The board, the staff, the administrator—Checks and balances in hospital government, *Trustee*, Vol. 18:2, February 1965.

The nation's hospitals—A statistical profile, *Hospitals: Journal of the American Hospital Association*, Vol. 45, Part 2, pp. 447–492, August 1, 1971.

2

Environmental
Services

INTRODUCTION

The services provided within a medical care facility for patients, staff, and visitors all have their own unique problems and methods for prevention of environmental health hazards. Although unique, they are considered very important links in the chain of effective institutional health protection. The unsafe and careless practice of environmental protection in the institutional services has and certainly always will endanger the health of the communities which the hospital serves as well as the institution itself. No service can be left without consideration. This chapter is designed to aid in the individual services' consideration for the safe practice of total environmental health.

2-1 BARBER AND BEAUTY SHOP SANITATION

2-1-1 Introduction

Hair and scalp may be the reservoirs of infection for fungal, parasitic and bacterial infection. This hazard is intensified by equipment, technique of the operator, condition of the skin and site of hair removal. In a medical care facility, these problems of disease and disease vector transmission become much more of a problem due to the existence of the patient-staff-visitor association within this particular service.

In some institutions, an actual shop for ambulatory patients, staff, and visitors or a combination of any two may exist or it may remain a single service to patients only. Whether these associations exist or not it is still imperative to retain good sanitation for the prevention of spread of disease to anyone. Regardless of the association, it may well be that the operator has a shop outside the institution and could bring in disease as

16

well as take it to the community. This situation should be either discouraged or at least acutely observed for disease potentials. The following is a guide in the proper methods of sanitation in this service.

2-1-2 Employees

A. Employees of barber and beauty services should fulfill the following requirements:
   1. Be free of communicable disease.
   2. Receive preemployment and periodic physical examinations to rule out communicable diseases.
   3. Always wear clean and sanitary outer protective clothing—as necessary when attending patients or customers.
   4. Wash hands in hot soapy water after each service.

2-1-3 Environmental Standards

A. Operator should not perform work in food service areas or sleeping quarters and the latter only when necessary for bed patients.
B. Should always have available an adequate supply of hot and cold water and proper methods of waste disposal.
C. Area should always be adequately lighted and ventilated.
D. Should maintain environment and equipment in a sanitary manner at all times.
E. The removal of cut hair from floors shall be done after each patient, or frequently, and by dustless methods such as by vacuum. Removal of hair from floors and other surfaces may be avoided by the use of vacuum clippers which immediately collect the hair as it is cut.

2-1-4 Sanitary Procedures

In the institution, hair cuts and hair sets may be given at the bedside or in a special room. In either case, the operator should use a special set of properly wrapped, clean and disinfected tools for each patient. Shaving should be preceded by a thorough washing of the skin with individual soap and towels. Aerosol shaving foam and single service razors and razor blades are indicated.

Preoperative shaving is done at the bedside within 18 hours of the operation. Hair removal of infected patients should be accompanied by strict isolation technique, special training in asepsis for the operator, sterilization of all equipment, and periodic health examinations for employees.

Health authorities should make periodic inspections.
The following are general recommendations for this service:

A. Only U.S.F.D.A. approved cosmetics, tonics, bleaches, etc. should be used.
B. Treating boils, ingrown hairs, etc. or any other therapy should be prohibited.
C. When using a head rest, it should be covered with a clean sheet of paper or towel for each person.
D. Only material approved by the hospital should be used to control capillary hemorrhage and be applied in the manner prescribed.
E. Brushes, dusters and shaving mugs should be replaced by the use of automatic dispensers or brushless shaving cream, and clean towels in place of brushes.
F. Separate neck bands should be used for each person.
G. In areas or cases of communicable disease, separate or disposable covering cloths shall be used.
H. Any and all shaving should be permitted only on the approval of the doctor or ward nurse and only by an approved operator.
I. Smoking should be prohibited while attending the patient.

2-1-5   Instrument Cleaning and Disinfection

The use of disposable instruments is recommended whenever possible. Nondisposable instruments and their parts should be thoroughly cleaned with soap and water, dried, individually wrapped and placed in a small instrument autoclave and sterilized prior to their use on the next patient.

If autoclaving is not possible then the next acceptable method is cold sterilization.

Nondisposable tools and instruments such as combs, brushes, and scissors should be cleaned thoroughly to remove all hair and other foreign material, washed with a detergent in hot water, rinsed under running hot water and finally placed in a container of a good quaternary detergent germicide or iodophor. The germicide should be changed between patients.

Instruments with nondetachable parts, such as electric clippers, should have their skin contact surfaces immersed and operated in a good quaternary detergent germicide and then allowed to air dry. It is also advised that the body and handle of such appliances be sprayed or wiped down with an appropriate disinfectant after each use. (Multiuse shaving brushes, mugs, and dusters are unacceptable.)

REFERENCES AND SELECTED READINGS

Conferences with noted surgeons concerning the effect of hair removal on the spread of infection, 1967.

Gordon, J. E., (Ed.) *Control of Communicable Diseases in Man.* New York: American Public Health Association, 10th ed., 1965.

Regulations Governing Operation and Conduct of Barber and Beauty Shops, Etc. Philadelphia, Pa.: Philadelphia Department of Public Health, 1956.

2-2 FOOD SANITATION

2-2-1 Introduction

The dietary department is similar to a large commercial food operation coupled with the many problems related to the patient and his infirmities, and its role in training of student nurses and student dieticians. The food service program contains the elements of purchasing, transporting, processing, storing, preparing, and serving of food.

2-2-2 Purchasing

High quality raw materials kept at proper temperatures and delivered frequently in a sanitary manner produces safe nutritional meals. A requirements contract should be established with suppliers who are inspected regularly by the local, state, or Federal government.

2-2-3 Transporting

Delivery should be made in clean trucks. Where refrigeration is required, the trucks must maintain the required temperature for 48 hours in case of mechanical failure of the truck. Upon arrival, the food should immediately be removed on clean vehicles to storing or processing areas. Upon arrival, all food should be inspected for damage, insect or rodent infestation or spoilage. If a problem exists, the material should be promptly segregated, returned, or destroyed.

2-2-4 Storing

Perishables need to be immediately refrigerated or placed in frozen food lockers. Dry foods require adequate ventilation, frequent rotation, proper stacking, and intensive pest surveillance.

Recommended Delivery Schedules and Storage Temperatures

Food Item	Frequency of Delivery	Storage Temperature
Meats, poultry, fish, shellfish	2–3 times/week	32–36°F
Fresh vegetables and fruits	2–3 times/week	45°F
Eggs, processed foods, pastries	2–3 times/week	40–45°F
Milk	3–4 times/week	40°F
Frozen foods	1 time/week	−10–0°F
Dry foods	1 time/week or 2 weeks	68–72°F

Hot foods stored at a minimum of 150°F for a maximum of a two hour period during the serving time.

2-2-5   Processing and Preparing

The scope of the operation varies from the production of baked goods and ice cream to special diets and mass feeding. Despite the multitude of activities, good quality control is realized through detailed specifications of production, efficiently planned operations, precision tools, well trained staff, effective supervision, and adequate cleaning and disinfection of utensils and equipment.

Equipment

Food service equipment in the broad sense includes complete kitchen installations as well as chinaware, glassware, kitchen utensils, silverware, and service items. No longer can the modern institution tolerate cast iron sinks, iron kettles, chipped enamelware, poorly constructed and badly used preparation equipment. Ease of cleanliness, size of equipment, and usability are of primary concern. The size of the kitchen, the layout, and the equipment will be based on the bed capacity plus the anticipated expansion of bed capacity for a 10-year period. The equipment includes but is not limited to, electric meat slicers, cutting boards, stainless steel sinks and drain board units, food carts or trucks, vegetable peelers, food choppers, cutters or slicers, mixers, baking bins, proof boxes, bakers' racks, bakers' scales, broilers, ovens, steam kettles, cabinets, deep fat fryers, food mixers, ranges, hoods, ventilator fans, removable grease filters, steam jacketed kettles, freezers, refrigerators, walk-in boxes, hot and cold patient food carts, conveyor belts, dumbwaiters, dishwashers, steam tables, soda fountains, trash cans, garbage cans, can washers, garbage grinders, ice cube makers, shaved ice makers, shelving, tables, chairs; milk dispensers, vending machines, food grinders and choppers, peelers, saws, tenderizers, knives, patty machines, meat blocks, toasters, french fry potato cutters, coffee makers, and coffee urns.

The following standards from the National Sanitation Foundation, Ann Arbor, Michigan should be part of the library of each hospital:

Standard #1   *Soda Fountain — Luncheonette Equipment and Appurtenances*, April 1969;

Standard #2   *Food Service Equipment*, July 1970;

Standard #3   *Commercial Spray-Type Dishwashing Machines*, April 1965;

Standard #4   *Commercial Cooking and Warming Equipment*, April 1970;

Standard #6   *Dispensing Freezers*, July 1970;

Standard #7   *Food Service Refrigerators and Storage Freezers*, July 1970;

Standard #8   *Commercial Powered Food Preparation Equipment*, July 1972;

Standard #12   *Automatic Ice-Making Equipment*, July 1972;

Standard #18   *Manual Food and Beverage Dispensing Equipment*, April 1966;

Standard #20   *Commercial Bulk Milk Dispensing Equipment and Appurtenances*, April 1966.

Common Food Service Problems

In some ways the food service problem within the institution is equivalent to the food service you find in any large restaurant or other food facilities. In other ways it differs because of the extreme susceptibility of patients to further infections and the seriousness of potential outbreaks of food-borne infection or poisoning. More stringent requirements are needed and yet in many cases practices are less stringent than in the commercial establishments. Good manpower is hard to secure and costly. Hospitals are in a position where they have to offer generally lower salaries than the surrounding communities. This plus inadequate supervision, because of financial problems and inadequate training, compounds the hospital food service problem. A series of problems will now be mentioned; however, it should be understood that some of these exist in some hospitals; many exist in some hospitals; all may exist in some hospitals. However, this listing is not all inclusive.

1. In many reconverted kitchens or old kitchens, there is an inadequate supply of light. This contributes to worker fatigue, increased possibility of rodents and insects, and inadequate removal of soil and food wastes.
2. Depending on the ability of the food service manager and the rigor with which he inspects his kitchen, many of the areas of the kitchen may easily become soiled. Accumulations of this soil leads to unhealthy conditions.
3. Soil, food particles, dirt, and dust may be found in and around all equipment, in drawers, between pieces of equipment such as cookers, stoves, ovens, deep fat fryers, etc. Food particles may also be found in mixers, slicers, can openers, cutters, conveyors, sinks, cabinets, shelves, storage areas, pots, pans, baking dishes, etc.

4. Surfaces easily become coated with greasy residues, soap films, or burnt on deposits. This gives off odors and causes freshly prepared foods to have off flavors.
5. Refrigerators become corroded with off odors, gaskets lose their elasticity.
6. Although new kitchens are constructed, old equipment still manages to find its way into the operation. These are usually in very poor shape and should be replaced as soon as possible.
7. Many dish rooms are very poorly ventilated. This condition at times causes unbearable working situations and contributes heavily toward improper dish and utensil cleaning.
8. Dishwashers become corroded because they are not cleaned properly and frequently enough. The spray-arms become clogged and therefore do not do an effective job of rinsing dishes.
9. In many older hospitals, steam pressure is very poor and for this reason it is almost impossible to obtain proper washing and rinsing temperatures. This can be corrected by the insertion of a booster heater in the line prior to the washing and rinsing cycle.
10. Chemical food poisoning though infrequent has resulted in the death of hundreds of patients in hospitals. It is essential that in the inspection of kitchens the food service manager, as well as, the environmental health person carefully segregate all chemicals, insecticides, cleaning materials, and other poisonous materials from food stuffs. These items should not be transferred from their original container into jars and bags. They should be very accurately labeled.
11. Hand washing facilities are generally inadequate or too far away from the preparation areas. Since a great deal of infection is transferred by the hands, it is essential that the handwashing facilities be appropriately located and used. Germicidal liquid soap is recommended.
12. Many outbreaks of disease which are food-disseminated can be traced back to the food handlers. All food handlers who have diarrhea, vomiting, boils, severe upper respiratory illness, etc., should be removed from service and have appropriate lab specimens taken. The results must be negative before the employee returns to work.
13. There is a tendency to save leftovers from one meal to another. This contributes to outbreaks of food-borne infection. Improper storage of foods in overlarge containers does not permit adequate rapid refrigeration of the mass of food. This type of problem has been known to lead to outbreaks of food-borne infection. Where food is reheated, the internal temperature of the food should be above 150°F for several minutes. Thawing of frozen food such as turkey, and other meats, outside of the refrigerator allows incubation of organisms on the surface of the product while the inner core is still defrosting. Chicken and turkey, etc., should be defrosted in the refrigerator.
14. The practice of defrosting foods in water is not approved since the trays

in which the food is placed, the hands of the employee, and the time-temperature relationship could lead to growth of bacteria and food-borne infection.

15. It is the practice in some institutions to place grinder heads, tenderizer blades, and other demountable working parts of equipment into the refrigerator instead of cleaning daily. This practice should be abolished.

16. Water carafes and glasses are of concern. The best procedure is to use disposable carafes and glasses which will be sent home with the patient. They should be dishwasher proof and should be put through the dishwasher each day. In contaminated areas, the carafes and glasses should be rinsed and washed within the room and then sanitized with chlorine or a quaternary ammonium chloride compound.

2-2-6 Service

Food is dispensed by means of centralized, decentralized and bulk tray service, and in cafeterias, snack bars, and vending machines. The type of service is determined by the size, layout, and function of the institution.

Centralized Tray Service

All trays are assembled in a kitchen and are transported by tray truck, dumbwaiter or conveyor to patient area, and returned the same way for washing. Major problems are that food tends to become cold, spillage occurs, and dirty utensils, dishes, and food remnants may contaminate the new trays.

Centralized Bulk Tray Service

The trays are set up centrally with cold foods and are then transported in bulk food trucks with heated and unheated compartments to serving pantries where hot food is added from heated insulated food conveyors. Major problems are the maintenance of proper temperatures in the food conveyor, its cleanliness and the protection needed for the partially set up trays.

Decentralized Tray Service

Most of the food is prepared in a central kitchen and is then transported in bulk food trucks with heated and unheated compartments to serving kitchens in the patient care areas. The trays are then assembled for delivery to the patients. Coffee, toast and eggs might be prepared in the serving kitchen. The problems are the same as in centralized bulk tray service plus the necessity for supervising additional food preparation areas.

Cafeteria

The cafeteria is provided for ambulatory patients in some institutions, employees and visitors. This facility offers a greater variety of food, more quickly and with fewer personnel.

Vending Machines

Vending machines may dispense any food from candy bars and coffee to sandwiches and hot meals. The major problems are the handling, storage, temperature control, dispensing of the food, and cleanup of the machines and food service areas.

Snack Bars

The operation and problems are similar to luncheonettes outside of the hospital, with the exception that it provides a ready means of securing food for patients and eventual storage of remnants in patient care areas.

2-2-7   Disposables

Disposable glasses, dishes, silverware, and trays are being used in many institutions. The advantage is in the reduction of washing needed and in the safe removal of food remnants and utensils from patients with communicable or infectious diseases. The disadvantage is the increased amount of storage and waste disposal facilities needed.

2-2-8   Disposal

Food remnants are insect and rodent attractants and may be vehicles of disease transmission. Food from patients' trays are scraped into garbage cans, which become dirty, encrusted and odoriferous. Use of plastic or waterproof paper liners and proper can cleaning daily with a detergent-disinfectant sprayed into the cans will eliminate this problem. Hospital garbage should not be fed to pigs, but rather should be destroyed by incineration or landfill operation, for the organisms which are endemic to the hospital might be transferred to the hog, and the hog may then become a reservoir of infection for the community. Trash which is generated during the food processing procedure is removed to trash holding rooms, Dempster dumpsters, or incinerators. Since the trash generally has food particles on it, it may act as an insect and rodent attractant.

2-2-9   Special Foods

Infant Formula Room

The function of the infant formula room in a hospital is to prepare and serve nutritious, wholesome food for the proper growth and health of infants. Milk, formula ingredients, baby bottles, and equipment must be free of debris, and sterile. Debris may cause mechanical damage or suffocation. Any bacterial invasion may be the cause of serious illness. The water which is used in formula preparation must be checked for chemical content. An excess of certain chemicals in the water could cause extreme damage to the infant. The formula room should be removed from general traffic to reduce contamination by visitors and personnel. A minimum amount of time should be spent in transporting the bottles. The room should be constructed of nonporous material (such as tile), painted in a light color, brightly lit, well ventilated, and free of cracks.

To prevent the inadvertent contamination of milk bottles or formula with detergents and cleaning supplies, these items when not in use should be immediately stored below the washing sinks in cabinets. Brushes must be of adequate design and size to aid in the physical clean-up of bottles and nipples. The bristles should be black, since a white bristle might get into the milk and cause suffocation of the infants. Sufficient shelves should be provided for storage of extra bottles and racks. When milkstone and water deposits cling to the bottle, nipples, or equipment, a special type of safe acid detergent should be used followed by a mild alkaline or neutral detergent and thorough rinsing. The formula room should be set up in two separate units. In the bottle washing room, all of the bottles, nipples, and caps should be preflushed, then soaked in detergent solution, scrubbed, and rinsed thoroughly. They should then be placed in racks and sent to the preparation room through a small opening. The preparation room should be used for preparing the formula, filling the bottles, cooking, sterilizing, and refrigerating.

Tube Feeding

Infection may result from preparation, handling, quantity of food stored, length of time in tube, and cleaning procedures. The liquid nature of the food whether it be a normal diet pureed, or milk-based formulas become excellent bacterial culture mediums. Bacteria have an opportunity for rapid growth since the food is served warm over a period of time. The practice of storing liquified foods in gallon jugs prevents the center of the food mass from reaching the appropriate temperature of 45°F quickly enough to retard considerable growth of microorganisms.

To prevent obstruction of the tube or obstruction in the patient, the food must be of proper consistency.

The tube feeding unit is made up of a levine tube, a septo syringe, which acts as the funnel and a spout cup.

The two main types of tube feeding are the intermittent type, in which food is given to the patient several times a day for periods of 10–15 minutes, and the constant drip type, in which the food is supplied on a continuous basis, 24 hours a day. The major problem is with food that remains in the tube for more than one hour and frequent proper cleaning and disinfection.

2-2-10   Cleaning Technique

Proper cleaning, with adequate tools and detergent-disinfectants, by trained personnel, well supervised, reduces the potential growth and spread of food-borne infections. Varying types of equipment create a need for a variety of cleaning procedures. However, since the section on detergent and disinfectants (*see* Chapter 7), amply and clearly discusses the various types of cleaning, the detergent-disinfectants recommended and the cleaning mechanism, it would be superfluous to detail individual cleaning techniques. Such information may be obtained from a variety of housekeeping manuals.

Dishwashing Techniques

Since adequate dishwashing is essential to eliminate dishes and utensils from becoming mechanical transmitters of disease, commercial mechanical dishwashers of the multiple tank variety should be used. They vary from conveyer dishwashers with prewashing to multiple tank rackless type to circular conveyor type. Joints and seams should be of intrical construction or intrically welded. Pipes should be kept to a minimum to prevent unnecessary loss of heat or temperature and should not obstruct excess openings or interfere with cleaning. The space beneath the dishwasher should be high enough to provide easy cleaning.

(This is one of the best areas for the propagation and growth of insects and rodents.) The machine should be easily cleanable and have thermostatic controls (automatic), so installed to provide the minimum temperature required, for washing and sanitizing of dishes. An easily readable thermostatic gauge should be located on the machine to show the temperature of the final rinse water. The thermostatic gauge shall be accurate to within, plus or minus, 3°F. A timing device which automatically times washing in cycles is required. It is strongly recommended that a prerinsing unit be used prior to the washing machine. The wash water should be 150°F. The rinse water should be maintained at not less than 180°F nor more than 195°F. At the entrance of the rinse manifold, the flow pressure should not be less than 15 pounds per square inch. (The very best material including diagrams on commercial dishwashers is *Commercial Spray-Type Dishwashing Machines*, Standard #3 by National Sanitation Foundation, April 1965.)

Pots and pans should be prerinsed with cool water, soaked in suitable size sinks with hot detergent water for several minutes, brushed out with bristle brushes or steel wool pads, thoroughly rinsed, and if necessary the process of washing and rinsing should be repeated until all visible soil is removed. Finally, rinse and then immerse in a sink of cool water with either chlorine at 100 ppm or quaternary ammonium chloride compound at 200 ppm, for two minutes.

2-2-11   Related Programs

The food service department does not operate in a vacuum. It is deeply concerned with housekeeping, insect and rodent control, and patient care. Division of responsibility in housekeeping activities can create serious problems unless proper coordination exists. The food service worker may contaminate the patient, or in turn be contaminated by the patient.

2-2-12   Self-Inspection Concept and Procedures

Consistent, unbiased evaluation of sanitation items requiring correction is essential to the improvement of a hospital food service program. A dual approach may be used. First, a self-inspection program based on the use of two forms; and, second, specialized training classes. The inspection forms provide an easy method of monitoring the sanitation level. The classes teach the food service staff about sanitation practice and theory.

The tool used is the Food Service Self-Inspection Form. (*See* Figure

2-1.) Supervisory personnel use the form to systematically inspect their own facilities; identify problem areas; determine whether improvements are being effected weekly; record the facts which can be used as a basis for budget requests, further study, program changes, changes in material and techniques, employee training, and necessary disciplinary action if assigned tasks are consistently not completed.

The form is arranged in such a manner that those items which may contribute the most to the spread of food-borne infection are listed first. The supervisor determines whether the item should be marked satisfactory, improvement needed, or poor. His inspectional techniques should be standardized by someone proficient in food service inspections.

Specialized training classes for supervisors and dieticians should be interwoven with the use of the form. Top level administration and various department heads should explain the role of food service in patient care. The food service director and her assistants attend all sessions to provide an opportunity for an exchange of ideas with members of her supervisory staff.

2-2-13   Recommended Training Program

Session 1	Introduction by Hospital Directors
*Session 2	Review of General Hospital Problems
*Session 3	Review of General Hospital Problems
Session 4	The Self-Inspection Form and Technique
Session 5	Field Experience in use of Form
Session 6	Field Experience in use of Form
*Session 7	Review of Food Service Department Problems
*Session 8	Review of Food Service Department Problems Initiate use of form on weekly basis
*Session 9	General Housekeeping Theory Discuss results of inspections
*Session 10	General Housekeeping Techniques Discuss results of inspections
*Session 11	General Food Service Equipment and Utensil Cleaning Techniques Discuss results of inspections

*Seminar type sessions. Gives each supervisor the opportunity to examine a general or specific problem and voice his opinion about possible causes and solutions. This technique gives the supervisor confidence in his ability to handle problems in the kitchen; helps him recognize that other supervisors have many of the same problems; allows the food service director to evaluate and review many ideas which may improve her operation.

2-2-14   Food-Borne Diseases

Diarrhea, abdominal cramps, vomiting, chills and fever all may be part of the clinical picture that the physician sees when his patient has a food-borne infection or intoxication. Food-borne bacterial infections are of two types. One type consists of those diseases which are transmitted by a variety of vectors or vehicles, of which food is but one, and whose clinical symptoms are not those usually associated with food poisoning. For instance, typhoid, paratyphoid fever, dysentery, cholera parasites and other enteric infections.

The second type of infection which is associated with the salmonella group, has a short incubation time, sometimes severe gastrointestinal disturbance, but of rather short duration and exhibits the typical symptoms of viral enteritis or food poisoning. These salmonella infections are much like a grass fire once they are introduced into the institution. They spread rapidly, occur in many places almost at once and can smolder for long periods of time. Many examples of outbreaks of *Salmonella Derby*, *Salmonella Infantis*, and other salmonella species are present in the literature. Some case histories follow:

An outbreak of *Salmonella Infantis* occurred in a newborn nursery in August 1966, in Kansas. The outbreak was traced to a dinner at which the then pregnant mother of one of the infants became ill. Several of the individuals attending the dinner became ill with gastroenteritis. The woman delivered three days after the dinner. Two days later she became ill with gastroenteritis and, a few days after that, six infants, beginning with her own child, developed febrile diarrhea. *Salmonella Infantis* was the infecting organism. A sample of pineapple cream pie was tested and *S. Infantis* was isolated. Seven additional cases of *S. Infantis* were found in persons who were in contact with the hospital acquired cases after they were discharged from the hospital.

An outbreak of gastroenteritis involving seven children and six adults occurred in October 1966, in a chronic disease hospital in Connecticut. Two deaths occurred among the severely debilitated children. *Salmonella Typhimurium* was isolated in the stools of six patients. Since the pediatric and adult wards are located separately, the only common factor was that all of the patients who became ill were receiving tube feedings. A specimen of the pediatric formula obtained from the ward was *S. Typhimurium* positive. All ingredients were cultured and found to be negative. However, swab technique demonstrated that two of the adults were contaminated. The organism was isolated from the chief cook who occasionally prepared the formula.

An outbreak of *S. Infantis* occurred in a hospital in Pennsylvania in August 1965. Seven hundred positives were identified. The initial case was probably a food handler with gastroenteritis who twice contaminated food. Removal of all infected personnel from duty plus strict environmental health measures brought the outbreak under control. No new cases were reported or cultured after 30 days.

Food poisoning may be classified as the result of individual idiosyncrasies; toxemia from naturally poisonous foods; foods into which poisons have been accidentally introduced; and foods containing poisons of bacterial origin, such as *Clostridium botulinum* and *staphylococcus*.

Epidemic diarrhea of the newborn is an acute, highly communicable, highly fatal, diarrheal disease of unknown etiology, occurring in the newborn in nurseries. The infective agent may be a virus. The mode of transmission is not clear. It may be either a direct or indirect person to person infection. Food, bottles, or nipples may be incriminated.

Infectious hepatitis is spread through fecal material which may contaminate shell-fish or other types of food.

Whenever a food-borne outbreak of disease is suspected, a detailed investigation should be made to try to determine the origin of the outbreak and modes of transmission. It is not necessary to wait for a final epidemiological report to make changes or introduce unusual environmental control measures into the food service operation and the handling of fecal material. The function of the study is different than studies carried out in the community at large, for most food-borne illnesses in the community at large, represent a single incident in time which may rapidly disappear. In institutions, the infection may go on and on. The patient is far more susceptible to food-borne disease and could suffer great hardships, maybe even death, from a Salmonella or Shigella infection. This is in sharp contrast to the average healthy person who may become moderately to violently ill but recovers rapidly. The following is a recommended procedure for the investigation and study of an outbreak of suspected food associated illness.

The definition of an outbreak of food-borne disease is any illness associated with intestinal upset resulting from the suspected ingestion of food containing certain chemical poisons, poisons derived from animals and plants, toxic products of several types of bacteria, and infections caused by several types of bacteria. This would apply whenever two or more patients or members of the staff are affected.

Procedures

1. Medical-nursing personnel should record on each shift all incidents mentioned under the definition.
2. The outbreak should be reported immediately to the Executive Director, Medical Director, Nursing Director, Administrative Services Director, Chairman of the Committee on Infections, Environmental Health Specialist and Health Department.
3. Stool samples should be taken in all cases where diarrhea occurs.
4. Any samples of food remaining from meals should be preserved for later analysis, and then taken to appropriate laboratories when indicated.
5. All patients and members of the staff who have become ill should be examined and case histories prepared. These case histories should include the types of food eaten in the last four meals, whether there was any unusual taste, color, odor, or means of presentation involved.
6. Employees should be referred to employees' clinic for examination and stool culture.
7. An immediate investigation should be made of food service facilities and procedures including storage, preparation, serving, transportation of food and any unusual occurrences, including time-temperature relationships.
8. All sick personnel should be removed from duty until their infection is cleared up. (They should be compensated for this time off as a service connected disability.)
9. Food Service, Nursing, and Medical personnel sick leave records should be checked immediately for a one month period prior to the outbreak, to determine if anyone had diarrhea or vomiting. (Investigate and culture all cases diagnosed as summer virus, viral enteritis, gastrointestinal upset, etc.)
10. An investigation of the initial case histories reported should be started as soon as possible after the outbreak of the illness.
11. If new cases are occurring, there should be a rapid implementation of emergency environmental health measures related to all preparation, service, storage and transportation of food; cleaning and sanitizing of utensils, equipment and food conveyors; removal, cleaning, and sterilization of bedpans and urinals. (Bedpan sterilizers are not adequate for this purpose.) Strict handwashing procedures using medical aseptic technique and intensive frequent cleaning and sanitizing of bathroom facilities are essential.

12. If many new cases are occurring, all members of the staff related to patient care including medical, nursing, and food service personnel should have their stools cultured at least twice (in case of false negatives).

13. All personnel with positive cultures should be removed from duty (service connected disability) until they have five consecutive negative stool specimens. In the event that medical or nursing personnel are badly needed, they should be allowed to return to work providing they exhibit no clinical symptoms and are not directly involved in patient care, or they have two consecutive stool specimens which are negative and do not perform oral procedures, give medication, perform operations, give injections or intravenous procedures until they have five consecutive negative cultures.

14. Preliminary decisions on the possible causes of the outbreak should be followed by the implementation of specific recommendations to help break the chain of infection and prevent further reoccurrence.

15. A final report should be prepared and correlated with laboratory data. This report should include as clear a definition of the problem as possible and concrete recommendations for the future protection of the patients and staff.

18. An appropriate form should be developed for data gathering, which includes:

> Name, age, sex, title, duties, date and diagnosis of patient's illness where pertinent. Symptoms include time of onset, date and hour, description of symptoms, character of stools, duration of symptoms, fever, last food eaten, last three meals and other foods and liquids eaten between meals. Summary of lab findings includes stool cultures, urine cultures, and food cultures.

2-2-15 Conclusions

There is an inseparable relationship between the management of a food service department, its operation, the purchase, storage, transportation, preparation, service, disposal, special foods, isolation techniques, use of disposables, sanitation, cleaning techniques, and the quality of food plus an avoidance of food-borne intoxications or infections. The fundamental object of the department is to provide high quality food in a sanitary manner from clean equipment. Cleanliness has a direct effect on food flavor. The sense of sight, the sense of smell, and the sense of taste become all important in the presentation and consumption of food. All of this is made possible by the proper use of food service personnel, the proper distribution of food, adequate lighting, adequate ventilation, proper design, construction and installation of equipment, utensils, and facilities, and the use of the services of the Environmental Health Hospital Specialist to conduct studies, prepare recommendations, institute emergency procedures when needed and develop training programs for supervisory personnel and food service workers.

2-2-16   Food Service Self-Inspection Form

Instructions

The Food Service Self-Inspection Form is a concise systematic means of self-inspection by food service supervisors, dieticians, and nursing supervisors. Regular use provides a complete overall view of conditions in hospital food service areas. It identifies problem areas, facilitating supervision and increasing motivation among employees.

General Guidelines

1. The form may be used for any food service area. The score is automatically controlled by what the rater actually checks. An entire food service area would be inspected and filled in on one form.
2. If any part of an area or item is unsatisfactory, a number "1" is inserted under points at that item. This indicates improvement needed. If several parts of an area or item is unsatisfactory a "0" is inserted under points at that item. This indicates, poor.
3. In order to emphasize the necessity for properly identifying the area, 4 points are added to the final score on the form.
4. Inspection techniques should be standardized by qualified environmental health specialists.
5. Weekly inspections are recommended.
6. The total score at the upper right hand corner is the sanitation grade. One hundred percent is perfect. However, the passing grade for a specific area should be established by the Food Service Director.
7. The summary sheet can be modified to fill the needs of the particular institution. It indicates individual ratings and total scores of all food service areas in the hospital. (*See* Figure 2-2.)
8. Fill out top of form completely.
9. Begin at item 1 and go down the list in order rating each item satisfactory (2), improvement needed (1), poor (0).
10. Scoring—add up the total number of points +4 for completing the form.

FOOD SERVICE INSPECTION REPORT

(Submit Weekly to Sanitation Officer)

_____ HOSPITAL
(name)
ENVIRONMENTAL SANITATION

KEY:
2 – Satisfactory
1 – Improvement Needed
0 – Poor

BUILDING NAME AND NO.	FLOOR	DATE	TIME	TOTAL SCORE

POINTS	ITEM
	1. Perishable foods used within a 2-hour period of preparation or immediately refrigerated.
	2. Perishable foods are not to be reused at anytime.
	3. All refrigerators kept below 45°F.
	4. Ice making machines clean and operating properly.
	5. Food carts washed and sanitized at ward kitchens.
	6. Food protected from contamination: Preparation Storage Transportation
	7. Hands thoroughly washed and cleaned after use of toilets and before preparation of food.
	8. Clean outer garments worn at all times.
	9. Soap, paper towels, and waste receptacles available at all times at handwashing sink.
	10. Lavatory facilities clean and in good repair.
	11. Dressing rooms, areas, and lockers kept clean.
	12. All food handlers with diarrhea removed from duty until negative stool culture.
	13. Food utensils, dishes, glasses, silverware, and equipment scraped, pre-flushed, and soaked.
	14. Silverware, dishes, and glasses clean to sight and touch.
	15. Silverware, dishes, and glasses sanitized.
	16. Dishwasher wash and rinse temperatures checked daily *(insert temp. rinse)* *(insert temp. wash).*
	17. Food utensils, such as pots, pans, knives, and cutting boards clean to sight and touch.
	18. Grills and similar cooking devices cleaned daily.
	19. Food-contact surfaces of equipment clean to sight and touch.
	20. Tables and counters clean to touch.
	21. Non-food-contact surfaces of equipment clean to sight and touch.
	22. Washing and sanitizing water clean.
	23. Single service food articles properly stored, dispensed, and handled.
	24. Containers of food stored off floor on clean surfaces.

34

25. No wet storage of packaged food.		
26. Sugar in closed dispensers or individual packages.		
27. Poisonous and toxic materials properly identified, colored, stored, and used; poisonous polishes not present.		
28. Clean wiping cloths used and properly restricted.		
29. All late trays served after 8 p.m. scraped, rinsed, and stacked in previously cleaned sink.		
30. Garbage and rubbish stored in metal containers with lids; containers adequate in number.		
31. All garbage removed from area at end of working day.		
32. Containers cleaned when empty.		
33. When not in continuous use, garbage and rubbish containers covered with tight-fitting lids.		
34. Garbage and rubbish storage areas adequate in size and clean.		
35. All outer openings screened.		
36. Absence of rodents.		
37. Absence of flies.		
38. Absence of roaches.		
39. Floors kept clean.		
40. Floors in good repair.		
41. Floors and wall junctures properly cleaned.		
42. Walls, ceilings, and attached equipment clean.		
43. Walls and ceilings properly constructed and in good repair; coverings properly attached.		
44. Walls of light color; washable to level of splash to shoulder height.		
45. Lighting adequate.		
46. Light fixtures clean.		
47. Areas clean; no litter.		
48. Ample quantities of cleaning supplies available.		

REMARKS:

_____

Signature of Dietician or Nursing Supervisor

Figure 2-1 Food service inspection report.

35

FOOD SERVICE INSPECTION SUMMARY

_____ HOSPITAL

(name)

ENVIRONMENTAL SANITATION

WEEK OF _____

ITEM	MED. 8-4	MED. 8-5	FOOD				SURG. 17-22-2	OB-GYN.		PEDS.		KITCHEN			PSYCHIATRIC					TOTAL
			9-2 DIET	9-2	9-3	9-4		21-1	21-4	26-1	26-2	27-3-59	27-3-21	27-4	27-5	27-6	27-6E	27-7	27-8	
1																				
2																				
3																				
4																				
5																				
6																				
7																				
8																				
9																				
10																				
11																				
12																				
13																				
14																				
15																				
16																				
17																				
18																				
19																				
20																				
21																				
22																				
23																				
24																				

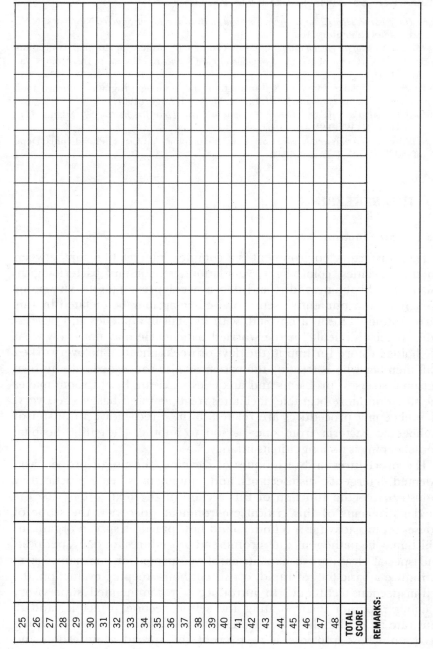

Figure 2-2 Food service inspection summary.

REFERENCES AND SELECTED READINGS

Films: *One Chance, How Clean is Clean, Spotlight on Breakage, Flying Saucers*, New York, N.Y.: Economics Laboratory, Inc.

Food Service Manual for Health Care Institutions, Chicago, Ill.: American Hospital Association.

Iowa State Department of Health, *Sanitation of Food Service Establishments*, Des Moines, Ia., April 1962.

Koren, H. and Blake, Mary E. Self-inspection and training programs improve food service sanitation, *Hospitals, J.A.H.A.*, Vol. 41, Part 1, August 1967.

National Communicable Disease Center, Salmonella Surveillance Report No. 59, Atlanta, Ga.: U.S. Dept. HEW, PHS, April 1967.

Regulations for Maternity and Newborn Services, Philadelphia, Pa.: City of Philadelphia, Dept. of Public Health, February 1963.

2-3 HOUSEKEEPING

2-3-1 Introduction

The satisfactory environment is a complex interrelationship between physical facilities, color, light, ventilation, asthetic and bacteriological cleanliness. Shabbiness, dirt and debris are depressing. Our views, our thoughts, even our entire sense of well-being may be dictated by our surroundings. Life in a hospital, with its built-in anxieties and depressions, is most difficult for the worried patient. He may not know what life holds in store for him in the days or weeks ahead. The overworked staff member who is treating the patient, is also concerned with his own personal stresses, problems and anxieties. A clean, bright room makes the situation more bearable, facilitates treatment and hastens recovery. Housekeeping procedures are related to the direct-indirect transfer of pathogenic bacteria from one person to another. Scientific hospital housekeeping is no longer in its infancy.

The procedures and techniques of cleaning, the use of proper task-oriented detergents, disinfectants, and equipment is being practiced by industry. It is the function of this section of the text to describe the special problems of this critical environment; to review the scope of housekeeping activities; to understand how practices spread organisms which may be pathogenic; to recommend procedures for daily, periodic, and special cleaning; to explain employee protection mechanisms; to introduce a basic tool of rapid, consistent housekeeping evaluation, the self-inspection technique; to introduce a recommended supervisory training program incorporating the self-inspection principle; and to integrate all of the above principles into a well balanced housekeeping program whose purpose is to prevent the spread of infection and promote health and safety in the hospital.

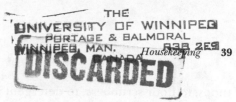
2-3-2 Special Problems

Housekeeping activities have to be suited to the main function of the hospital, good patient care. It has to be adapted to the scheduled and unscheduled visits of the medical staff, nurses and other auxiliary medical personnel. Some rooms are crowded with essential equipment, others are too small for the number of patients residing. Food spillage, dripping urine, broken glass, silver nitrate (used for burn victims), cigarette butts, chewing gum, and litter increase the problem. In contaminated areas, special precautions must be taken in the use of the equipment, the removal of infected material, and the handling of contaminated mops, buckets, water, cloths, etc. The cleaning person and his equipment must not become a vehicle for the transmission of infection.

Certain high risk areas such as the labor and delivery rooms, nurseries, operating rooms, and reverse isolation rooms have to receive intensive care. The infant, the new mother, the patient who has undergone the severe trauma of surgery, critical illness or burns is not capable of protecting himself from infection as well as the healthy individual.

The limited amount of time in the operating room between cases dictates a procedure which has to be both swift and comprehensive.

2-3-3 Scope of Housekeeping Problem

The institution is a vast conglomeration of buildings and areas, floors, corridors, windows, and assorted rooms used for a variety of functions. The areas include: nurses' stations, bathrooms, utility rooms, hopper rooms, ward dining rooms, ward pantries, wards, pathology, morgue, record room, laboratories, animal rooms, administration, doctors' and nurses' homes, X-ray clinics, outpatient care areas, storehouse, food service, linen exchange, laundry, powerhouse, offices, garages, sidewalks, roads, and outside grounds.

The detergent-disinfectants used, manpower needed, and the specific problems of special areas such as the O.R., labor and delivery rooms, nurseries, and isolated areas will be evaluated in other parts of this book.

Surfaces and Cleaning Methods

The types of floors or floor coverings to be cleaned include rugs, terrazzo, tile, rubber tile, rubber, cork, cement, wood, and composition, as well as conductive flooring. The walls include tile, brick, painted surfaces, and wood paneling. The age and use of each area may vary considerably. Cleaning is complicated by the number and variety of individuals and activities which are present at any given time. The cleaning methods vary from the use of wiping cloths, to bucket and mops, to floor scrubbers, to detergent spraying and mop or wet vacuum pick-up systems. Removal of waste and laundry, and cleaning of waste, laundry cans, and chutes are usually time consuming and ineffective.

Housekeeping Subsidiary Program

Housekeeping is also responsible for the moving of furniture, the securing of equipment and supplies, insect and rodent control, odor control and removal of snow. These unscheduled events interfere with the housekeeping program. Terminal cleaning after the infected patient is gone is necessary but can be very time consuming.

2-3-4   Spread of Pathogenic Organisms

Infections usually make their appearance in the forms of boils, furuncles, carbuncles, sties, abscesses, impetigo, pneumonia and other respiratory infections, diarrhea, vomiting, malaise, and pus. The sources of contamination include toilet seats, bedpans, urinals, bath tubs, hand towels, drinking glasses, chairs, beds, and linens of the infected individual. Improper handling of dressings is another source of contamination. Waste of any kind, especially dressings and disposable needles or syringes, are hazardous. The housekeeping department spreads these organisms through the improper use of dry mops, dirty wet mops and dirty water, pieces of equipment, improper waste disposal, improper cleaning of contaminated areas and poor timing. Since all linens must be considered to be contaminated, the improper handling of these linens tends to distribute large quantities of these organisms. Electric lights, cords, curtain rods, door-facing tops, door hinges, and corners are places often missed in routine housekeeping. Orderlies or hospital aides who perform housekeeping functions are serious contributors to the spread of infection, if they do not wear a cover gown during housekeeping and dispose of the gown plus perform a medical scrub before attending to the patient's needs.

2-3-5   Recommended Daily, Periodic, and Special Cleaning Procedures

The material in this section is meant to be examples rather than specialized cleaning methods for every type of situation. There are many fine manuals, old and new, that present specific cleaning techniques for all types of equipment and areas. The section on detergents and disinfectants specifies the type of material to be used in all hospital situations.

SPECIFIC FUNCTIONS OF THE HOUSEKEEPING DEPARTMENT

General Daily Cleaning

Materials and Equipment Required

1. 20 in. special mop tool
2. Disposable treated dust cloths
3. Polyethylene bags for waste disposal
4. Steel wool
5. Pump-up spray can on wheels
6. Clean sterile mop
7. A clean single pail and mop press
8. Detergent-disinfectant
9. Clean cloths
10. Toilet swab with disposable head
11. Toilet acid detergent

Procedure #1   Main Ward — Floor Cleaning

A. 6:30–6:35 a.m. Check in and go to location.
B. 6:35–7:10 a.m. The entire ward area should be swept with the dusting tool and disposable dust cloth. Trash should be bagged.
C. 7:10–7:20 a.m. Equipment and material should be made ready for floor washing.
   1. One bucket on a dolly containing hot water and detergent-disinfectant.
   2. A clean sterile mop.
   3. A pump-up spray can with detergent-disinfectant.
D. 7:20–8:50 a.m. Main ward and nurses cubicle.
   1. The custodian will spray the floor along the covings or baseboard, starting with the far end of the room. He will pick up the solution with the mop and rinse in the pail. After a given number of feet of floor area, which will be determined by actual practice, he will spray again and repeat the procedure. He will continue this practice one area in front of another until one half of the length of the floor is completed.
   NOTE: Frequent rinsing of the mop is essential.
   2. He will repeat the procedure on the other side of the ward.
   3. Where the floor is heavily soiled (especially in corners) use the heel of the mop for scrubbing.
   4. Move beds on one side of room each day.
   5. Return the beds when the floor is dry.
   6. Spray and mop the other side of the ward with figure 8's to within a foot of the wall.
   7. The following day the other side of the room will be given the same detailed washing procedure.

Procedure #2   Solarium — Floor Cleaning
  A. 8:55–9:05 a.m. The entire solarium area will be swept with a treated dust cloth.*
  B. 9:05–9:25 a.m. Floor washing. (*See* Procedure #1D.)
  C. 9:25–9:35 a.m. Wash buckets and mops thoroughly.
  D. 9:35–9:45 a.m. Break.

Procedure #3   Policing of Bathrooms — 9:45–10:00 a.m.
  A. Linens will be removed from the floor into a linen bag.
  B. Trash will be swept up with a treated dust cloth.
  C. Pieces of soap will be thrown away.
  D. Where needed, paper towels, toilet paper, and soap will be placed.

Procedure #4   Hopper Room — 10:00–10:30 a.m.
  A. Trash cans and equipment will be removed and the floors swept.
  B. Wash walls to shoulder height with a detergent-disinfectant, hot water, and cloths every third day.
  C. Wash radiators with detergent-disinfectant.
  D. Clean sinks with an acid detergent and rinse with a detergent-disinfectant.
  E. Wash floors with hot water and detergent-disinfectant. (*See* Procedure #1 for method.)

Procedure #5   Linen Closet
  A. 10:30–10:45 a.m. Linen carts will be removed and clean linen picked up and delivered to ward.

Procedure #6   High Dusting
  A. 10:45–11:05 a.m. One-half of the ward walls will be dusted with a treated mop each day. One-half of the curtain rods and other high places will be dusted each day with treated cloths.
  NOTE: Caution should be taken not to scatter dust. If mop or dust rag is dirty, use another one.

Procedure #7   Central Corridor Floor
  A. 11:05–11:25 a.m. Wash central corridor and one-half of waiting room floor. (*See* Procedure #1D.)
  11:30–12 Noon. Custodial Workers will have lunch.

Procedure #8   Bathroom — 12:15–12:40 p.m.
  A. The bathrooms will be washed thoroughly and patients will not be permitted to go in unless they really have to use the toilet.

---

*If this area is an isolation area, special isolation technique must be followed by the custodian. This includes: masking, gowning, hand washing, and the placing of the treated mop head in a plastic bag after use.

B. All toilets and urinals should be flushed.
C. Acid detergent should be placed in the toilets and urinals and allowed to stand for at least five minutes.
D. Scrub the toilets and urinals with a toilet swab and rinse with a detergent-disinfectant from the spray can.
E. Clean the sinks with an acid detergent and then rinse thoroughly with a detergent-disinfectant from a spray can.
F. Wash the outside of the sink and wall around it with a detergent-disinfectant.
G. Wash one half of the walls and partitions with a detergent-disinfectant, each day.
H. Wash the floors with a detergent-disinfectant. (*See* Procedure #1D.)
I. The custodian will then wash his hands thoroughly with soap and running hot water for at least two minutes.

Procedure #9   East Wing
12:40–1:40 p.m. Clean floors, walls, etc. as outlined in the previous procedures for the main ward area.

Procedure #10   West Wing
1:40–2:40 p.m. Clean floors, walls, etc. as outlined in the previous procedures for the main ward area.

Periodic cleaning is heavy duty cleaning performed by several individuals in an empty ward (all beds or other equipment having been removed). It includes the cleaning of windows, walls, and floors with mechanical equipment. All other duties mentioned under general cleaning are performed. The wax and/or sealer is stripped off the floors, which are then thoroughly scrubbed, rinsed, dried, resealed, and refinished. The amount of manpower needed depends on the speed with which the ward must be returned to active service. This procedure should be performed once every three months in heavily used areas, once every six months in moderately used areas and once a year in lightly used areas.

Special cleaning refers to terminal cleaning in rooms after the patient with an infection or contagious disease has been transferred, gone home or died and to areas like the operating room, delivery room, nurseries, and reverse isolation.

Terminal isolation cleaning is similar to heavy duty cleaning with the following modifications:

1. All equipment, beds, etc. remain in the room until the procedure is completed.

2. The housekeeping personnel must mask, glove, gown, wear caps and booties.
3. After completing the procedure they must discard the outerwear properly, and then perform a two minute medical scrub of forearms and hands.
4. All equipment must be disinfected before leaving the contaminated area.

The important concept to remember is that the major amount of organisms in the soil is removed by thorough scrubbing and rinsing, and that the application of a germicide is added protection. The concept of terminal cleaning through germicidal fogging is unsatisfactory since it does not provide for intensive soil removal from all parts of the contaminated area. Fogging of even very lightly soiled surfaces results in virtually no removal of organisms.

The cleaning of operating and delivery rooms is a two part process. Between operations the procedure should include:

Part I
1. Emptying of all waste receptacles outside of operating room.
2. Spraying of all equipment (with detergent), including counters, tables, stands, O.R. tables, sponge racks, etc. and then wipe off with clean cloths.
3. Emptying and cleaning of suction bottle and change of tubing.
4. Spraying of floor with detergent-disinfectant under pressure and then picking it up with freshly cleaned mop or wet vacuum.

Part II
1. At the end of the day follow procedures in Part I but carry out assignment more rigorously.
2. Spot clean walls.
3. Clean top of lights, vents, etc.

In the case of a septic or contagious case carry out the Part II recommendations plus leave the O.R. vacant for at least eight hours. Personnel should follow recommended isolation technique.

In nurseries or reverse isolation follow procedures in daily general cleaning with the following additions.

1. Use increased dust suppressive procedures, that is, dust frequently but gently with treated clean cloths.
2. Use isolation technique.
3. Use clean or new equipment only.
4. Exclude employees with any type of infection from a simple cold to a carbuncle.

Employee Protection Mechanisms

Employee protection mechanisms are discussed in isolation nursing as well as in the section on the role of occupational health in the hospital setting.

2-3-6   Housekeeping Evaluation Techniques

To determine housekeeping practices, the condition of the institution, and the potential spread of infection, it is necessary to first determine if the areas are clean, if the equipment is clean, and if the procedures are carried out in an appropriate manner. Many approaches may be used. It is possible to walk through parts of the institution and physically observe whether or not areas are clean or dirty. This approach is deceiving, for the black and white of the situation is rarely presented. The many grey areas cannot be measured and evaluated thoroughly. One could compile and measure complaints. However, the more vociferous individual would complain more frequently, whereas the timid would not complain at all. Many situations would go unnoticed and unattended because personnel would not complain for a variety of reasons. One can question the staff of the various services to determine the scope of the existing problems. The information that is gathered by this method is only partially factual, because the feeling of the individual influences his power of observation and his interpretation of what he has seen. The value of this technique is that it offers some general insight into the existing problems.

Another technique is the microbiological sampling of various parts of the environment. This approach is only satisfactory if an extremely large amount of samples can be taken, otherwise a statistically valid analysis cannot be made. At best, this analysis only indicates the bacterial load at the time of collection of the samples. This approach is costly and a rather indirect method for determining housekeeping problems. Its major value is as an educational and motivational tool.

Another approach is to make inspections on a limited basis. This would give accurate information, but since inspections cannot be made very frequently, it would only be a small sampling of existing conditions.

The best approach is the use of self-inspection technique. It is possible to compensate for the limited amount of time the Environmental Health Specialist can spend in the housekeeping program by training custodial supervisors in the use of self-inspection techniques and requiring weekly inspections. This method automatically increases the available manpower needed for sanitation inspection from one to many.

2-3-7   The Housekeeping Self-InspectionProgram

The self-inspection program includes a new inspectional procedure, the use of check sheets on a weekly basis and evaluation of reports (*see* Figures 2-3 and 2-4). The philosophy of the program is that specific studies made by trained line supervisors will provide a concrete picture of housekeeping problems and needs. Group and individual participation would stimulate *group* and *individual* interest and lead to more rapid improvement of existing inadequacies in the housekeeping program.

The self-inspection sheet will become the supervisory tool which will be used by all nursing and custodial supervisors to determine specific problems. This sheet, and instructions which are on pages 51–56, was developed, in 1964, at the Philadelphia General Hospital and revised at least seven times during its use. The final product is a concise, organized approach to inspections. When one uses it, one will observe a flow pattern that would be similar to an inspectional flow pattern. The observer first looks at the floors, then the walls, window sills, radiators, door ledges, ward sinks, etc. If he finds one part of an area unsatisfactory, he marks it all unsatisfactory. Individual judgment concerning levels of cleanliness is controlled, since the inspectional techniques are uniform and the supervisors are trained in a uniform manner. The technique is standardized by the Environmental Health Specialist. The area codes on the form are important since they indicate where the specific problems exist. The repair section of the form acts as a check on requisitions which are submitted to the Buildings Maintenance Department.

The trained observer can make an inspection of a 40 bed ward, with all of its side areas, in approximately 45 minutes. This inspection is to be completed at different times on different days, on a weekly basis. The total score at the upper right hand corner of the form indicates the level of compliance with acceptable standards of cleanliness. The rating report is used in several ways.

The form itself is an educational tool. It constantly reminds the supervisor of the various component parts of the housekeeping environment. The layout of the form is such that when it is followed chronologically, it will indicate the proper way of making an inspection. The supervisor uses the form as a work order. He has an effective means of evaluating one ward against another and a ward against itself over a period of time. In this way he can determine if all of his employees are performing either above or below standard and can attempt to standardize performances within this section. He can also compare his group's results to the work of other custodial supervisors and note the unsatisfactory conditions found in his area. He can, therefore, make corrections before the next weekly inspection.

The entire group of forms from the hospital at large represents a concrete picture of the status of the housekeeping program in the institution on a week to week basis. In this manner it acts as a tool for the Executive Housekeeper and for administration to judge whether there is a general improvement or a general decline in good housekeeping practices.

The problems which are mentioned in the rating report can be judged either as isolated or general ones. Those problems which are isolated can be handled by specific corrections. Problems which are of a general nature can be investigated further. The lack of either manpower, materials, supplies, proper planning, or supervision can be determined and necessary recommendations can be made.

Compilation of Data

To compile the information from the housekeeping self-inspection forms the secretary to the Environmental Health Specialist makes a series of lines on Figure 2-4 to represent all unsatisfactory conditions. She then tabulates each item on the horizontal lines and arrives at the percentage of compliance per item. Then she arrives at the percentage of compliance for all inspections. This compilation takes approximately one and one-half hours for each 120 inspection reports. This data is then available for review and distribution. After several months' experience it is possible to get a more concrete idea of what is occurring in the housekeeping phase of patient care and then it is possible to develop means of improving the housekeeping programs based on fact.

2-3-8   General TrainingPrinciples for Custodians

The best training is that in which the student participates fully and has an opportunity to state his problems. The classroom should be well ventilated, sessions should not last longer than one hour, and courses should not last longer than one week. Coffee which is furnished by the institution should be planned for morning and afternoon breaks. All details of the job, and the job of the first level supervisors should be explained to the custodians. Small group teaching of 10–20 at a time is preferred. The smaller the group, the better individual training each employee receives.

The course should have the following recommended format:

1st morning   Lectures, Demonstrations, Films, and Discussion
1. Greetings from Administrative Services Director
2. Greetings from Executive Housekeeper
3. Importance of Housekeeping
4. Housekeeping Procedures Manual
   (*General Hospital Policy*)
   Sick leave, lunch, breaks, time to report to work, cleaning procedures, reasons for disciplinary action, reasons for promotion
5. Basic Floor cleaning procedure
   a. Treated mop sweeping
   b. Spray mop method

1st afternoon   Field work
1. Tour of work area
2. Demonstration of sweeping with treated dust cloths
3. Spray and mop method — demonstration and trial

2nd morning   Lecture and Discussion
1. Review previous day's material — by a student
2. Very fundamental explanation of spread of infection
   a. Inoculate blood agar plates with cough, fork, finger prints, hair, dirty mop, wash water, air, dirty dressing, dirty tissue. Keep control plate which is properly marked
   b. Incubate all plates
3. Isolation technique — have nurse teach it

2nd afternoon   Field work
1. Observe actual and potential sources of infection
2. Practice isolation technique under nursing supervision
3. Practice floor washing procedure

3rd morning
1. Review previous day's work — by a student
2. Discuss and see film strips of other cleaning procedures such as policing of areas, high dusting, bathroom cleaning
   a. Discuss hazards to patients
   b. Discuss hazards to employees
3. Introduce and discuss concept and practice of work schedule

3rd afternoon   Field work
1. Demonstration and practice of:
   a. Policing of areas
   b. High dusting
   c. Bathroom cleaning

4th morning
1. Review previous day's work — by a student
2. Discuss and see film strips on:
   a. Waste handling, removal and cleaning of containers

  b. Laundry handling, removal and cleaning of containers
3. Discuss role of nurse and housekeeping department — by Executive House-keeper and Nursing Supervisor
4. Discuss safety as a way of life

4th afternoon
  1. Practice bathroom cleaning
  2. Practice waste handling, removal and cleaning of containers
  3. Practice laundry handling, removal and cleaning of containers

5th morning
  1. Review of previous day's work — by student
  2. Observe blood agar plates and discuss implications of spread of infection
  3. Discuss personnel hygiene — protection for self, family, and patient
  4. Review isolation techniques
  5. Discuss role of supervisor, self-inspection technique

5th afternoon
  1. One hour written examination on material
  2. Two hour field experience examination

Follow-up with close supervision for one month. Retest after field experience. Give certificate indicating successful completion of course at general meeting of housekeeping staff. Give close supervision for the rest of a 6–9 month probationary period

2-3-9 Supervisory and Administrative Training

The main purpose of this course is to train individuals in a new supervisory technique, self-inspection. The subsidiary purposes are to re-emphasize existing hospital procedures and introduce new ones. The desired ultimate result is to provide a clean, bright, safe environment where hospital acquired infection would not flourish. The material discussed includes principles of the spread of disease, basic bacteriology, the self-inspection program, proper cleaning techniques, inspectional techniques, basic supervision, techniques of supervision, elements of supervision, and specific supervisory problems. It also includes decontamination and asepsis, isolation techniques, proper cleaning of contaminated areas, safety, and employee training. The relationship of the nursing supervisors and the custodial supervisors are discussed thoroughly. This is an excellent way of making sure that channels of communication are open and therefore the work of the hospital in this area should proceed more smoothly.

Several general discussions are held concerning specific housekeeping problems. These problems are noted on the self-inspection sheet. Priority items are those which are either of very serious nature or appear frequently on inspection sheets. Although supervisors are somewhat hesitant in the beginning to discuss problems in their area for fear that it might reflect upon them, they soon learn that their problems are not unique and that other supervisors are faced with the same situations. Because this free flow of ideas could take place, many good recommendations are made, and subsequently several procedures may be changed.

Group interest is usually so high that the two hour seminar is generally over before the discussions can be brought to a close. Initially, two two hour seminars are scheduled. Actually, a third or fourth two hour seminar may be scheduled to cover more of the material disclosed on the self-inspection sheets.

The teaching staff should include the Chief of Environmental Health, or the local or state Environmental Health Supervisor, the Executive Housekeeper, and the Chief Custodial Supervisor. Special topics should be presented by guest lecturers who would include the Executive Director, Medical Director, Administrative Services Director, Nursing Director, and the Assistant Administrative Services Director of the hospital. Topics should also be presented by outside specialists such as the Chief of Accident Control, and the Chief of Training of the proper Public Health Department. The training courses should be two hours long and given bi-weekly to nursing and custodial supervisors. In a large institution the nursing program on housekeeping differs only in that basic information on asepsis and decontamination is not included in the course. They are excused from this session; however, they may attend if they so desire. The training is fully integrated with the self-inspection program and part of the session should be conducted in a seminar type manner. During the seminar individual problems noted on the self-inspection sheet will be discussed and suggestions will be made by the participants who should show great enthusiasm and interest, for their problems and pet gripes will be aired with fellow supervisors and administration. This approach contributes to the resolution of many incipient problems that have been bothering the supervisors for long periods of time. It also helps develop the need for further study.

There are many fine courses available in supervisory and administrative training. Since all supervisory and administrative personnel of the housekeeping department should have a familiarity with good housekeeping techniques, it would be well to obtain and study some of this course material in addition to the supervisory and administrative training.

2-3-10   The Well Balanced Housekeeping Program — A Summary

The Housekeeping Department strives to attain the goals of a safe, aesthetically, microbiologically clean environment that contributes to the main function of the institution, the best patient care available for the least cost. It is based on the knowledge of the principles of management, supervision, scheduling, training, work procedures and time studies, actions of detergents and germicides, tools and equipment, special precautions in highly critical areas such as communicable disease wards, infection units, operating and delivery rooms, nurseries, and areas of reverse isolation. It is vitally concerned with the control of the spread of infection and the prevention of accidents to patients and employees. It possesses and uses an excellent means of rapid analysis of the Housekeeping Program, "The Housekeeping Self-Inspection Form." It reviews and analyzes the program as needed.

In 1957, MacEachern in his famous textbook on *Hospital Organization and Management* said that scientific housekeeping is just being recognized. Now we say that it has arrived with the assistance of the Environmental Health Hospital Specialist and modern concepts of detergency and cleaning. It has only to be implemented!

2-3-11 Housekeeping Sanitation Checklist Instructions

The Housekeeping Sanitation Checklist is a concise, systematic means of self-inspection by executive housekeepers and supervisors. Regular use provides a complete overall view of conditions throughout a hospital, pinpointing problem areas, facilitating supervision and increasing motivation among employees.

General Guidelines
1. The form can be used for any type of building or floor — large or small. The score is automatically controlled by what the rater actually checks. Typically, an entire floor would be inspected and filled in on one checklist form.
2. If any part of an area or item is unsatisfactory, the entire area or item gets rated unsatisfactory. For example, if you are inspecting the fifth floor of the hospital and one lavatory wash bowl is dirty, then all are rated unsatisfactory.
3. Naturally, some raters will be stricter than others, but discussion between raters and the Executive Housekeeper can provide practical standards.
4. Weekly or twice monthly inspections are suggested.
5. The total score at the upper right hand corner of the form is the "cleanliness grade." One hundred percent is perfect. However, what the "passing grade" for a specific area should be is up to the Executive Housekeeper.
6. The summary sheet shows individual ratings and total scores floor by floor for the entire hospital.

Specific Instructions
1. Fill out top of form completely.

HOUSEKEEPING SANITATION CHECKLIST
PREPARE IN DUPLICATE

This form based on a design by Herman Koren, R.S., M.P.H., Chief of Environmental Health and Safety at Philadelphia General Hospital, Philadelphia Dept. of Public Health. Printed and distributed by Economics Laboratory, Inc., 250 Park Ave., New York, N.Y. 10017.

BLDG. NAME AND NO.	FLOOR & NAME	DATE	TIME
SUPERVISOR MAKING INSPECTION (Sign)		CUSTODIAN OR HOUSEKEEPING AIDE (Sign)	

RATINGS

U – Unsatis. (0)
S – Satis. (1)
N – Not apply

TOTAL SCORE

$$\frac{S's}{S's + U's} \times 100 = \quad \%$$

Fill in all parts of the form. If the item is "Unsatisfactory" show a "U" under the **RATING** and the code under the **AREA CODE**. If an item is "Satisfactory" show an "S" under the **RATING** and nothing under the **AREA CODE**. For example, if the floors are found dirty in the Nurses Station, Laboratory, and Supply Room, put a single "U" under **RATING** on line #2 (*Floors—dirty*). Then list N.R., Lab. #3, and S.R. Use "N" if the item is not applicable. Under **TOTAL SCORE**, count up all the S's, then divide by the S's plus the U's to give you the percentage grade.

AREA CODES:

W. – Ward – Give #	U.T. – Utility Rm.	S.A. – Storage Area	A.R. – Animal Rooms	L.D.R. – Labor & Del. – Give #
So. – Solarium	T.R. – Treatment Rm.	W.R. – Wait. Rm. & Lobby	K – Kitchen	O.R. – Operating Rm. – Give #
P.R. – Patient Rm. – Give #	E.R. – Exam. Rm.	Of. – Offices – Give #	S.R. – Supply Rm.	
N.R. – Nurses Station – Give #	J.S.C. – Janitor Supply Closet	Co. – Corridor	I.C.R. – Instr. Cleaning Rm.	
B.R. – Bathrooms	L.C. – Linen Closet	Lab. – Laboratory – Give #	A.U. – Autoclave Rm.	
	S.S.C. – Sterile Supply Closet	L.R. – Locker Rooms	M.R. – Miscellaneous Rm.	

FLOORS	AREA CODES	RATING	LAVATORIES	AREA CODES	RATING
1. Dust			32. Toilet Paper		
2. Dirty			33. Wash Bowls		
3. Litter			34. Soap		
4. Spillage			35. Paper Towels		
5. Stains			**HOPPER ROOM**		
6. Warning signs			36. Dirty		
WALLS			**JANITORIAL SUPPLY CLOSET**		
7. Dust			37. Adequate supplies		
8. Splattering			38. Clean		
9. Cobwebs			39. Equip. stored properly		
10. Dirty			**PAILS**		
WINDOW SILLS, VENTILATORS			40. Dirty		
11. Dust			**MOP WATER**		
12. Spots			41. Dirty		
RADIATORS			**MOP HEADS**		
13. Dirty			42. Dirty		

52

DOOR LEDGES & FRAMES, TOPS OF CABINETS		43. Poor Condition	
14. Dirty		**REPAIRS**	
WARD SINKS		44. Repair reported below	
15. Wash bowl		**INSECT AND RODENT CONTROL**	
16. Wall		45. Mice	
17. Soap		46. Roaches	
18. Towels		47. Ants	
WASTE RECEPTACLES		48. Flies	
19. Need emptying		**LIGHTS**	
20. Dirty		49. Fixture dirty	
EQUIPMENT		50. Bulbs need replacement	
21. Dust		**WINDOWS AND SCREENS**	
FURNITURE		51. Dirty	
22. Dust		**STAIRWAYS**	
23. Spillage		52. Litter	
LAVATORIES		53. Dust	
24. Walls and windows		54. Spillage	
25. Partitions		55. Needs repair	
26. Floors		56. Needs bulbs	
27. Tubs		**ELEVATORS (Give number)**	
28. Showers		57. Floor	
29. Urinals		58. Walls	
30. Toilet Seats		59. Tracks	
31. Toilet Bowls		60. Doors	

44. REPAIRS REPORTED	LOCATION	44. REPAIRS REPORTED	LOCATION
a. Wall needs repair		k. Wash basin faucets leaking	
b. Broken window		l. Wash basin stopped up	
c. Broken or missing window screens			
d. Ceiling needs repair			
e. Peeling paint			
f. Floor tile loose			
g. Floor tile broken			
h. Broken lighting fixtures or burnt out bulbs			
i. Stopped up floor drains			
j. Hopper broken or stopped up			

Figure 2-3 Housekeeping sanitation checklist.

HOUSEKEEPING SANITATION CHECKLIST SUMMARY

BUILDING

NAME OF RATER

DATE

ITEM	SUB-BASEMENT	BASEMENT	1ST FLOOR	2ND FLOOR	3RD FLOOR	4TH FLOOR	5TH FLOOR	6TH FLOOR	7TH FLOOR	8TH FLOOR	TOTAL
1											
2											
3											
4											
5											
6											
7											
8											
9											
10											
11											
12											
13											
14											
15											
16											
17											
18											
19											
20											
21											
22											
23											
24											
25											
26											
27											
28											

29																														
30																														
31																														
32																														
33																														
34																														
35																														
36																														
37																														
38																														
39																														
40																														
41																														
42																														
43																														
44																														
45																														
46																														
47																														
48																														
49																														
50																														
51																														
52																														
53																														
54																														
55																														
56																														
57																														
58																														
59																														
60																														
Total Score																														

Figure 2-4   Housekeeping sanitation checklist summary

2. Begin at item 1 and go down the list in order, rating each item as "S" (satisfactory), "U" (unsatisfactory) or "N" (not applicable).
3. If a "U" rating is given, fill in the area code in the "Area Code" column space to identify the trouble spot. Leave the area code column blank if "S" or "N" is filled in. Area codes may be found at the top of the checklist. If more than one area has the same problem, fill in the other area codes beside each other in the same space in the area code column.
4. Where repairs are needed, put a "U" beside item #44 on the form and then fill in the area code next to the appropriate repair description at the bottom of the sheet.
5. Scoring:
   When figuring the score, count up all the "S" ratings and then all the "U" ratings. Ignore "N"'s—they do not count. Then fill in the total number of "S"'s and "U"'s into this formula:

$$\frac{S's}{S's + U's} \times 100 = \ \% \text{ grade}$$

In other words, divide the total number of "S" ratings plus "U" ratings into the total number of "S" ratings and multiply by 100 to get the percent grade.

For example, after an inspection you may find you have 40 "S"'s and 10 "U"'s. Filling in the formula you have:

$$\frac{40}{40 + 10} \times 100 = \ \% \text{ grade}$$

your percent grade comes out to 80%.

REFERENCES AND SELECTED READINGS

A Series of Housekeeping Lectures, New York: Economic Laboratories.

CDC Training Program, *Selected Material on Environmental Aspects of Staphylococcal Disease*, Atlanta, Ga.: U.S. Dept. of HEW, PHS, January 1959.

Feldman, E. B. *Industrial Housekeeping: Its Technology and Techniques*. New York: MacMillan, 1963.

Housekeeping Manual for Health Care Facilities, Chicago: American Hospital Association, 1966.

Koren, H. Housekeeping self-inspection program, *Hospitals, J.A.H.A.* Vol. 42, pp. 107–113, February 16, 1968.

Loftus, J. T. and Roan, A. J. Modern Management Edu-Text Series International Textbook Company, 1966.

MacEachern, M. T. *Hospital Organization and Management*. 3rd ed. revised, Chicago: Physicians Record Company, 1957.

Management Techniques for the Hospital Executive Housekeeper, Chicago: National Sanitary Supply Association, Inc., 1965.

Many conferences with Miss Rita Fennwick, Director of Nursing, Phila. General Hospital, Dr. Evelyn Carpenter, Director of Food Service, Phila. General Hospital and their staffs.

Many conferences with physicians and surgeons from University of Penn. Medical School, Jefferson Medical School, Temple University School of Medicine, Hahnaman Medical School, Women's Medical College.

Pfiffner, J. M. and Fels, Marshall. *The Supervision of Personnel.* Englewood Cliffs, N.J.: Prentice Hall, May 1965.

2-4 ICE SANITATION

2-4-1 Introduction

Ice is used in institutions, as elsewhere, for cooling drinks and food to make it more palatable and safer. It is used for a variety of therapeutic procedures: ice water enemas and ice water sponges, which reduce high temperatures, for packing around gangrenous legs before amputation, in ice bags used on patients to reduce swelling, and in tubs of ice to reduce extremely high temperatures.

Potential pathogenic organisms which are water borne are not killed by freezing; therefore, ice may act as a means of transmission of these organisms.

2-4-2 Production

Ice comes in three forms: natural ice, which is harvested from naturally occurring bodies of water; manufactured ice, which is made by freezing water in containers; and cubed or flaked ice, which is made in a variety of machines which are located within the institution.

Natural ice is subject to impurities and contamination from air, soil, dust, snow, and flooding. Although a natural purification takes place by means of the ice formation, i.e., ice goes downward and therefore leaves suspended and dissolved materials near the surface, it cannot be considered to be pure.

Manufactured ice is made by filling cans with pure water, placing them in a brine tank, enclosing a copper pipe called a needle, and freezing. The copper pipe conveys compressed air, which bubbles up constantly to prevent the water in and around the center from freezing. The water in the core contains most of the impurities and salts. The needles are then removed and an instrument is used for sucking out the contaminated center. Fresh water is then added to the core and frozen. The freezing period takes from 40 to 50 hours and is usually done at 14–20°F.

Cubed ice is made by passing a few quarts of water across a special freezing plate continuously, thereby carrying away water impurities. A clear sheet of ice builds up to selected thickness. This sheet of ice is transferred to ice cutting grids which divide it into cubes. Cubes then drop into a bin and are stored until used.

Chipped or flaked ice is formed by passing water over an evaporator plate and then subjecting it to an auger, which resembles a corkscrew. The ice then drops into a bin. Chipped ice is somewhat heavier than flaked ice, because it contains more ice crystals. Flaked ice resembles snow.

The latest ice making machines are self-contained wall production and storage units which drop the ice automatically into the vessel on demand. The quantity of ice used within the institution varies with the time of day, season of the year, temperature and humidity, and the particular hospital department. It is necessary, allowing for this reason, to base the purchase of ice making machines on the maximum amount used. This allows some reserve for emergencies. For planning purposes, a rough estimate of ice needs would be six pounds per bed per day and four to six pounds per person per meal per day in a cafeteria type operation. However, only the individual experience of a particular hospital will provide the administrator with fairly accurate information concerning ice needs. (*See* Section 2-4-4 and Figure 2-5.)

2-4-3   Ice — The Potential Disease Hazard

There have been few instances of the spread of disease traced to ice. (*See* Rosenau's *Preventive Medicine and Hygiene.*) However, the potential is ever present because of poor techniques of transportation of commercial ice and poor practices of storage and distribution of commercial as well as cubed ice. Although extremely desirable, it may be very costly and impractical to place an ice making machine in each area of the institution. Therefore, employees, usually hospital aides or food service workers, will have to go from their assigned area to the area in which the ice is produced. This means that the ice will be handled by many personnel and transported in a variety of containers. The handling and transportation introduces unwanted organisms which contaminate the product. The container which may vary in type and size becomes contaminated through use, and therefore creates a cleaning problem.

The storage bin of the ice making machine is a further source of contamination. When personnel dip into the ice to remove the amount they need, they contaminate the remainder. Some personnel have the bad habit of storing food, blood specimens, or other laboratory specimens in the ice. A recent unpublished study indicated that 88% of all commercial ice used in an institution was contaminated with *E. Coli*. Since the ice making plant was sanitary, and the procedures good, the contamination had to be attributed to transportation and storage. It is suspected that studies of cubed and flaked ice would also reveal contamination.

2-4-4   Ice Survey

It is necessary to survey an institution to determine the condition in which the ice reaches the patient (*see* Figure 2-5). Pitchers, glasses, ice storage boxes, and ice makers are inspected for cleanliness. Their condition is noted and proper locations are determined for existing units, as well as new units. Ice needs, distribution patterns, and manpower utilization are measured.

The condition of the ice reaching the patient can be ascertained by physical observation of the ice itself, and the containers in which it is transported. Once it is determined that the ice and the appropriate containers are clean, then it is well to conduct limited microbiological studies to make sure that other types of unseen contamination are not entering the ice supply.

The condition of ice machines is most essential, since poor condition leads to contamination and reduces ice production, which in turn raises the demand for manufactured ice. Manpower evaluation can help the hospital save time in ice distribution duties; limit contamination by reduced handling; and thereby help the hospital aides concentrate more profitably on patient care.

Distribution patterns and needs of specific areas are assessed by determining the amount of ice each nursing unit uses during the summer and winter. New machines are placed in areas which can conveniently serve adjacent nursing departments.

2-4-5   Recommendations

Based on the surveys and studies which are made at the institution, new machines, such as flakers, cubers, and storage equipment, should be purchased and placed in those areas which are most readily accessible, to satisfy the needs of the nursing departments. Ice making machines, as any other machine, have a specific life. When machines become dilapidated, they should be replaced. It would be well to institute a program which would replace each machine over five years old.

Ice machines should be cleaned twice a week or when contaminated. A monthly maintenance cleaning and emergency service contract should be made with a reputable organization. A yearly contract is usually less expensive than a service on demand contract. All visits by the service organization should be recorded and their emergency number should be listed on the machine in order that they can be reached immediately when needed.

Proper distribution of ice can be maintained if one or two individuals are assigned the task, rather than sending a representative from each nursing department. The scoop should be stored on the outside of the machine and washed before use with hot water and detergent, rinsed with hot water and then finally with cold water. Glasses and carafes should be washed each day in automatic dishwashers. A final rinse of hot water of 180°F is essential. In some institutions disposable carafes and glasses are used. This is a more acceptable procedure, if the carafe or glass is washed daily. Names should be put on in indelible ink. In some areas of the hospital, it might be more feasible and cheaper to install water coolers. This could reduce the ice drain, especially during the summer months.

Training programs should be developed for nursing and food service personnel to teach them how to handle ice, clean utensils and equipment. Where sufficient funds are available, a new type of ice making machine which produces the ice and delivers it to a distribution or storage unit automatically should be purchased. An acceptable unit is a 450 lb/24-hour capacity machine with a 350–400 lb storage unit.

2-4-6   Summary

There may seem to be a disproportionate amount of material presented in this area compared to more important programs, however, the reliance on ice might increase sharply as power failures due to overload occur, and water coolers and ice makers become partially or totally inoperative.

2-4-7   Care of Ice Making Machines

Where hospitals perform their own cleaning, the following procedures should be followed:

1. *Daily Care*
   a. Once, each third day, turn off the machine, clean out ice cubes, and thoroughly clean all exposed surfaces of ice machine, inside and out, with standard quaternary detergent-disinfectant or iodophor solution ($\frac{2}{3}$ oz

per gallon of water). Use a good nylon brush to clean crevices and a sponge for the flat surfaces.

b. Rinse the inside of the machine with clear water.

c. Using a standard quaternary detergent-disinfectant or iodophor solution, sanitize all inner surfaces using a sponge.

d. These operations should be performed at a time when ice is in small demand. Do not put ice removed at the start of the cleaning operation back into the machine.

ICE SURVEY REPORT

NAME OF INSTITUTION	NAME OF INVESTIGATOR	DATE	TIME

AREA CODES:

W. – Ward – Give #	U.T. – Utility Rm.	S.A. – Storage Area
So. – Solarium	T.R. – Treatment Rm.	W.R. – Wait. Rm. & Lobby
P.R. – Patient Rm. – Give #	E.R. – Exam. Rm.	Of. – Offices – Give #
N.R. – Nurses Station – Give #	J.S.C. – Janitor Supply Closet	Co. – Corridor
B.R. – Bathrooms	L.C. – Linen Closet	Lab. – Laboratory – Give #
A.R. – Animal Rooms	S.S.C. – Sterile Supply Closet	L.R. – Locker Rooms
K – Kitchen	L.D.R. – Labor & Del. – Give #	O.R. – Operating Rm. – Give #
	S.R. – Supply Rm.	I.C.R. – Instr. Cleaning Rm.
	A.U. – Autoclave Rm.	M.R. – Miscellaneous Rm.

CONDITION OF STORAGE CONTAINER

1. Clean = C
2. Sanitized = S
3. Dirty = D
4. Slimy = Sl

TYPE OF STORAGE

Stainless Steel = S
Galvanize = G
Canvas Bags = C
Wooden Buckets = W
Plastic Containers = P

TYPE OF ICE
Natural = N
Manuf. = M
Cubed = C
Flaked = F

AGE OF MACHINES
Show number of
years from date
of installation

CONDITION OF MACHINE
Excellent = E
Good = G
Fair = F
Poor = P
Not Working = NW

Amount of Ice Required
Show Winter and Summer quantities as <u>x lbs winter, y lbs summer</u>

Build. Name #	Floor & Name	Area	Type of Ice	Age of Machine	Type of Storage	Cond. of Storage Container	Amt. of Ice Required	
							Win.	Sum.

COMMENTS:

Figure 2-5   Ice survey report.

e. The ice scoop should never be left (sitting) on top of the ice cubes. Between uses, it should be kept immersed in a weak clorox or iodophor solution (one teaspoon, or one capful of clorox, if the quart bottle of clorox is used, in one quart of cool water, provides about 250 ppm available chlorine). Change the solution daily at the same time the machine is cleaned.

f. Personnel, before removing ice, should wash their hands.

2. *Monthly Care — Deliming*
   a. Once a month, or oftener if needed, defrost the ice making machine and dismantle.
   b. Use a solution of one ounce mild acid detergent per quart of water, brushwash all parts of a machine, using a good nylon-bristled brush.
   c. Make sure all holes where water is flowing are completely cleaned. Use a test tube or catheter brush, if needed.
   d. Rinse thoroughly with clear water, and inspect major parts. Reassemble machine for normal operation.

REFERENCES AND SELECTED READINGS

Personal conferences with nursing personnel concerning the use of ice in therapeutic procedures, 1965.

Rosenau, M. *Preventive Medicine and Hygiene.* Kenneth F. Macy (Ed.), 8th ed., p. 1234, 1956.

Sanitarian's Handbook, Theory and Administrative Practice, Ben Freedman, M.D., M.P.H., p. 1060.

Unpublished studies on Bacteriological Analysis of ice in an institution.

Unpublished studies on Ice Sanitation—Transportation, Storage Distribution, Sanitation, Quantity and Quality of existing ice makers and recommendations based on need.

2-5 ILLUMINATION, COLOR, AND CALL SYSTEMS

2-5-1 Introduction

Illumination is a factor of primary importance in the hospital environment. The ever increasing development of new medical techniques and intricate equipment demands proper levels of illumination. Light levels may vary from a fraction of a footcandle for night-lights to 2500 footcandles for intricate surgical procedures.

The role of light is to promote efficiency, sanitation, safety, and comfort. Poor lighting results in eye and then body fatigue, decreased service, increased irritability, poor housekeeping, accidents, and low patient and staff morale.

Good illumination is the accumulated effect of quantity and quality of light, direct and reflected glare, brightness ratios, color of surfaces, contrast between walls and door jambs, cleanliness of fixtures, and individual idiosyncrasies.

In patient areas during the day general lighting should be about 10 footcandles. Higher levels may produce direct or reflected glare. Routine nursing care can be carried out at this level, but it is insufficient for detailed reading of thermometers, charts, instruments and other data which needs additional light. A bedside lamp should be provided for these purposes, and for examination of the patient by the doctor. When patients sleep or rest a night-light of a low level of illumination should be used to help the patient orient himself to his surroundings. This light should not disturb other patients.

The usual cause of complaints from patients are glare from bright light sources and reflecting surfaces. Excessive variations in light may cause discomfort. Heat generating from reading lights can cause annoyances. The hospital staff usually complains about insufficient general illumination for routine nursing care, housekeeping, examinations, intravenous injection and wound dressing.

A detailed discussion on lighting for hospitals may be found in *Illuminating Engineering*, June 1966. Tables of recommended footcandles for all hospital areas from the autopsy room to the storage rooms are presented.

2-5-2   Wiring

Proper lighting is intimately related to the electrical wiring system and emergency lighting system. Electric call systems must also be considered.

Modern existence demands the use of air conditioners, special electrically operated equipment and increased voltage bulbs. Old buildings unless renovated are unprepared to service this demand. The result is shut down in service or fires from short circuits.

The necessity for emergency electrical systems with automatic switch on gear to provide power for heat, light, food services, and emergency facilities such as operating, delivery and emergency rooms, fire alarms, call systems and exit lights, was amply demonstrated during the massive power failures in parts of Eastern United States, November 10, 1965 and June 5, 1967. The emergency source of electricity is usually provided by gasoline or diesel driven generators.

2-5-3   Lamp Maintenance

Dirt accumulations on lamps reduce available light by 50%. This negates all of the efforts directed toward improving the quantity of available light for important tasks. Burnt out lamps have the same effect.

It is important to clean lamps and replace blocks of lights on a routine basis determined by survey.

2-5-4 Special Electrical Problems

Lights on the nurses' monitoring station in coronary care are most essential. Sudden changes represented by fine graph lines on a tape, or a pulsing line on a screen can represent life or sudden death. If the nurse is unable to read these recorded heart beats quickly and accurately, disaster may follow.

A new concept in lighting is necessary for the intensive care unit, since the area serves as a combination examination, treatment room, emergency room, nurses' station, and patient ward. The light must be distributed to serve a multiplicity of functions ranging from emergency minor surgery, to quiet bed rest for patients. The environment must combine visual control, and efficiency with thermostatic and humidity control.

Bathrooms without electric call systems are a hazard to patients and employees. These signals should register on a call board in the nurses' station. The call system should also be installed in bedrooms, and should have a visual as well as audible signal.

2-5-5 Program

A study program should include the proper use of light materials and the determination of the quantity and quality of light, the maintenance of lights, color of walls, and electric call systems. This study should be carried out once every six months. *See* Study Form Figure 2-6.

Discussion

Illumination is such a complex subject that environmental health people could spend all of their time in this particular area, and still not be proficient. Specialists who are illumination engineers can determine for the hospital how to get the best results for specific problems, and how to set up proper lighting facilities. The function of the environmentalist is to determine where the problem exists, and to advise the administrative staff in order that they might secure competent help.

2-5-6 Summary

Proper illumination is the key to our modern society, and therefore the key to the modern institution. Where electrical systems fail institu-

LIGHT STUDY FORM

DATE	TIME	RATINGS S = Satis. (1) U = Unsatis. (0) N = Not apply	TOTAL SCORE $\dfrac{\text{S's}}{\text{S's} + \text{U's}} \times 100 =$ %
PERSON MAKING STUDY			

AREA CODES:

W. – Ward – Give #	U.T. – Utility Rm.	S.A. – Storage Area
So. – Solarium	T.R. – Treatment Rm.	W.R. – Wait. Rm. & Lobby
P.R. – Patient Rm. – Give #	E.R. – Exam. Rm.	Of. – Offices – Give #
N.R. – Nurses Station – Give #	J.S.C. – Janitor Supply Closet	Co. – Corridor
B.R. – Bathrooms	L.C. – Linen Closet	Lab. – Laboratory – Give #
A.R. – Animal Rooms	S.S.C. – Sterile Supply Closet	L.R. – Locker Rooms
K – Kitchen	L.D.R. – Labor & Del. – Give #	O.R. – Operating Rm. – Give #
	S.R. – Supply Rm.	I.C.R. – Instr. Cleaning Rm.
	A.U. – Autoclave Rm.	M.R. – Miscellaneous Rm.

	AREA CODE	RATING
WIRING SYSTEM		
1. Does the electric wiring system meet the local, state or underwriters' standards?		
2. Is there any loose wiring?		
3. Are octopus connections used?		
4. Is there a system overload? (Name electrical appliances & location)		
QUANTITY		
1. Is there an adequate quantity of light for the task? (Indicate actual footcandles)		
QUALITY		
1. Is there an adequate brightness ratio for the task?		
2. Is there uniform distribution of light?		
3. Are colors distorted?		
4. Is there a source of direct glare? (Name source)		
5. Is there a source of indirect glare? (Name source)		
MAINTENANCE		
1. Are there any burnt out units?		
2. Are the fixtures dirty?		
3. Is there a scheduled replacement program of lights?		
4. Is there a scheduled cleaning program?		
COMMENTS:		

Figure 2-6   Light study form.

tions immediately stop operating in an efficient and effective manner. Electric power failures have demonstrated in recent years how much we depend on electricity. Hospital illumination poses many problems involving a wide range of conditions. Comfortable illumination must be provided for doctors, nurses, technicians, employees, patients, and visitors.

REFERENCES AND SELECTED READINGS

Griffin, N. L. *Hospital Electrical Facilities*. U.S. Dept. HEW, PHS Pub. #930-D-3, U.S. Gov. Printing Office, Washington, D.C. June 1963.

Lighting for hospitals, *Illumination Engineering*. 61, June 1966.

Lighting for Hospital Patient Rooms. U.S. Dept. HEW, PHS Pub. #930-D-3, U.S. Gov. Printing Office, Washington, D.C. June 1963.

Lighting hospital patient rooms, *Architectural Record*. 134, November 1963.

2-6 INSECT AND RODENT CONTROL

2-6-1 Introduction

The very nature of the hospital makes it a place where rodents and insects cannot be tolerated, yet where conditions are favorable for the entrance and multiplication of such pests. Their normal propensity for transmitting disease is markly increased by the substantial quantity of virulent organisms present in the environment.

A pest control program includes comprehensive studies; organization, scheduling and training of exterminators; elimination of food, harborage and points of entrance for insects and rodents; and the coordinated efforts of the entire hospital community.

Breeding Habits and Life Cycle of Insects

Roaches

Oriental Roaches
1. Breeding Habits. Moisture needs to be present. Usually unsanitary conditions exist, but can be present under very clean conditions if moisture and minimum food are available. Nocturnal in habit. Found in crevices behind moldings, and door and window frames, in cabinets and closets, in asbestos covering of hot water lines, in corrugated paper, and under general debris.
2. Food. Cereals and baked goods, small amounts of grease, glue, starch, wall paper binding, fecal material, and dead animals.
3. Life Cycle. Varies from 7 to 30 months. Adult longevity averages three months. Each female produces an average of 14 egg cases, each containing 14 eggs.

German Roaches
1. Breeding Habits. Same as Oriental.
2. Food. Same as Oriental.
3. Life Cycle. Varies from 3 to 9 months. Adult longevity averages four and one-half months. Female produces an average of 7 egg cases, each containing 37 eggs.

American Roaches
1. Breeding Habits. Same as Oriental.
2. Food. Same as Oriental.
3. Life Cycle. Varies from 3 to 18 months. Average adult life is 14 months. Female produces average of 58 egg cases, each containing 15 eggs.

Bedbugs
1. Breeding Habits. Temperature should be around 70°F. No eggs are laid below temperatures of 50°F.
2. Food. Blood from man, rats, poultry, and other animals.
3. Life Cycle. From 2 to 4 eggs are laid per day. The egg hatches in 6–17 days. Development takes from 3 to 8 weeks. Adults may live from 6 to 8 months where there is favorable temperatures and ready food supply.
4. Description. The adult bedbug, *Cimex Lectularis* is $\frac{1}{5}$ in. long, $\frac{1}{8}$ in. wide and reddish brown in color. The flattened oval body is adapted for hiding in narrow crevices. The head bears a pair of four segmented antennae and piercing-sucking mouthparts which fold to lie between the first pair of legs. The wings are represented by pads. The body may become greatly enlarged and blood red in color during the taking of a blood meal.

Ants
1. Breeding Habits. The most common ant breeds beneath pavements, in foundation walls, under wooden floors.
2. Food. Scraps of food in the kitchen, particularly sweet and fatty foods.

Flies (Housefly is most common type)
1. Breeding Habits. Any fresh, moist organic material, such as wet cereal grains, animal manure, and garbage.
2. Food. Sugar and starch are needed for energy and proteins are needed for egg production.
3. Life Cycle. Eggs hatch within 12–24 hours. Development of the three larval stages takes about 4–7 days in warm weather. After completing this part of the development, the larvae migrate to dryer portions of breeding media to pupate. Pupal stages are completed in 4–5 days. Adult then emerges and after one day is capable of mating.

Rats and Mice
1. Breeding Habits. Protected areas near food and water. Out-of-doors, they will breed in a burrow or in debris. In-doors, between walls, between stacked boxes, and in unused places.
2. Food. Rats and mice eat almost any food that man eats.
3. Life Cycle. The period of gestation in the Norway rat averages 22 days and mating can take place as soon as two days after young are born. Four to six litters are produced a year, each with from 8 to 12 babies in it. Sexual maturity is gained about three months after birth in the rat and between 6 and 8 weeks after birth in the mouse.

2-6-2   Study Techniques

Infestation may be measured by sanitary surveys, analysis of records and procedures, special studies, and interviews of the hospital staff.

Sanitary surveys determine the location, extent, and severity of infestation, probable routes of travel or transportation, and causes for the presence of mice, rats, roaches, ants, and other insect pests. They also determine the housekeeping and maintenance problems by location, extent, and type (*see* Figure 2-3). Existing pest control measures are analyzed by the use of available records; by the observation of procedures, techniques, and chemicals used for chemical control; and the observation of procedures and techniques used for the physical control of insects and rodents. Special time studies determine the amount of work completed, time used by the present exterminating crews and the amount of manpower needed to conduct a satisfactory control program.

Interviews determine staffing patterns of units in relationship to the amount and type of supervision of housekeeping, food services, and nursing personnel; areas of cleaning responsibility; areas of food service responsibility; and the type of services offered by the hospital exterminating crew or private exterminator. Interviews also help identify certain problem areas, and test the efficacy of certain recommendations. Since it is impractical to examine every part of a given area in the hospital, once a pattern of infestation has been established, additional studies may not be necessary.

2-6-3   General Sanitation and Housekeeping

Food Area

This includes preparation, serving, storage, and dishwashing areas and equipment. In preparation and serving areas of kitchens and pantries, crumbs and food residue may be found between sinks and walls, on the bottom of shelves, under tables, under equipment, behind stainless steel shelves and walls, stoves and steamers, in sinks, in ice chest wells, in garbage and trash cans, and on floors in corners. Butcher shops have a large accumulation of sawdust and organic matter from meat cutting. In storage areas, accumulations of spillage of flour, sugar, and beans may be found on shelves, on floors, and in corners. Food may be stored against the wall. In ward pantries and kitchens, large quantities of unprotected bread, bananas and other food may be seen at night. They should be stored in roach and mouse proof containers. Food remnants from late trays may be left standing for several hours in the dishwashing room and in ward kitchens.

These conditions may be corrected by establishing proper schedules of cleaning and tray removal, reinforced by good training courses for food service employees and close supervision of problem situations to insure compliance.

Ward Area

Food residue from the evening meal, visiting time, and nourishment periods may be left on floors, in bathrooms, in encrusted stepcans and uncovered waste baskets all night long. Baby formulas, milk, and other foods may be dumped into ward sinks and the sinks may not be washed out thoroughly. A bedside table may contain accumulations of all types of food and crumbs, it may be cleaned infrequently or just when the patient leaves the hospital.

Food from Visitors

It is recognized that it is virtually impossible and probably psychologically undesirable to stop the patients from receiving food from visitors. Therefore, it should be stipulated that all food be eaten at once, or discarded. Hard candy may be kept in cans or bottles. All patients and visitors should be notified in writing about this rule. Nurses should then be given authority to discard any food improperly stored. Bedside tables should be inspected and cleaned out by nursing personnel each morning.

Janitorial Assignments

Some custodians will have to work a shift from 12–9 p.m. to remove trash from waste containers, and utility rooms; clean floors under beds and radiators; after the dinner, visiting and nourishment periods. This will eliminate a major source of food for pests.

Nurse's Station

Roach problems in this area can generally be eliminated by cleaning up spilled syrupy medication and removing cracker crumbs, snacks and coffee containers from drawers or waste baskets.

Clinic Areas

Clinic patients may eat everything from snacks to almost full course meals in various waiting rooms, bathrooms, and examining rooms. Crumbs and food residue may be found on the floors, under benches and under radiators. Waste cans of the self-closing type are not roach proof. Food wrappers and food residue may be found in open waste baskets. It is essential that these areas be cleaned, trash removed, and waste containers emptied before the hospital settles down for the night.

Informal Staff Lunchrooms

It is probably impractical to attempt to eliminate the informal staff lunchrooms. Therefore, the cleanliness, food storage, and disposal of waste from these rooms must be the direct responsibility of the unit supervisor and he must be held accountable for any breaks in technique.

Nurses' Home

Student nurses' living quarters that are cluttered or contain food or food remnants attract pests.

Animal Laboratories

Animal laboratories provide excellent sources of food and harborage for insects and rodents. Roaches live in the channels between cages and feed on the animal food which is always available. Food spillage, improper storage of animal food in bags instead of metal cans with lids and leftovers from employees lunches increase the food supply for pests. Unfortunately, these areas usually receive a minimum amount of cleaning. Proper daily cleaning, waste removal, improvement in employee habits, and frequent rotation and cleaning of cages coordinated with use of insecticides can eliminate the pest problem.

Conveying Equipment and Shafts

Food conveyors, tray carts, laundry carts, and other vehicles may contain food accumulations, dust and dirt, roaches, ants, and mice. Plumbing and elevator shafts may contain paper, food wrappers, and other litter. Pests use this material as a source of food.

The Morgue and Autopsy Room

The morgue and autopsy room are usually not cleaned as thoroughly as other hospital areas. Quantities of blood and bits of tissues near the weighing scales, autopsy tables, or storage tables act as a powerful attractant to roaches, flies, and rodents.

The Laundry

In the laundry, large quantities of lint, dust, and dirt may be found on floors, under, behind, and on equipment, walls and ceilings. Cleaning may be grossly inadequate, especially in older laundries because of layout and construction. Uncovered trash cans may contain food accumulations from employees lunches and snacks. Used, soiled and blood-encrusted linens are a powerful attractant for insects and rodents. Screening is essential. Laundry carts which transport clean linens may contain large quantities of dirt, dust, etc. The cloth containers in old-fashioned carts may either be infrequently washed or not washed at all.

A regularly scheduled program of cleaning, intensive housekeeping, proper storage of dirty linens and rapid washing needs to be planned and implemented to reduce this pest attractant and place of harborage. Laundry carts should be cleaned daily.

2-6-4   Refuse and Garbage Storage and Disposal

Metal cans used for trash and garbage storage tend to become encrusted with dirt and organic material. Where the quantity of trash exceeds the capacity of the containers, cardboard boxes or bags, although unsatisfactory, may be used. All garbage and waste containers need plastic liners and should be scoured weekly. The last trash removal in an institution usually takes place at the end of the day shift (between 3:00 and 4:00 p.m.). Since this is prior to dinner, visiting time and nourishment periods, substantial quantities of trash remain in patient areas overnight. Improperly packaged surgical and isolation waste create hazards. Where Dempster dumpsters are used they usually have accumulations of trash and food around them. They are subject to damage during transportation. Even when Dempster dumpsters are structurally sound, the doors are usually left open, and the unit is permitted to overflow. Where incinerators are used, the residue of incomplete combustion and noncombustables are usually not hauled away quickly enough to prevent infestations.

Outer Premises

Garbage and trash may be stored or scattered in many areas. Especially during nice weather, employees tend to eat lunches outside. Bird feeding may occur.

2-6-5   Construction and Maintenance

Holes and openings of almost any size provide means of ingress and egress for pests. Holes may be present in floors, walls, and ceilings where repair work has been done. Piping conduits in floors serve as areas of harborage and as runways for mice and in some locations for roaches. The metal collars around steam pipes and water pipes leading to fixtures and which lead to radiators, may frequently be missing or not tightly secured. In many cases where cement is used to seal the holes between the steam pipes and the walls, the cement may shrink and create a new opening. Mice or roaches find ready access through all of these openings. Radiator covers may be so constructed that cleaning and inspection cannot take place without the removal of several metal screws. Partitions in rooms may be double walled and therefore permit harborage. There may be openings around electrical switchplates, in the grouting between the wall tiles, and behind metal strips and coving at the base of walls. False ceilings act as hiding places for roaches and possibly mice. The molding between walls and ceilings is not always tight fitting. In certain buildings or areas, there may be inspection ports in shafts containing utility lines which either are not tight fitting or covered at all. There may be false housings enclosing the piping behind water coolers. This is an area of roach and mouse harborage, and a place to accumulate junk and debris. Basements are plagued by broken windows and accumulations of junk.

Corrective measures involve the proper type of seal for each opening, a continuous surveillance program, preventive maintenance and immediate, although temporary, closing of all emergency openings in floors, walls, and ceilings. All inspection ports, metal covers and metal housing should have spring type clips for easy removal. Tight metal collars should be placed around all pipes. All cracks should be sealed with cement and checked periodically.

2-6-6   Problems of New Construction

Demolition of buildings and new construction contribute to the spread of pests by disrupting their nesting areas. Other migration occurs from uncapped sewers, especially at night. Food is provided by construction workers who indiscriminately discard their lunch bags. Liquid is provided by any standing water at the construction site. Mosquitoes may grow in this water. Pest problems may be resolved by intensive poisoning before demolition or ground-breaking, strict enforcement of rules concerning disposal of food waste, closing of sewers at night and removal of standing water.

2-6-7   Pest Control

Only the most common pests will be discussed since the type of pest may vary. from area to area. However, this material with modifications will apply to other insects and rodents.

Control Measures for Rats

Red squill should be mixed with corn meal, ground corn or oats, and corn oil. The formula should be 1 part fortified red squill concentrate to 9 parts bait and 3 gallons of corn oil to 100 pounds of mixed bait. A pound of the mixed bait should be placed in all burrows and in other locations where rats may harbor. If control with red squill becomes unsatisfactory, an anticoagulant rat poison (Warfarin, Fumarin, or Pival) should be substituted and used in the formulation of 1 part to 19 parts bait plus corn oil. Water bait stations of liquid anticoagulant are an excellent adjunct to the dry bait. Although many other types of rat poison are available, they are too dangerous to use in the institution.

Control Measures for Mice

Several types of poisons such as 50% DDT tracking powder, strychnine seeds, strychnine with bacon and peanut butter and 1% warfarin dust are effective for mouse control. Special applicators and a respirator should be obtained for this activity. The DDT tracking powder may be used in dry areas at mouse runways and entrances in areas other than wards and food preparation areas. The strychnine seeds may be placed in plumbing shafts and in holes along utility pipes immediately prior to sealing the holes. Strychnine with bacon and peanut butter may be used in the storehouse, in the food service building away from food preparation areas, and in the animal laboratories away from traffic. Mouse traps may be baited with bacon, peanut butter or ground meat, raisins, corn meal, gum drops, nuts, small sardines, but not with cheese. Four unit mouse traps should not be used. Mouse traps should be placed perpendicular to walls where mice are running, with the trigger adjacent to the wall. The bait should be secured with thread. Mouse glue boards (a 6 × 6 inch firm felt base thickly covered with a non-drying adhesive) should be used in locations where dusts, poisons, or traps might be hazardous.

The reason for a variety of mouse control measures is that under the ideal conditions which exist in the hospital, mice may only travel a 20 foot radius from their shelter for food, and because mice are dedicated nibblers. A frequent change in the diet may reduce bait shyness. Where fresh bait is used, it will be necessary to change it each day.

Control Measures for German, American and Oriental Roaches

The German roach has developed a resistance to commonly used insecticides. For this reason, special formulations must be used to control this insect. A 2% baygon roachicide bait has proven very effective as a specific control. Other types of roaches and other insects, however, are amenable to control with the same insecticide. Treatment for roaches should be performed on a bi-weekly basis.

Nonpatient Areas

In hospital areas not directly related to patients, such as bathrooms, hopper rooms, utility rooms, laboratory areas, records rooms, morgue, residence areas, admissions, X-ray clinics, and linen exchange, a 1% diazinon spray should be used. It should be applied by handsprayer at the rate of 1 gallon to 250 square feet of surface area so that the surface is dampened, but the spray does not run off. The diazinon should be mixed with #2 fuel oil at the rate of two ounces of 4S concentrate diazinon to one gallon of oil which will then equal 1% oil base solution. After the first application, it is recommended that the concentration of diazinon in sprays be reduced from 1% to $\frac{1}{2}$%. This will reduce the danger from this insecticide but still maintain effective control. Caution must be exercised against possible fire hazards during spraying and for about six hours after the application because of the oil. Two percent diazinon dust should be puffed into hard-to-get-to places such as the interior of the shell of water coolers, and in electrical switch plates. A dust applicator should be used for this purpose. Kepone paste bait mixed with peanut meal or peanuts may be used to supplement the spray and dust, and should be placed in cracks and crevices. The concentration of kepone in the bait is 0.125%.

Kitchen Areas

Kitchen areas should be fogged with a pyrethrum insecticide, after food service activities have been completed. This should be immediately followed by steam cleaning of cracks, crevices, and other hiding places. The roaches should then be swept up and placed in roach proof containers and destroyed. A 1% diazinon solution should be sprayed carefully on the under surfaces of all food service equipment, which have been wiped dry prior to such application. In addition, the diazinon should be sprayed on an area approximately one foot each way from the junction of walls and floors, behind steamers and stoves. Kepone bait and diazinon dust should be used in the false ceilings of the kitchen. Caution must be exercised in the use of the dust. It should be determined if the false ceilings are tight before the dust is applied. After fogging, spraying, or any use of insecticides in kitchens, and prior to the preparation of food, all food contact surfaces must be thoroughly scrubbed to remove any possible spillage of chemicals. This scrubbing must be very closely supervised by dietary supervisors.

Ward Areas

Bedside tables should be removed to the solarium every other week. The drawers should be removed by nursing personnel. Pyrethrum spray should be used in the channels and sides of the drawers where the metal overlaps. These areas should then be painted with an oil base diazinon solution. In the wards, diazinon oil solution should be sprayed on the wall for a two foot radius around sinks. In wards housing acutely ill patients, only kepone paste bait should be used.

Nursing Stations

Medicines and drugs should be removed for a period of one day from cabinets. The shelves and walls should be thoroughly cleaned, then sprayed with diazinon and the entire cabinet fogged with pyrethrum. After one day, a lining should be placed on the shelves, and the medicines and drugs may be returned. After one week, the lining may be removed and all shelves and walls thoroughly scrubbed.

Other Areas

In the laundry, a water emulsion of diazinon 4E concentration should be used. The water emulsion is prepared by adding two and one-half ounces of 4E concentration to one gallon of water. In addition, kepone baits should be used. The morgue should be fogged extensively with pyrethrum and a water emulsion of diazinon spray should be used. In basements, diazinon dust should be placed around the rodent bait, since roaches will feed on the rodent bait. Kepone paste should be used.

Control Measures for Flies

Flies are controlled by the removal of breeding places; prompt, thorough cleaning of waste receptacles and waste storage areas; screening of all windows, doors, fan openings, etc., and the use of self-closing mechanisms on doors. Propping open of doors by employees is a nasty problem that should be punishable by forceful disciplinary action.

In nonpatient areas, fly baits, fly traps, DDVP strips, fogging with Pyrethrin and Piperonyl Butoxide may be used. After all food has been removed it is possible to fog food service areas with Pyrethrin. (All dead and dying flies should be swept up and removed and all food contact services thoroughly scrubbed.) In some patient areas it is possible to use a fly bait, which is concealed. However, this must be closely supervised by competent people.

There is a great need for research in safe chemical procedures to be used in patient care areas.

Control Measures for Ants

The ant colony which includes the queens and young should be sought out and destroyed. Ants in and around houses can be controlled with 2% chlordane oil solution, or emulsion spray, or kepone paste bait, placed in cracks and crevices in baseboards, under sinks, etc. Ant colonies outside can be destroyed with 2% chlordane solution.

Control Measures for Bedbugs

It is necessary to first find where the bedbugs are hiding. They may be in the seams of the mattress, cracks and crevices of the bed frame. Spray in any hollow place in the bed frame, baseboard, wood trimming on walls, pictures, etc. They can be spotted because they leave stains. Five percent DDT spray should be applied to mattress, bed frames and other cracks and crevices to eliminate the bedbugs.

Control Measures for Lice

Ten percent DDT dust should be rubbed into the head and sifted about the body and clothing, especially the hair. The clothing should be placed into a plastic bag with the DDT powder, thoroughly shaken and then allowed to stay for 24 hours.

It is recognized that other pesticides are constantly being introduced. However, they should only be used when the present measures prove ineffective.

2-6-8   The Program

The program should be in two parts: an intensive campaign of poisoning, trapping, cleanup and pest proofing; then, a permanent preventive program. Accurate records of activities and complaints are a useful tool in program evaluation.

Scheduling

The work of the exterminators must be done at such a time that it will not interfere with the normal operation of the hospital departments and will aid, rather than detract from, patient care.

The exterminators must be prepared to move to other areas at the request of the head nurse if problems occur. Certain areas should be treated only by the exterminator foreman. Other crucial areas should be treated only with the consent of the specialist in environmental health. Schedules which are based on severity of infestation and the nature of the critical area, must be reevaluated every three to six months to determine if changes are necessary. The program in pest control is preventive, and therefore all areas must be serviced regularly. Although complaints must be serviced, to do all of the work necessary to eliminate an infestation and then afterward work only on a complaint basis, leaves the institution wide open to renewed infestation that may be more serious than the original one, since the environmental balance has been disturbed.

Special Safety Precautions

The chemicals used for pest control have to be chosen very carefully, since many of them are extremely toxic. Even those with limited toxicity can be used only in certain parts of the hospital because of the type of patient or patient condition. For instance, traps cannot be used in psychiatry wards, for the triggers could be dangerous. Any type of bait, no matter how nontoxic, cannot be placed on shelves or within reach of children in the pediatric ward.

Precautions must be taken in food handling areas, for any chemical that will eliminate insects must of necessity be toxic. Apparatus powered by gasoline or fuel oil should not be used indoors with the exception of insecticidal fogging machines. All indoor applications should be by hand, compressed air, or properly grounded, electrically operated devices.

Extreme caution must be exercised in and around sterile areas. Close supervision of exterminators by their supervisor or the nursing staff should be mandatory.

The Exterminating Crew

The size of the exterminating crew varies with the size of the institution. It is suggested that one exterminator should be allocated for every 300 beds. An exterminator foreman should be available for every institution. In the institution with less than 300 beds the exterminator foreman can also act as the exterminator.

The sole job of the exterminating crew should be the control of insects, rodents and noxious birds. This crew should report directly to the Executive Housekeeper. It should be a special unit whose function is not diverted to other janitorial services. Pest control of necessity is a continuing and permanent process in all of its phases. There cannot be any reduction in service.

The Exterminator Foreman

An exterminator foreman should be hired to supervise the crew and the extra assistants. He should have several years of experience in the inspection and control of rodents, insects, and noxious pests, including two years in a supervisory capacity, and education equivalent to a high school diploma.

His duties consist of supervisory and training work concerned with the year-round insect and rodent control program, supplemented during the summer months by a program for the control of mosquitoes, flies, and other insects. He makes comprehensive studies of the institution for insect and rodent control problems under the supervision of an Environmental Health Specialist. He must use considerable judgment in working with the medical, nursing, and administrative staff, and must be able to make a field determination, subject to review by the Environmental Health Specialist, whether a specific area can be sprayed for insect work. This is determined by the type of treatment given to patients, by the nature of the patients' illnesses, and by environmental conditions such as the use of oxygen and anesthetic gases.

2-6-9   Training Program

The men hired for exterminating work at the hospital should be at the level of custodian. The requirements for the job include the ability to read and write English and to follow orders. The individuals chosen should be interested in learning a new field and be willing to adapt to new responsibilities. It is believed that an inexperienced person, trained

Sample Schedule for Exterminators for Routine Program

Time for Exterminator's Service	Area to be Serviced	Frequence of Service Per Month				
		Roaches	M..ce	Rats	Flies	Others
Noon to 9 p.m.	Nurses' stations	2	12	Every day when problem exists	Three times a week during fly season	On demand as needed
Noon to 9 p.m.	Bathrooms	2	12			
Noon to 9 p.m.	Utility rooms	2	12			
Noon to 8 p.m.	Hopper rooms	2	12			
7:30 p.m. to 9:30 p.m.	Ward dining rooms	4	15			
7:30 p.m. to 9:30 p.m.	Ward pantries	4	15			
Noon to 9 p.m.	Wards	4	15			
Anytime	Pathology	4	12			
5 p.m. to 9 p.m.	Record room	2	4			
5 p.m. to 9 p.m.	Laboratory floors	4	12			
5 p.m. on	Administration	2	8			
Noon to 5 p.m.	Doctors' and nurses' homes	2	8			
5 p.m. on	X-ray	2	8			
5 p.m. on	Outpatient care areas	4	12			
5 p.m. on	Storehouse	2	15			
Anytime	Office building	2	8			
8 p.m. to 4 a.m.	Food service	4	30			
5 p.m. on	Linen exchange	2	15			
5 p.m. on	Laundry	4	15			
Anytime	Powerhouse	2	8			
Anytime	Outside grounds	—	8			
Anytime	Basements	2	8			

by the Environmental Specialist, is more valuable than a trained person who may have numerous bad habits and may be complaint-oriented.

Course Content

The course consists of lectures supplemented by demonstrations and field trips in the following subject areas:

1. Rodents: their relationship to public health and the hospital; biology of rodents; recognition of rodent signs; and basic principles of rodent control.
2. Insects: their relationship to public health and the hospital; mixing and formulation of insecticides; equipment use; hazards and safety measures.
3. Types of insects: American and German roaches; flies, ants and silverfish; bedbugs, fleas, and ectoparasites of rodents and birds; scabies, mites, and lice; food product insects.
4. Safety problems and sterile areas in the hospital.

At the conclusion of a week of training, a difficult written examination as well as a practical field examination should be given. Exterminators are then given seven additional weeks of closely supervised field experience before they are allowed to perform in the hospital.

2-6-10 Summary

Through careful study insect and rodent problems can be clearly identified. Specifications and schedules can be developed, programs for housekeeping and maintenance formulated and control procedures enacted. The coordinated efforts of the hospital staff, patients, visitors, and others will lead to a pest-free environment.

REFERENCES AND SELECTED READINGS

Davis, V. T., M.D. (Director of the Division of Mental Health and Hospitals, New Jersey.) Control of rodents and other animal pests, *Sanitarians Manual, Standard Operating Procedures for Institutions and Agencies.*

Koren, H. A coordinated program for pest control, *Journal of American Hospital Association.* Vol. 40, October 1966.

Koren, H. and Good, Dr. N. E. A study of the continuing effective killing power of red squill, *Pest Control Magazine,* Vol. 32, No. 8, August 1964.

Mallis, A. *Hand Book of Pest Control: The Behavior, Life History, and Control of Household Pests.* 4th ed., New York: MacNair-Dorland Company, 1964.

Pest Control Record for a Given Area at Designated Hospital

PEST CONTROL RECORD

NAME OF HOSPITAL: _____ BUILDING: ___ FLOOR: ___ AREA: ___

ENVIRONMENTAL SANITATION

Date	TYPE OF SERVICE						TIME			TYPE OF CONTROL																		REMARKS	EXTERMINATOR
	Complaint	Routine	Mice	Roaches	Ants	Flies	Other	Start	Finish	Paint	Spray	Fog	Traps	A-c Liq.	A-c Dry	DDT Pwdr.	Red Squill	Diazinone	Chlordane	Pyrethrum	D.D.T.	Dead mice	Still mice	Still roaches	Other pests found		

Form Developed for Hospital Control Survey

ENVIRONMENTAL INVESTIGATION RECORD FOR INSTITUTIONS

U = UNSATISFACTORY   Cleanliness   R = ROACHES   O = OTHER INSECTS (specify)
S = SATISFACTORY   M = MICE   X = NEEDS REPAIR
                                                 □ INDICATES HEAVY INFESTATION

BUILDING NAME AND NO. _____ DATE _____

FLOOR _____ TYPE OF AREA OR FACILITY _____

1. FOOD
2. Receiving Platform _____
3. Storage Room _____
4. Kitchen (Main) (Ward) (Pantry) _____
   (Coffee Shop) _____
5. Stoves _____
6.   Under & Behind _____
7.   Inside _____
8. Canopies & Exhaust Systems _____
9. Steam Tables _____
10. Sinks _____
11. Grease Traps _____
12. Floor Drains _____
13. Food Conveyors _____

30. PATIENT FACILITIES
31. Sick Room Furnishings _____
32. Beds _____
33. Other _____
34. Bed Side Table _____
35.   Clean _____
36.   Food Present _____
37. Trash Containers _____
38. Walls _____
39. Ceilings _____
40. Floors _____
41. Waiting Rooms _____
42. Toilet Facilities _____
43. Storage Areas _____

59. OTHER FACILITIES
60. Floors _____
61. Walls _____
62. Ceilings _____
63. Files _____
64. Desk & Cabinets _____
65. Closets _____
66. Waste Disposal _____
67. Dead Storage _____
68. Toilet Fac. _____

69. BASEMENT AREAS
70. Crawl Spaces _____
71. Runways _____

14. Food Storage Areas
15. Refrigerators
16. Dry
17. Walls
18. Ceilings
19. Floors
20. Equip. & Utensil Storage
21. Dishwashing Equip.
22. Garbage & Trash Storage
23. Other
24. Transportation of Food

25. LAUNDRY
26. Hoppers
27. Laundry Chutes
28. Soiled Linen Storage
29. Clean Linen Storage

44. HOUSEKEEPING FACIL.
45. Storage
46. Linens
47. Cleaning Materials
48. Equip. Closets
49. Utility Sinks
50. Trash Units
51. Other

52. REFUSE STORAGE & DISPOSAL
53. Garbage
54. Trash
55. Contaminated
56. Dressings
57. Materials
58. Human

72. Heating
73. Water
74. Electrical
75. Equipment
76. Drains
77. Plumbing
78. Storage

79. GROUNDS
80. Type of insect or rodent observed

81. OTHER
82. Water Coolers

ITEM

COMMENTS:

2-7 LAUNDRY

2-7-1 Introduction

The laundry is a large service unit within the total hospital complex. It provides an adequate quantity of clean and sanitary linens routinely, but must also be flexible enough to furnish emergency supplies when needed. The laundry is usually operated by a manager and assistants.

Linen is usually distributed by the housekeeping department. The modern trend is to maintain the laundry manager but put the laundry function under the Executive Housekeeper.

2-7-2 Physical Structure and Flow

In numerous hospitals, the laundry is located on the ground floor in one of the older parts of the physical plant. It may lack adequate light and ventilation. The laundry equipment, the washers, dryers, extractors and ironers, may be old and subject to numerous breakdowns.

The location of the soiled linen room and the flow pattern of the linens affect the potential spread of infection. Soiled storage and sorting areas should be under negative pressure and completely separated from washing, extracting drying and ironing areas, which are under positive pressure. Linens should flow in a straight line from one operation to another without backtracking (*see* Diagram 2-1). Although washing removes organisms, extraction of water, and air contamination may add new ones.

2-7-3 Laundry Chutes

Exhaust air from laundry chutes have been shown to contain staphylococcus. An outbreak of staphylococcus infection in a hospital nursery was traced back to the laundry and refuse chute. Employees leave the chute open after depositing bags. The falling bag causes a piston effect which results in the spread of bacteria throughout the institution. A natural draft or chimney effect also occurs.

This situation may be greatly improved upon by immediately closing the door, and applying exhaust ventilation to linen chutes of about 0.40 inches of water static pressure with the doors closed. Plastic innerlinings further reduce bacterial levels. The chutes should be spray cleaned and disinfected weekly. Special equipment is available for this task.

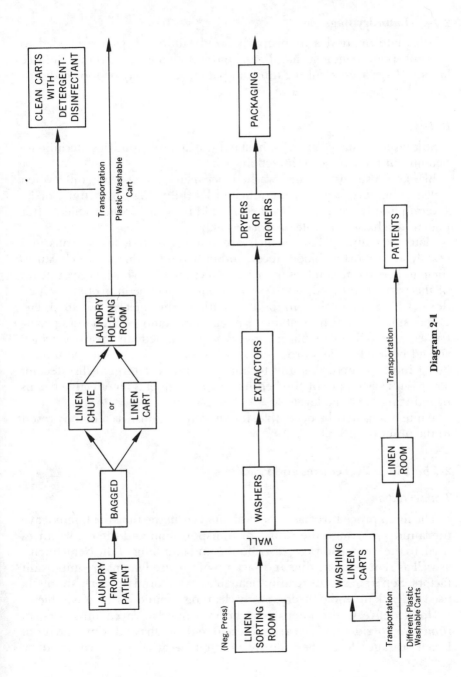

Diagram 2-1

85

2-7-4   Laundry Bags

Adequate quantities of properly sized laundry bags are needed to prevent poor bagging, handling, and ultimately, infections. Soluble laundry bags are useful for infected patients, but may be too costly for normal usage.

Bedding

Studies in military barracks, hospital wards, and laundries incriminate bedding in the spread of infection.

Blankets usually are not washed between patients, but only when soiled. They are heavily contaminated by the patient over time, or by several patients. Synthetic blankets should be washed when soiled, after patient discharge, or at least twice weekly.

Mattresses and pillows, which are not plasticized, are porous and readily absorb urine, blood, feces, and other contaminants which causes them to become serious reservoirs of infection. Upon discharge or death of the patient, the bed, mattress, and pillow may be improperly wiped down with a soap solution, iodine solution, phisohex, green soap, etc. Organisms are smeared about, rather than removed. Enclosing mattresses and pillows in plastic covers is an immediate measure which should be used while a program of replacement with plasticized units is being implemented. A spray technique using a detergent-disinfectant along with scrubbing of the bed unit by personnel is an effective means of reducing bacterial levels.

White linens may be deceptive, for virulent organisms could be present in the absence of visible soil.

2-7-5   Linen Procedures and Practices

Transportation

The linen procedure has to be evaluated from the time the linens leave the laundry, through the routes of transportation and the conveyances used, to the wards. Storage, distribution and handling of the clean linens, as well as removal, bagging and pick up of the used linens are important factors. Separate sets of readily cleanable carts stored properly should be used for pick up and delivery. Spray cleaning techniques are advisable.

Upon delivery, the linens may be improperly placed on floors, in rooms, or corridors, which are subjected to dust, dirt and contamination. Linen storage closets become overstuffed because of hoarding; dirty because of neglect; and a depository for old equipment, materials and junk.

Bedmaking

Beds are generally stripped with some vigor, which causes the organisms on the linens and in dust to become airborne. Clean linen should only be exposed to the dirty linens when the patient cannot be moved from the bed.

Washing Procedures

Adequate washing procedures are available in the literature. The most authoritative source is The American Institute of Laundry. Briefly, the washing procedure should consist of subjecting the soiled clothes to a series of sudsings and rinsing operations in a rotating washer called a "wheel." This is usually preceded by the flushing and breaking operation, and may be followed by bleaching, souring, and bluing. The final rinse treatment may contain a quaternary ammonium compound. This is followed by adequate drying or ironing.

2-7-6   Housekeeping

The laundry should be swept several times a day with treated mops and all trash should then be removed. Eating should be prohibited. Once a week the laundry ought to be vacuumed to remove excess lint.

2-7-7   Commercial Laundries

There are several potential dangers in the use of the commercial laundry vs. the hospital laundry. The same trucks may be used for the removal of contaminated linen and the delivery of clean linen. Unless the sorting, washing, extracting, drying, packaging, and shipping of hospital linens are separate from the rest of the commercial laundry business, it is quite possible to spread the hospital bacterial flora, which might be quite virulent into another environment, the community at large. Where a virulent strain of organisms exists because of a current outbreak of infection, the risk is multiplied manifold.

At best, laundry personnel even within the hospital setting inadequately protect themselves from infection. What might nonhospital oriented laundry personnel do?

If a commercial laundry is used, it should be carefully surveyed and

LAUNDRY STUDY FORM

Name of Hospital

DATE	TIME	RATINGS	TOTAL SCORE
		S = Satis. (1)	
PERSON MAKING STUDY		U = Unsatis. (0)	$\dfrac{\text{S's}}{\text{S's} + \text{U's}} \times 100 =$ %
		N = Not apply	

AREA CODES:

L – Laundry	D.L.S. – Dirty Linen Sorting	W – Ward – Give #
So. – Solarium	P.R. – Patient Rm. – Give #	B.R. – Bathrooms
T.R. – Treatment Rm.	L.C. – Linen Closet	K – Kitchen
L.D.R. – Labor & Del. – Give #	O.R. – Operating Rm. – Give #	

Complete in duplicate: Original to the Hospital Adm., Duplicate to Laundry Manager.

	AREA CODE	RATING
SORTING		
1. Are dirty linens sorted in such a way as to protect the operator from becoming contaminated?		
2. Is there a special sorting room?		
3. Are contaminated linens handled separately?		
LAUNDRY CHUTE		
4. Is the linen chute clean?		
5. Is the linen chute washed thoroughly at least once a week?		
6. Is the linen chute free of cracks and seams?		
TRANSPORTATION		
7. Are clean linens protected during transportation to ward areas?		
8. Are clean linens transported on the same truck as dirty linens?		
TRANSPORTATION EQUIPMENT		
9. Are the laundry trucks and carts cleaned daily?		
10. When not in use, are the trucks stored in an area which is free of gross contamination?		
WASHING PROCEDURE		
11. Does the procedure clean linens?		
IRONING		
12. Is a high temperature used for drying and ironing?		
CONTAMINATED LINENS		
13. Are infected linens placed in disposable plastic bags which dissolve during the washing procedure?		

Laundry Study Form (*Continued*)		
	AREA CODE	RATING
14. Are all linens from infected patients placed in a specially marked laundry bag and closed at once?		
15. Do all linens from infected patients receive special handling?		
16. Are laundry bags from isolation placed in clean outer bags?		
CLEAN LINENS		
17. Are the clean, ironed linens exposed to the dirty linens in such a way that there may be a transfer of pathogenic bacteria?		
18. Are linens stored in a clean linen closet?		
19. Are the clothes immediately packed?		
PATIENT PROTECTION		
20. Are all linens, blankets, and other bed covers gently removed from beds to prevent air dispersion of bacteria?		
21. Are all blankets sterilized before reuse?		
22. Are mattresses washed with a detergent between patients?		
23. Are pillows washed with a detergent between patients?		
24. Are beds washed with a detergent between patients?		
25. Are nonporous covers used for mattresses and pillows?		
REPAIRS		
26. Is all the equipment repaired by list and complaints when repairs are needed?		
27. Is there a continuous maintenance problem?		

Instructions for Form

1. Fill out top of form completely.

2. Begin at item 1 and go down the list in *order*, rating each item as "S" (satisfactory), "U" (unsatisfactory) or "N" (not applicable.)

3. If a "U" rating is given, fill in the area code in the "Area Code" column space to identify the trouble spot. Leave the area code blank if "S" or "N" is filled in. Area codes may be found at the top of the checklist. If more than one area has the same problem, fill in all of the area codes.

COMMENTS:

Figure 2-7 Laundry study form.

licensed by the state or local health department. Specific rules, regulations, procedures, and practices should be established, taught to laundry personnel, and rigidly enforced.

Health of Laundry Personnel

Laundry personnel processing contaminated linen should follow aseptic techniques. All personnel should be cautious and practice good handwashing techniques before touching processed linen and after working with any soiled linen. Those personnel who have infections should be removed from duty until the infection is controlled.

2-7-8 Study Technique

The potential problem that has been discussed can be related to the specific institution by conducting a comprehensive study of the sorting, transportation, washing, ironing, and handling of linens. This study should include the laundry chute, vehicles of transmission, blankets, mattresses, pillows, and beds used by the patients. It should be carried out in several areas, or several buildings of the institution. A model laundry study form is shown in Figure 2-7.

2-7-9 Summary

Linens and bedding are closely associated with the patient and his bedside care. They can either serve as a means of promoting health, or as a vehicle for the spread of infection. Proper transportation, storage, distribution, handling, and cleaning procedure will make this determination.

REFERENCES AND SELECTED READINGS

Control of Cross Infection, New York: Research Department, Hospital Bureau, Inc., May 1966.

Environmental Aspects of Staphylococcal Disease-Selected Materials, C.D.C. Training Program, Ga.: U.S. Dept. of HEW, PHS, January 1959.

Hughes, H. G. Chutes in hospitals, *Journal Canadian Hospital Association*, Vol. 41, No. 9, September 1964.

Klenzade Hospital Environmental Sanitation Handbook. 3rd ed., Beloit, Wisconsin: Klenzade Products, 1961.

Le Riche, Harding, W., Balcom, Carolee E. and Belle, van G. *The Control of Infections in Hospitals*. Springfield, Ill.: Bannerstone House, 1966.

Michaelsen, G. S. *Design of Linen Chutes to Reduce the Spread of Infectious Organisms in Hospitals*. Minneapolis, Minn.: University of Minnesota, October 1963.

Proceedings of the National Conference on Institutionally Acquired Infections. Minneapolis: University of Minnesota Press, U.S. Dept. HEW, Atlanta: Public Health Service, September 1963.

The Hospital Laundry. U.S. Dept. of HEW, PHS, Pub. # 930-D-24, U.S. Gov. Printing Office, Washington, D.C., November 1966.

2-8 MAINTENANCE DEPARTMENT

2-8-1 Introduction

The Maintenance Department is responsible for the maintenance and operation of the physical plant of the hospital. The size of the department and the line of responsibility varies with the size of the hospital. In the smaller hospitals it is common practice to employ an engineer whose main job is to manage the power plant, and to supervise the maintenance of buildings and grounds. Housekeeping and laundry services may be placed under his authority. This department is usually supervised by the assistant administrator of the hospital. In a large hospital its staff is composed of stationary firemen, oilers, engineers, heating maintenance managers, steam fitters, electricians, refrigeration mechanics, plumbers, welders, carpenters, brick masons, roofers, gardeners, locksmiths, plasterers, painters, and air-conditioning mechanics. In small hospitals any one of the above services might be contracted out, based on need.

2-8-2 Function of Departments

The Power Plant, under the supervision of the Chief Power Plant Engineer, is responsible for the uninterrupted supply of steam for heating and sterilization for the entire hospital, and generation of direct current for electric power for elevators in the hospital, equipment in the laundry, and current for special shops. It operates steam driven water booster pumps in the event of fires.

The electrician turns all inside and outside lights on and off. He performs emergency calls, directed to the Electrical Shop by the Night Supervisor of Nursing Service, Hospital Telephone Operator, or other authorized personnel. When not answering or servicing emergency calls, the electrician performs bench repairs in the shop on electrical equipment, such as fan motors, electric clocks, electric lamps, toasters, centrifuges, incubators, etc. The Night Electrician on duty, upon receiving calls for contractual services, such as elevators and air conditioning, investigates areas in question, and then calls the proper contractor for required services. He makes at least one or more visits to the Main Power Sub Station.

The Mechanical Shop is responsible for all phases of heating and plumbing work throughout the hospital and the powerhouse.

The Carpenter Shop is responsible for a wide range of work including all branches of carpentry, repairing of metal equipment, masonry, roofing, and plastering throughout the hospital. The engineering group is responsible for preparing plans, estimate of costs, structural changes, or equipment purchases for the hospital.

The Maintenance Department services complaints. It provides and keeps records of keys issued to authorized personnel. These keys are "Grand Master Keys" which fit most locks; narcotics cabinet keys; medicine cabinet keys; and psychiatric ward keys.

It services emergencies such as overflowing plumbing units, loss of electrical power, and hazardous structural defects. It provides a continuous maintenance program for all equipment and facilities in the institution. It can use the summary of the "Repairs Needed" section of the Housekeeping Self-inspection Form as a tool of program evaluation or problem identification.

2-8-3   Relationship to Environmental Health

The Environmental Health Specialist has direct and indirect contact with the maintenance department. The success of his program depends on the repair of equipment and the state of repair of the physical structure of the hospital. For instance, if the dishwashers are not functioning properly the rinse temperature on the final cycle of washing dishes may be too low. The maintenance department would be responsible for correcting this equipment in order that it might produce sanitary dishes.

If the hospital had an insect and rodent problem the routes of entry might well be through holes in the wall, or openings around metal pipe collars. The final elimination of these pests would be contingent on the correction of structural defects.

2-8-4   Summary

The function of the buildings and grounds department is intertwined with the function of the environmental health programs.

REFERENCES AND SELECTED READINGS

MacEachern, M. T. *Hospital Organization and Management.* 3rd ed. revised, Chicago, Illinois: Physicians' Record Company, 1957.
Personal conferences with directors of maintenance departments — 1967.

2-9   PHYSICAL THERAPY

2-9-1   Introduction

Under-water physical therapy is part of the curative procedures used to improve the physical condition of patients. They may perform exercises, use the water in motion to stimulate muscles, slough off dead skin or debrid decubiti ulcers.

Infection may be transmitted from person to person; or person to water or equipment to person. Contamination comes from dead skin, body waste, saliva and draining wounds. The organisms may be small in number but extremely virulent. They enter the host because of the stress of heat loss due to the water, which conducts heat away from the body 25 times faster than air.

2-9-2   Equipment and Operation of Therapeutic Pools

The equipment and operation of therapeutic pools is similar to other indoor pools with the addition of certain lifting and carrying devices, including water stretchers, handrails, suspensions, body slings, wading harnesses, body hammocks, headrests, etc.

The physical therapist should clean and operate the pool, since the pool's irregular use would negate the hiring of a full time maintenance man.

Inspections should be made monthly by competent environmental health people. Study forms should be used and records should be checked.

2-9-3   Cleaning Techniques — Therapeutic Pool

Therapeutic pools should have an adequate filtering system which operates 24 hours a day. Weekly, the pool should be vacuumed, the hair catcher emptied and the filters backwashed. Daily, the decks should be washed and all equipment should be thoroughly cleaned.

After a patient with a known infection uses the pool, it should be emptied, scrubbed down with a good detergent-disinfectant, thoroughly rinsed and then refilled. Cleaning of the hair catcher and backwashing of filters is part of this process.

Hubbard and Other Physical Therapy Tanks

Cleaning and disinfecting physical therapy tanks manually is time consuming, laborious, and unpleasant. Complete disinfection may not occur. Effective cleaning may be carried out in an automated manner.

Procedure   after each use
1. Empty tank.
2. Turn on hot water or a precision device for injection of detergent-disinfectant into hose or pipe line.
3. Hose down the inside of the tank carefully, flushing debris and solution toward the drain.
4. Saturate a clean cloth with solution from the hose and wash down the top six inches of the tank and rim.
5. Use a small squeegee to push puddles of solution into the drain.
6. Be sure to hose off stretchers and other equipment.
7. Rinse tanks thoroughly.
8. Clean outside of tank by wiping down with cloth saturated with solution.
9. Once a week, delime tanks with a mild acid detergent—follow steps 1–7. The final rinse is very important.
10. Refill with water and add 0.4 ppm chlorine.
11. Moist air cabinets, furniture, exercise equipment, tables, arm leg rests, etc.,—follow step 8.

2-9-4 Safety Hazards

Drownings may occur. Falls, cuts, abrasions may be due to improper movements near walls and protruding appurtanences. Slippery floors around hubbard tanks and whirlpool baths may result in falls.

Separation of Patients

Patients with infections should be treated in a separate room. Normal isolation procedures should be followed.

Reverse isolation patients should be kept in a separate clean room. They should be removed to their room promptly upon completion of therapy. Proper reverse isolation procedures should be followed.

2-9-5 Summary

Although a substantial risk of infection occurs in physical medicine, it has not been well recognized and therefore inadequately treated.

REFERENCES AND SELECTED READINGS

Ehlers, V. M. and Steel, E. W. *Municipal and Rural Sanitation*. New York: McGraw-Hill Inc., 1965.
Klenzade Hospital Environmental Sanitation Handbook. Beloit, Wisconsin: Klenzade Products Inc., 1961.
Koren, H. Role of the sanitation officer in promoting environmental health, *Hospitals*, *J.A.H.A.*, Vol. 39, October 16, 1965.

2-10   PLUMBING AND CROSS-CONNECTIONS

2-10-1   Introduction

Plumbing represents a potential, and often unsuspected, threat to the sanitation of every hospital.

Public health records report many epidemics whose spread was a puzzle until a plumbing system — in some instances in a hospital — was investigated.

While every home owner and apartment dweller has a vital interest in plumbing systems, medical care institutions, and particularly hospitals must be especially on guard against faulty or incorrect plumbing.

Every type of organism which can spread contagion can be found in most general hospitals at one time or another. Notably, disease organisms found in body waste which can be water-borne, including some of the viable viruses highly resistant to chlorine, may be present. Minor enteric disturbances are seldom reported unless food poisoning of several people is suspected.

Providing "transportation" for these disease breeders, hospitals have more piping than almost any other type of building. To name the common piping systems: cold potable water; chilled and recirculated drinking water; distilled water; fluid suction systems; vacuum cleaning systems; oxygen; fire sprinkling and standpipes; lawn irrigation; air-conditioning and refrigeration systems; recirculated cooling water; drainage systems; soil, waste and vent; storm water systems, and building sewers.

Since the adoption of its comprehensive ordinance in 1943, the city of Detroit requires a survey of the plumbing of existing buildings by the Bureau of Plumbing Inspection of the Department of Buildings and Safety Engineering. Hazardous installations, uncovered by this survey, must be corrected by the building owner. The information developed through these surveys, and the conditions they uncovered, may be of some help to hospital administrators, mechanical superintendents, and maintenance personnel. This ordinance is typical of most cities and towns across the country.

Foundations of a New Science

Interest in modern plumbing's health hazards dates back to the late 1920s, when some sanitary engineers tried to warn health officers and the plumbing industry that systems, fixtures, and equipment of that era could easily and unpredictably contaminate water supplies within buildings. Contamination could move so quickly — at the regular flow velocity of 2–20 feet per second—that chlorination had little opportunity to destroy the organisms, they pointed out.

These warnings generally went unheeded until the amoebic dysentery epidemic of 1933, during the Chicago World's Fair (as reported in a U.S. Public Health Service bulletin of 1936). Briefly, more than 1400 cases were found scattered through 400 cities in 43 states, Hawaii and three Canadian provinces. About two-thirds of the victims had visited the Fair, and 75% of this group had stayed or eaten at one of two adjacent hotels. The two hotels, one an annex of the other, had an interconnected water supply. During the last six months of 1933, 160,000 people had contact with these two hotels. The disease, which claimed 98 lives in this period, was found frequently among hotel employees.

Chicago plumbing inspectors and health officials, working with the Public Health Service, pinpointed the hotel's plumbing system as the cause of the epidemic. Part of the problem was poor maintenance, without adequate supervision. However, there were so many possibilities of contaminating potable water with sewage through cross-connections and interconnections that it was impossible to cite a single point as the focus of contamination.

Health and building officials throughout the country were shocked into activity, at least partly because of unfavorable newspaper publicity. Sanitary and mechanical engineers, associations of plumbers and manufacturers, and epidemiologists began a searching study of existing and planned plumbing systems. Hasty, stopgap methods and equipment were employed immediately, but it took years of research before effective solutions and devices became widely available.

When the survey program began in Detroit, personnel were shocked at the evident lack of understanding of the hydraulics, pneumatics, and mechanics of plumbing systems among people who managed and maintained buildings. Indeed, contacts with specifying engineers, designers, and contractors of new installations and the agents and engineers of plumbing manufacturers, revealed some amazing gaps in their knowledge of plumbing science.

As an educational aid, the Detroit Bureau of Plumbing put a demonstration and testing laboratory into operation in 1937. At the start of the survey program, groups of hospital administrators and mechanical superintendents were invited to view the demonstration and hear the explanations. This served to enlist their cooperation and ease the task of the inspectors.

Much of what follows is based on the materials used at the demonstration laboratory.

Definitions of Terms

To make certain we are speaking a common language, the first step is to sketch some basic definitions and theories.

Plumbing includes the materials, fixtures, devices, apparatus and equipment which either receive potable water or discharge wastes, or both; it includes the piping of all potable water, either hot or cold, and the drainage, waste and vent piping of any premises; it includes the appurtenances and devices necessary to fasten the plumbing to the building, make the entire system or any part thereof safe and sanitary, and includes the mechanical skills and knowledge necessary to place all parts of the plumbing system from the water main or private well to the public sewer or other acceptable disposal terminal for sewage. It includes repair, maintenance, and replacement of parts which wear out, break or otherwise fail to function in a safe and sanitary manner.

A cross-connection is any potable water point of discharge which can be or is submerged in any liquid other than potable water.

There are two kinds of cross-connections: (1) the connection between a piping system used to distribute potable water and another piping system which carries nonpotable liquid under pressure, and (2) the connection between potable water piping and some other part of the plumbing system, such as fixtures, appliances, drains, sewers, tanks and vats, which carry nonpotable liquids. This latter type of cross-connection often is called an interconnection.

Potable water piping systems normally are under positive pressure, derived either from pumps or from elevated tanks or reservoirs. Pressure is measured in pounds per square inch, while the "head" is discussed in feet or inches. The terms are interchangeable but their measurements require conversion factors.

Backflow occurs when the pressure on a potable system drops below the pressure on a cross-connected nonpotable system. The most common example occurs in a pressure-fed tank or vessel where the potable water connection is below the rim or overflow; if the pressure fails in the potable system, the tank contents backflow into the potable piping.

Back-siphonage takes place when less than atmospheric pressure occurs in potable water piping whose discharge end is submerged in nonpotable water or other liquids. The liquid in the receiving tank or vessel is back-siphoned through a cross-connection. Pressure reductions or failures which cause back-siphonage can be due to pump failure, breaks in the piping, or unusual and excessive demands on the main supply, such as those imposed by a fire pumper or pressure pump to an elevated tank.

A secondary water supply system taps an uncertified source, such as a lake, river or well, or any recirculated system whose contents may be rendered nonpotable. Examples are air-conditioning cooling water from a cooling tower, recirculated swimming pool water, which passes through filters, heaters and chlorinators.

Principles Illustrated

A few simple diagrams and explanations will demonstrate how these theories operate in practice. The starting point is a simple siphon, as shown in Figure 2-8.

A bent tube with liquid (F) is inverted, its short leg (B) with the open end (D) submerged in the liquid (F) in a container (E).

The liquid in the long leg of the tube (A) begins to fall (point G). This tends to create a vacuum (negative pressure) at the bend of the tube (C). Atmospheric pressure on the surface of the liquid (F) in the container

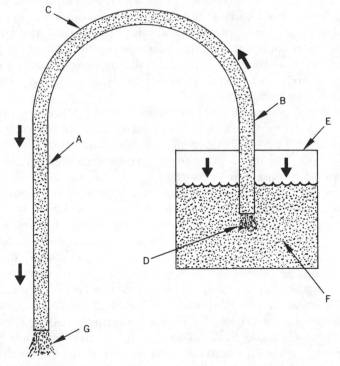

Figure 2-8 A simple siphon in which air pressure at right and gravity at left cause "reverse" flow out of beaker.

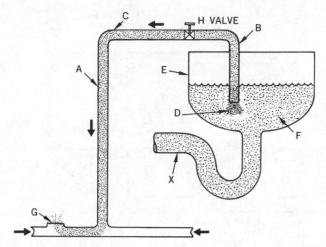

Figure 2-9 Schematic diagram or typical lavatory in which the waste stoppage occurs at X and break in the water supply piping occurs at G, creating a typical simple siphon situation: contaminated water is back-siphoned through cross-connection D and contaminates the water in piping from points D to G.

(E) causes a flow into the short leg (B) to the reduced pressure area (C). Gravity then causes the liquid to move into the long leg (A). This process continues as long as the level of the liquid in the container remains above the opening of the tube (D).

Theoretically, this process, operating at sea level, can lift pure water at 60° to a height of 34 feet. Practical limits are 28–30 feet because of head losses due to pipe friction, actual atmospheric pressure, and orifice head losses.

Figure 2-9 is a sketch of a lavatory flooded because of a waste pipe stoppage. The faucet supply valve is open and its discharge opening is below the rim of the lavatory. At the same time, a break occurs in the supply piping. All conditions illustrated in Figure 2-9, the simple siphon, now are present.

The basin represents the container (E); waste water is the liquid (F); the submerged faucet end is the end of the inverted tube (D); the long leg of the siphon is the piping from A to G; short leg of the siphon is the faucet (B); top of the siphon is at C; the waste stoppage is at X; the break in the water supply piping, at point G, could be caused by repair operations or installation of a potable branch.

In this situation, the nonpotable water in the lavatory is back-siphoned through cross-connection D and the piping from D to G is contaminated.

Figure 2-10 shows a condition where backflow is possible.

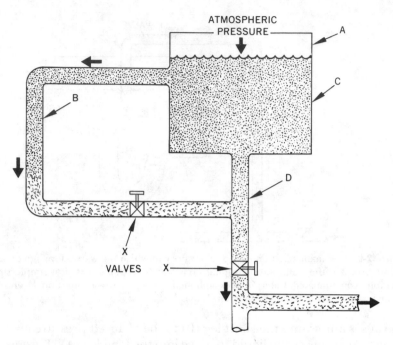

Figure 2-10 Nonpotable solution (C) here will backflow into potable system if pipe pressure drops in either fresh water pipes B or D.

The vat (A) contains a nonpotable solution (C) which requires periodic dilution with potable water through connected pipes (B or D). The full agitating velocity of the pressure flow from the supply is desirable. However, if pressure in the supply pipe is reduced below the atmospheric level, or if it fails, the nonpotable solution backflows into the water supply.

The serious problem which can be created by these seemingly simple situations can be appreciated by observing one statistic: In one 12 month period, between July 1, 1959, and June 30, 1960, the Department of Water Supply of the city of Detroit recorded 1056 main breaks. These breaks caused 11,136 interruptions of water supply to buildings in the area from the main tap to the main distribution line on the building side of the meter. In addition, there is no way of determining the number of times plumbers and maintenance men interrupted pressurized water supplies as they made repairs, replacements, additions or alterations.

The total number of interruptions is startling. The potential or actual cross-connections to be found in unsurveyed and uncorrected plumbing systems is an important factor in appraising the danger to public health.

Application to Hospitals

As this discussion indicates, each cross-connection is a hazard requiring individual protection. The importance of this conclusion to hospitals can be seen from a brief survey of equipment.

Many devices in hospitals are supplied with live steam to sterilize, distill or aid in cleansing. In closed vessels, such as sterilizers, which require steam under pressure of 15 p.s.i. or more, steam is allowed to condense and drain to the waste system. As cooling occurs, condensation creates a vacuum in the sterilizer. If the drainage from the sterilizer is directly connected to a soil or waste pipe, the contaminated contents of the trap can be drawn into the chamber of the sterilizer.

All water closets and urinals with siphon jets have channels concealed in the pottery which discharge below the seals. All water closets, when flooded, have flushing rim openings submerged. All flush valves permit back-siphonage. All water closet flush tanks of the low, close-coupled or integral types can be contaminated by using a plunger. All water supplied by ball cocks, either with hush tubes or if completely submerged, requires protection against backflow and back-siphonage.

All equipment and apparatus connected by means of hose threads on the faucet or bib are potential hazards.

All faucets whose discharge openings are less than one inch above the spill rim are potential hazards.

Drain air and sewer gas may be discharged into buildings through unsealed fixture traps, open cleanouts, or open and unused fixture openings. Drain and sewer air may be toxic. If the air contains hydrogen sulphide, there may be undesirable reactions with metallic paint, pigments, and metals commonly found in buildings.

Broken, chipped, cracked, corroded or blistered plumbing fixtures can harbor dirt, filth, and pathogenic organisms. Such conditions cannot be repaired; replacement is necessary.

Cafeterias, lunch rooms, and kitchens are often found with vats, cookers, serving tables, and dishwashers which contain plumbing hazards.

It is possible to determine in advance whether a cross-connection should be incorporated in an existing plumbing system. For example, consider the typical single cold water supply riser diagram shown here (Figure 2-11). It is proposed that a water cooled compressor, for air conditioning, be connected to the riser in the basement; the compressor will require a continuous flow of 10 gpm.

PROBLEM: to determine whether the present riser, one and one-half inches at its base, will serve without increasing its size. The piping is

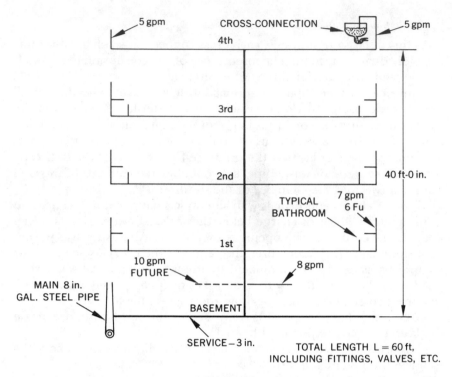

Figure 2-11

galvanized steel pipe 15 years old. Therefore, tables for fairly rough pipe are used to determine frictional losses.

The method used is that described in the Detroit Plumbing Code, namely, the WFU (water fixture unit) demand system.

H = Elevation — basement floor to 4th floor branches = 40 ft.

P = Normal static pressure at base of riser = 32 p.s.i.

L = Total length of pipe from basement floor to highest outlet including equivalent length in feet allowed for fittings, valves and so forth = 60 ft.

P_r = Residual pressure at highest fixture outlet = 8 p.s.i.

WFU Tabulation:

Six bathrooms on 1st, 2nd, and 3rd floor at 6 WFU = $6 \times 6 = 36$

Two 5 gpm demands at 4th floor at 4 WFU = 8

Basement fixtures, one tank water closet and laundry tub $1 + 5$

$$WFU = \frac{6}{50}WFU$$

From probability of simultaneous usage graph: 50 WFU = 30 gpm
From friction loss table: 30 gpm has 6 p.s.i. per 100 feet for

$$1\tfrac{1}{2}\text{ in. pipe } \frac{Lf}{100} = \frac{60 \times 6}{100}$$

To determine pressure design factor,

$$pP - \left(H \times 0.434 - P_r - \frac{Lf}{100}\right) = p$$

Substituting:

$$32 - \left(40 \times 0.434 + 8 + \frac{60 \times 6}{100}\right) = p$$

$32 - 28.6 = 3.6 = p =$ pressure design factor
10 gpm of continuous flow = 10 WFU
New WFU total = 50 + 10 = 60 WFU − 35 gpm

$$35 \text{ gpm} = \frac{60 \times 8}{100} = 4.8 = f$$

or

$$p = 3.6 - 1.2 = 2.4 = p$$

Surges in demand beyond the riser base may drop pressures at the base of the $1\tfrac{1}{2}$ riser 10 p.s.i. or more. Main pressures may vary and drop below normal as much as 15 p.s.i.

This illustrates that to decrease frictional losses it would be advisable to increase the $1\tfrac{1}{2}$ inch pipe from the continuation of the 3 inch service to the connections at the first floor. A tee $\tfrac{3}{4} \times 2 \times \tfrac{3}{4}$ with the 2 inch bushed to $1\tfrac{1}{4}$ on top is advisable.

It also is apparent that no cross-connection can be tolerated because of variations in main pressure and fluctuations in peak demands within the building.

2-10-2   Hospital Plumbing Survey Techniques

The reader should understand the foregoing definitions of terms which pertain to the work of the plumbing team and review the theory and illustrations Figures 2-9, 2-10, and 2-11.

PERSONNEL: Not less than two people should be assigned as a survey team. One should be a mechanic or supervisor from the maintenance staff of the institution. He must know the plumbing system and furnish guidance as to any limited access areas from a time or policy basis.

The other member of a survey crew may be a plumber employed by the hospital, a plumber employed by a plumbing contractor who is hired or contracted by the hospital, to find and correct any and all plumbing hazards in the institution. The other may be a plumbing inspector employed by the governmental unit responsible for inspection, survey, and reinspection. If the institution exceeds 30 beds, an additional member would be recommended, making a three man crew.

One person, preferably an inspector or a contractor's representative, should be designated as the recorder. The other members designate areas, wings, floors, sections or rooms, and provide the recorder with the information needed to determine whether any part of the plumbing system is or is not hazardous. Both correct and incorrect plumbing will show on the survey record.

Each survey man should have a flashlight, six foot folding rule, an eight or twelve inch pocket tape, a torpedo level, an inspectional mirror; and the recorder should also have a clip board to take $8\frac{1}{2} \times 14$ inch foolscap or sketching paper, pads of $8\frac{1}{2}$ or 14 inch foolscap and drawing paper, a twelve inch rule, and a small compact drawing tool that incorporates both 45°, 60°, and 90° right angle triangles, as well as openings so common plane geometrical figures may be drawn. The recorder should have a briefcase or kit in which these tools for use in making surveys are carried.

General Duties of Survey Crew

All plumbing piping must be traced. This includes both cold, hot, and recirculating water piping, chilled or distilled water, and all other piping, such as oxygen, gas or "gunk." Also, all drainage piping, soil, waste, vent, storm irrigation, and any special system. All plumbing fixtures, appliances, devices, or apparatus which are supplied with potable water or discharges to the drainage system, or both. In hospitals we must check operating rooms, recovery rooms, autopsy rooms, cafeterias, kitchens, scrub-up rooms, utility rooms both clean and soiled, and laundry piping identification.

The task of a survey crew is greatly reduced if the various piping systems are color coded or otherwise positively identified. If piping systems are not color coded, it is the duty of the survey men to trace the water distribution system from its entrance into the building to each point of usage. Also, the drainage and venting piping should be traced.

The survey crew should order any unidentified piping to be color coded or otherwise identified. A USASI American Standard, A-31-1-56 for color coding is available, price $1.50, as of 1964.

If the building being surveyed has its own scheme of piping identifica-

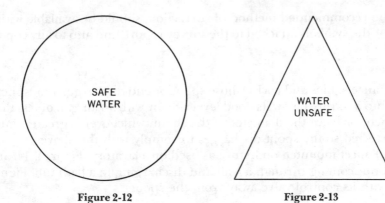

Figure 2-12   Figure 2-13

tion, this scheme should be posted in the office of the superintendent of maintenance, a copy directed to the office of the local plumbing inspector, and a copy issued to the survey crew. If complete painting is not used, bands of color on the pipe on each side of any partition, floor, ceiling, or wall should be made on each kind of pipe which passes through the structural separation, and at distances along the pipe of not more than 25 feet.

Shaped tags as shown in Figures 2-12 and 2-13 are used, particularly if colors could be easily faded. They should be of corrosion resistant material, such as aluminum or plastic, and bear a legend of their use and hung on the pipe at intervals as stated above.

It should be apparent to the reader why we insist on the survey recorder to accurately take notes which positively identify and locate the plumbing items surveyed.

The survey crew should also locate any water or drainage piping which is broken, leaking or improperly installed.

2-10-3 The Location and Means of Correction, Interconnections, and Backflow Connections

The survey crew must observe the discharge orifice of every potable water supply pipe, regardless of whether it is a hot or cold supply to a fixture, an appliance, a device or an apparatus.

Should the terminal orifice discharge below the spill rim of the unit surveyed, or be connected solidly to a drain or waste pipe, it is a crossconnection and must be so noted on the survey.

To avoid more voluminous notes, sketches and drawings, a symbol sheet which names the type of cross-connection, the fixtures, devices, and the recommended method of correction, should be available with a copy of the symbols attached to the survey report, and also to any copies.

Air Gaps

All faucets, bibs and cocks whose spout or end discharges atmospherically into a fixture below its flood level rim, or with an air gap of less than one inch, or twice the diameter of the spout, whichever is greater, must be corrected so the spout discharges to comply with the above.

See: Faucet mounted on fixture as used on a lavatory, Figure 2-14, and of a spout coming through a wall and discharging to a bath tub, Figure 2-15, with its control valve away from the spout:

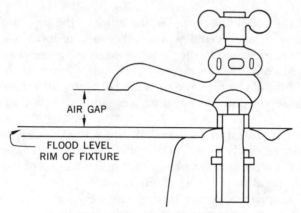

Figure 2-14 Air gapped faucet.

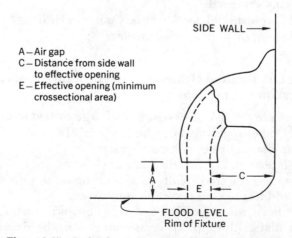

Figure 2-15 Bath tub spout near wall influence on air gap.

Since it is usually impossible for an inspector or plumber to know the minimum cross sectional area within a faucet, and since the faucet's tailpiece is usually concealed, the best practice is to take the diameter of the terminal end of the faucet or spout. If the discharge end is not circular, then use the diameter of a circular pipe whose area would be equivalent to that of the noncircular discharge end.

If the plane of the faucet or spout terminal is not parallel to the surface of the water in the fixture, the air gap should be measured from the spill rim of the fixture to the center of the orifice if it is 45° or less with the horizontal. If the plane of the faucet or spout terminal is more than 45° to the horizontal, then the measurement shall be made from the lowest point of the spout to the spill rim.

The distance which a vacuum will lift water or waste across an air gap is greater if one or more vertical walls are as close as three times the diameter of the discharge spout. Therefore, with single walls the air gap must be increased 50%.

If the faucet is set so the walls of a right-angle corner are as close as two inches or less to the faucet orifice (inner edge) then the gap must be four times the diameter of the discharge opening of the supply faucet or spout.

A list of fixtures and equipment which can be corrected by making a safe air gap are:

> Lavatories, bathrooms, scrub rooms, operating rooms, etc.
> Bath tubs, laundry trays
> Hydrotherapeutic devices which are of the soak type
> Sinks: kitchen, pantry, clinic, diet, etc.
> All open tanks, vats, receivers, and serving counters
> Soup kettles
> Janitors' sinks
> Drinking fountains and beverage dispensers
> Laboratory, sinks and lab tables

Should any faucets or spouts have a hose thread end or a serrated tip, additional protection is necessary and will be discussed later.

Pipe Applied Atmospheric Vacuum Breakers

Many types of fixtures, appliances, apparatus and equipment demand water to be discharged into the unit under pressure. Among these are:

> Flushometer valve water closet
> Flush valve urinals
> Flush tanks for urinals

Flush tanks for water closets
Bidets
Commercial laundry machines
Development tanks for X-ray and other films
All types of hydrotherapeutic swirl baths
All tanks used for dilution, solution, tempering or rinsing with
   potable water

Individual protection against backflow and back-siphonage with all such fixtures and other uses of potable water are to be protected by an atmospheric vacuum breaker, provided back to and including the vacuum breaker there is no back-pressure.

All vacuum breakers of the atmospheric type shall be installed so the critical level (C-L), or if no critical level is shown on the vacuum breaker, the base of the vacuum breaker is six inches above the spill rim of the unit it is protecting. The critical level is a point marked on the tail-piece of body of a vacuum breaker and represents the maximum height to which the liquid in the fixture may be lifted when under vacuum.

These breakers are of two types: the straight through type with the control valve tail-piece—the vacuum breaker and the spud connection to the fixture are in vertical alignment. The others are angle types with bottom inlets and side inlet. *See* Figures 2-16 and 2-17.

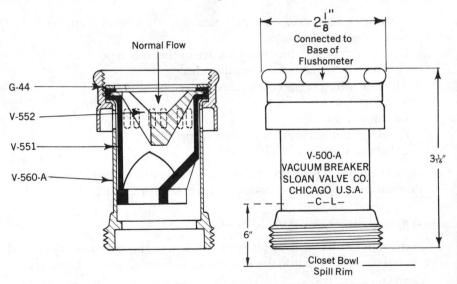

Figure 2-16 A vacuum breaker is installed at the outlet of the flush valve to prevent back-siphonage of the fixture. (Courtesy of Sloan Valve Co.)

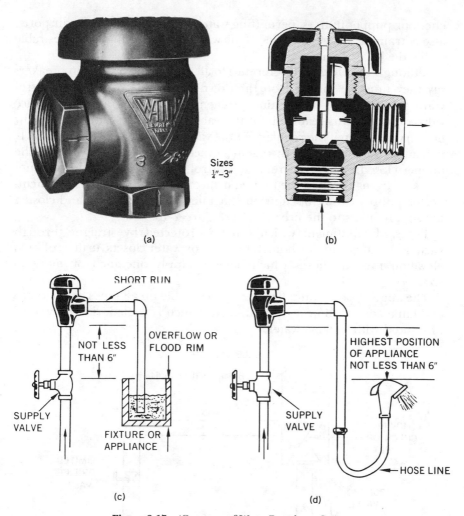

Figure 2-17   (Courtesy of Watts Regulator Co.).

It can be observed that these devices all have a moving check or poppet which closes the vent opening on the vacuum breaker and allows water to be discharged to the unit protected.

If the control valve (flushometer, gate, or angle valve) is closed, or pressure in the fixture supply branch fails or becomes negative, the check valve or poppet drops, or swings open, opening the vents on the vacuum breaker and closing the water inlet to the breaker.

In some cases the normal water demand may be only a trickle and the check or poppet flutters, permitting water spillage through the air ports; also entraining large quantities of air which might be highly undesirable in the device or fixture.

Although the rules with reference to all pipe applied vacuum breakers say they must be installed on the downstream side of the last control valve, we may solve the spitting problem by installing a limited orifice valve on the downstream side of the vacuum breaker. During very low flow in gpm, even if the regular control valve is wide open — giving nearly maximum static pressure through the vacuum breaker — it will keep the poppet closed. When the regular control valve is closed, the vacuum breaker drains through the limited orifice valve and the checking member or poppet drops, opening the air inlets on the breaker and closing the supply inlets to the breaker. *See* Figure 2-18.

Types of equipment which can be protected by straight through vacuum breakers are flushometer valves for water closets, urinals of high elevation flushing hoses which have a supply one inch or more in size.

The angle type vacuum breaker is acceptable on all types of open vats and tanks, on machinery or equipment which is cooled, rinsed, washed or diluted with potable water.

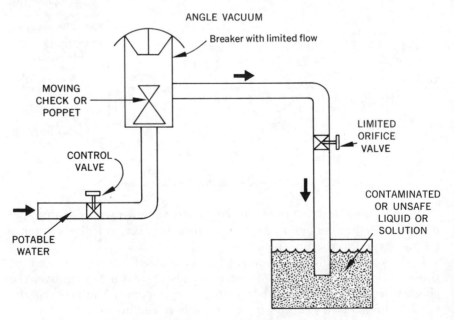

Figure 2-18 Very low volume.

Water Closet and Urinal Flush Tanks

The water supply to the fixture is usually connected to a spud in the bottom of the tank. The water flows through the spud into a vertical riser which terminates in a valve controlled by a float arm and hollow float ball. The incoming water moves up through the control valve with the majority discharging down through the hush tube—a second vertical pipe whose discharge end is near the bottom of the flush tank. Also, a second orifice on the downstream side of the ball cock valve has a connected tube which discharges into a standing vertical overflow. The tank overflow discharges to the water closet bowl through the base fitting of the tank which opens into the water closet bowl. This supply to the overflow is called the "refill tube." After a water closet is flushed, the siphonic action of the integral trap of the water closet bowl sucks the contents of the bowl, including most of the water discharged into the bowl from the flush tank, and discharges into the sanitary drainage system. While the flush tank is refilling through the hush tube, the refill tube is discharging into the tank overflow and the bowl water level (seal) is restored. Depending on the configuration of the various makes and types of water closets, the refill volume varies from one to four pints. The water level may be raised from one to three inches during the refill.

Any water closet flush tank can become contaminated by air-borne organisms or by lifting the lid of the flush tank and dropping discarded small objects into the tank. Also, bowls which are of the siphon-jet close coupled type can be contaminated when a force cup (plumber's friend) is used to clear a clogged bowl. The pressure exerted on the force cup is applied through the siphon-jet opening below the water seal of the water closet, as well as on the discharge passage to the bowl. The pressure on the siphon-jet opening may, and usually does, force the rubber flush ball up and off its seat, and the unsanitary contents foul the tank, the bottom of the flush ball, and the flush tank overflow.

Nearly all closet tank ball cocks allow the riser from the spud-inlet to pass through the water of the tank and very few manufacturers have felt it necessary to protect this water pipe which is in potentially contaminated liquid in the flush tank. However, we know such tubes are corroded by corrosive water so they may leak in a few months. This is an unfortunate condition, but even though this condition can be corrected, the unsafe ball cocks are still being sold to the unsuspecting public without warning.

Note that the vacuum breaker protects only against back-siphonage from the hush tube and refill tube. A single wall supply riser tube which

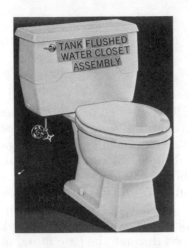

TANK FLUSHED
WATER CLOSET
ASSEMBLY

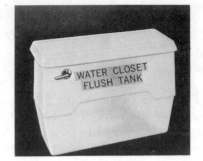

WATER CLOSET
FLUSH TANK

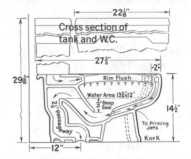

Cross section of
tank and W.C.

22⅛"

27⅝"

29⅜"

Rim Flush

Water Area 13½×12"

2¼" passageway

¾" Deep Seal

2"

14½"

To Priming Jets

12"

K or K

BALL COCK FLOAT VALVE

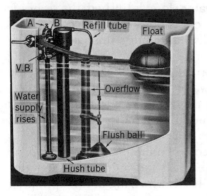

A   B   Refill tube   Float

V.B.

Water supply rises

Overflow

Flush ball

Hush tube

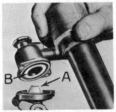

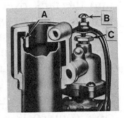

An important feature is the china seat (A) which is not affected by water. Seat and seat washer are easy to get at when necessary.
(B) Volume control.

(A) Vacuum breaker is of the non-mechanical, atmospheric type.
(B) Screw to adjust float rod for proper water level.
(C) Adjustment for volume control.

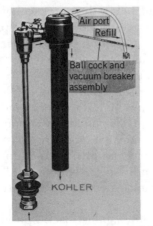

Air port
Refill

Ball cock and vacuum breaker assembly

KOHLER

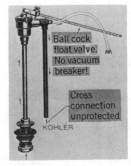

Ball cock float valve. No vacuum breaker!

Cross connection unprotected

KOHLER

Figure 2-19 (Courtesy of Kohler Co.).

becomes a leaker is not protected from sucking the contents of the flush tank back into the potable water distribution system of the building and the public main or well.

Pressure Vacuum Breakers

There are many kinds of water supplied devices which have no automatic cycle of opening-closing of the water supply control or which have no attendent who manually opens or closes the supply valve. The equipment may be under continuous flow pressure for days, weeks or months. Any atmospheric vacuum breaker if installed under such conditions may have its moving parts or the seats changed by physical-chemical action, such as corrosion, scaling, swelling, or chemical migration of components, so that if and when the normal water pressure fails, the atmospheric vacuum breaker may be unable to function.

Under such conditions on supply branches from $\frac{1}{4}$ to 2 inches diameter, pressure vacuum breakers may be a better choice. The moving parts have springs which aid them in moving in the proper direction so airports are opened or closed according to whether the pressure is positive, zero, or negative. The same principle applies to the poppet or check which is supposed to close the supply inlet to the vacuum breaker. *See* Figure 2-20.

Reduced Pressure Zone Backflow Preventives

In order of safety, the preferred methods of protecting individual supply branches against backflow or back-siphonage are, first, the air gap; second, the atmospheric vacuum breaker; and third, the pressure vacuum breaker. The second and third methods have the common requirement that no back-pressure shall be exerted against the vacuum breaker. However, there are conditions where back-pressure conditions may be unavoidable. For instance, a secondary system of water supply used for stand-by purposes where the pressure developed by the pumps on the secondary source are sometimes greater than the pressure on the potable system of water supply at the point of stand-by connection of the two systems of water supply. Another instance is possible if the potable system is at an elevation lower than one or more supply points with pressure required through the units supplied without interruption or undue reduction in pressure. A pressure failure or pressure drop on the inlet side may develop so that the elevation head in the supply riser to the higher points of usage is greater than the potable system pressure at the branching point of the supply riser. This is known as back-pressure caused by elevation head.

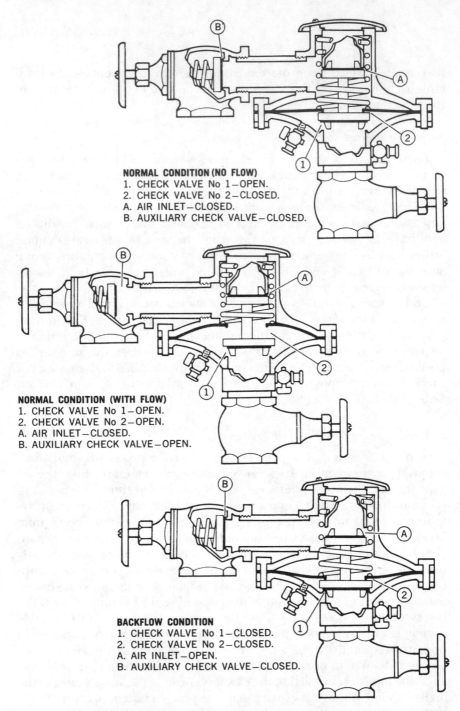

NORMAL CONDITION (NO FLOW)
1. CHECK VALVE No 1 – OPEN.
2. CHECK VALVE No 2 – CLOSED.
A. AIR INLET – CLOSED.
B. AUXILIARY CHECK VALVE – CLOSED.

NORMAL CONDITION (WITH FLOW)
1. CHECK VALVE No 1 – OPEN.
2. CHECK VALVE No 2 – OPEN.
A. AIR INLET – CLOSED.
B. AUXILIARY CHECK VALVE – OPEN.

BACKFLOW CONDITION
1. CHECK VALVE No 1 – CLOSED.
2. CHECK VALVE No 2 – CLOSED.
A. AIR INLET – OPEN.
B. AUXILIARY CHECK VALVE – CLOSED.

Figure 2-20 Pressure vacuum breaker. (Courtesy of Febco Inc.).

Sometimes several points of similar usage are found which are supplied through a common branch from the potable system, and there are no supplies off this common branch to potable water, such as drinking fountains, lavatories, etc. It has been deemed possible and feasible to isolate this portion of the water system, label all water pipe in the isolated system as being nonpotable; thus plumbers and maintenance personnel are warned against making future connections for potable water usage to the piping labeled "nonpotable," or "unsafe water."

There are several methods of isolating such systems or preventing backflow from nonpotable stand-by systems.

Usually, the most costly and difficult, in either new buildings or correction of plumbing hazards in existing structures, is the installation of a receiving tank, with an air gapped potable supply, a pump or elevation head sufficient to restore lost pressure to the supply branches at lower elevations. If it is a stand-by system, the potable supply has a three way valve downstream from the main supply branch with a removable spool piece which is manually connected if the necessity of using the stand-by nonpotable system arises. When the potable system can be restored to usage, the spool piece is removed, the three way valve is opened and the main control is opened. Lawn irrigation systems and water for cooling refrigeration and air-conditioning compressers are common uses for stand-by systems.

A more convenient method of isolation or protection is the Reduced Pressure Zone Backflow Preventer (RPZ). It consists of a system of spring-loaded differential check valves; one on the inlet supply to the reduced pressure zone of the unit; another on the discharge to the equipment usage on the discharge side of the RPZ-E, and a third on the discharge to atmospheric on the lower side of the RPZ. The springs and the check valve areas are designed so that a preestablished pressure differential of from two or more pounds per square inch exists in RPZ.

If the preestablished pressure zone develops a pressure from the downstream side (back-pressure) of more than the inlet pressure, then the diaphragm to which the atmospheric discharge check is connected is lifted and water runs from the RPZ until the pressure drops in the RPZ below the pressure exerted by the spring. The differential pressure in the RPZ is reestablished with no backflow to the potable inlet.

It is recommended that an instructor, or plumbing supervisor, or mechanic secure the test reports, on a Beeco Unit, made by the Atomic Energy Commission Engineers at Oak Ridge, Tennessee. *See* list of references and suppliers, and illustrations Figure 2-21a and b.

The design features of the Beeco may be licensed to other manufacturers, but regardless of whose unit is specified, the pressure drop

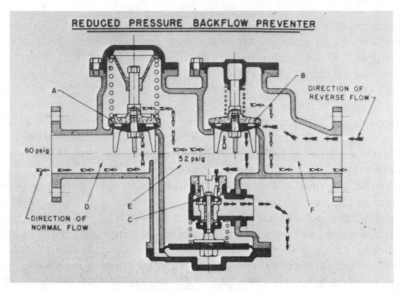

Figure 2-21(a) Reduced pressure backflow preventer. (Courtesy Hersey Products Inc., Dedham, Mass.).

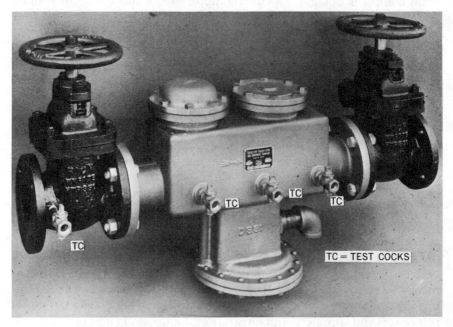

Figure 2-21(b) (Courtesy Hersey Products Inc., Dedham, Mass.).

through the unit must be studied. The manufacturers catalogs carry pressure drop figures for the various pipe sizes of the inlet supply connection, and the demand in gpm through the unit. The pressure drop through RPZ BFP may be as much as 25 p.s.i. without consideration of pressure drops due to friction in pipe and fittings, or elevation head.

Barometric Loop

In some installations it is possible to use a barometric loop or a modified barometric loop in a main supply or large branch supplying several demands. It is based on the theory that a perfect vacuum under ideal conditions can lift water only 34 feet. In nearly all instances 28 feet is considered the practical lift which may occur in piping.

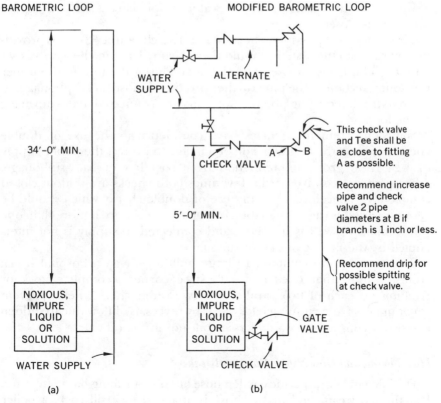

Figure 2-22 Barometric loop and modified barometric loop. (This type of installation must be approved by the Administrative Authority.)

Modified Barometric Loops may be used in locations where ceilings are too low to rise 34 feet.

A system of check valves which open under normal pressure and close under negative or zero pressure, as illustrated in Figure 2-22, are called modified barometric loops. From the supply, the first check is located in the horizontal piping of the loop. At the change from horizontal to vertical, a 45° branch open to atmosphere when the third check is open is installed. Under normal pressure, the third check is open, a drop pipe is installed on the downstream side of the atmosphere or third check to contain any spitting through the movement of check #3.

The second check is installed in the horizontal run to the units containing nonpotable liquid. A gate valve between check #2 and the unit is installed.

The operation is as follows:
Under positive pressure in the water supply checks #1 and #2 are open; #3 is closed.

Under negative pressure, checks #1 and #2 close and #3 opens providing air relief to the system, should there be any leaks in check valves #1 and #2. The five foot rise from the flood rim of the unit to the upper horizontal section of the pipe further protects against back-siphonage.

No fixtures requiring potable water may be connected to the down leg of the loop.

Some enforcement agencies have confidence in the use of double check valves on the building side of a meter to protect the public supply or well from gross contamination from backflow or back-siphonage. After such devices are used a few times both checks are seldom closed completely. Therefore, the only use of double checks which should be recommended is their installation on each water service if more than one public main or well is installed, and connected so supply is not interrupted by the failure of one of the mains.

Two services are common to large buildings, e.g., a hospital which fronts on more than one street—at a street corner, a complete block, or fronting on each of two parallel streets. Double checks, here, prevent water meters from running backwards by reversals of flow due to sudden pressure drops in one water service but not in the other.

Hose Thread and Hose Nipple Vacuum Breakers

Flexible rubber or plastic garden hose or rubber tubing has many uses. But the upstream end of the hose is attached to a sill cock, a boiler drain, a hose with a threaded connection to a faucet or rubber tubing

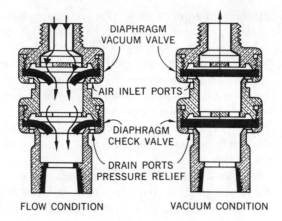

DIAPHRAGM
VACUUM VALVE

AIR INLET PORTS

DIAPHRAGM
CHECK VALVE

DRAIN PORTS
PRESSURE RELIEF

FLOW CONDITION   VACUUM CONDITION

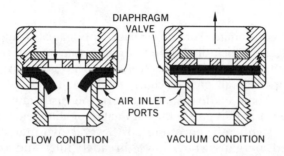

DIAPHRAGM
VALVE

AIR INLET
PORTS

FLOW CONDITION   VACUUM CONDITION

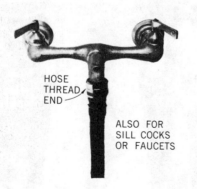

HOSE
THREAD
END

ALSO FOR
SILL COCKS
OR FAUCETS

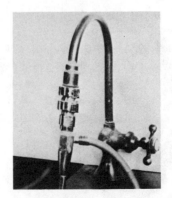

FOR SERRATED TIP
e.g. LAB TABLE

Figure 2-23   (Courtesy Videl Company, Grand Rapids, Michigan).

connected to serrated and tapered outlets for water supplies at laboratory tables, etc. The discharge end of a hose may be in a puddle on the lawn, a floor drain, a janitor's sink, a beaker, a vat, pail or can. It has been feasible to use hose vacuum breakers on threaded supply terminals and tapered hose nipples. These devices may be spring-loaded, or they may depend on resilent diaphragm check valves which under zero or negative pressure are closed. but open with positive pressure, and if either back-pressure or vacuum occurs on the vacuum breaker, a spring forces a check valve to close the opening to the faucet and vents to air are opened by the movement of the check.

In the hose thread and serrated tip vacuum breakers shown in Figure 2-23, the opening of the flexible diaphragm varies from a trickle under very low pressure to full capacity of the diaphragm orifice size when maximum flow demand occurs.

Use of Air Breaks

Protection of equipment from direct back-siphonage through supplies connected to drains which discharge to drain, waste or vent piping, also waste from steam sterilizers, gas sterilizers, autoclaves, etc. An air break must be developed on all such discharges. These may be fabricated on the job, but the home-made installations are too easily tampered with, resulting in the proper air gap being eliminated or changed. Also. splash and spray are frequently encountered. Several manufacturers have developed fixed air gaps which have threaded inlet and outlet con-

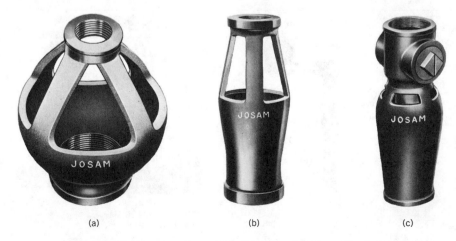

(a)   (b)   (c)

Figure 2.24   (Courtesy Josam Mfg. Company, Michigan City, Ind.).

nections with the basket type air break with adequate openings to atmosphere, so no negative pressure is applied to the discharge end of the fixed air gap.

The fixed air gap is the remedy for this hazard (*see* Figure 2-24a, b, and c).

2-10-4   Autoclaves and Other Steam Sterilizers (Figures 2-25a, b, and c)

It used to be common practice to connect the chamber drain condensate solidly to a plumbing drain or trap. As the steam in the unit condensed, a vacuum formed and the contents of the traps or drain were sucked back into the sterilized items in the autoclave or other type of sterilizer.

Another problem with sterilizers is that steam condensate or any liquid should never discharge to a drain at a temperature in excess of 140°F. This means in a central sterilizing room containing more than one autoclave, a unit to chill the condensate below 140°F is necessary. The unit consists of a small tank containing cold water coil which condenses and cools the steam. The cold water supply must be protected by an air gap or vacuum breaker.

If the steam in the space between the jacket of a sterilizer and this chamber is returned to the boiler, care must be exercised that the steam return is lower than the autoclave. Condensers are used on single autoclaves.

Vats and Tanks

Any assembly as observed in Figure 2-26, e.g., developing tanks, mixing tanks, cooling or dilution tanks, is protected. Note the distinction between the air gap and the air break.

Autopsy Tables

The potable water supplies, both hot and cold, to an autopsy table from the point where they come into the autopsy room shall rise within six inches of the ceiling. A vacuum breaker shall be installed at the top of the supply loop on the down leg of the supply loop. The supply to all hose connections, bibs, faucets, or rim flushed floor drains shall be taken from the protected supply. No potable supplies for drinking fountains, toilet rooms, or scrub sinks shall be taken off the downstream piping from the high vacuum breaker.

Wastes from the autopsy table shall be indirectly wasted and usually

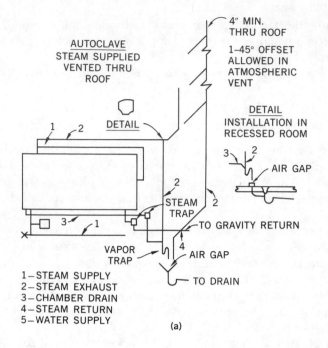

AUTOCLAVE
STEAM SUPPLIED
VENTED THRU
ROOF

4" MIN.
THRU ROOF

1–45° OFFSET
ALLOWED IN
ATMOSPHERIC
VENT

DETAIL

DETAIL
INSTALLATION IN
RECESSED ROOM

AIR GAP

STEAM
TRAP

TO GRAVITY RETURN

VAPOR
TRAP

AIR GAP

TO DRAIN

1 – STEAM SUPPLY
2 – STEAM EXHAUST
3 – CHAMBER DRAIN
4 – STEAM RETURN
5 – WATER SUPPLY

(a)

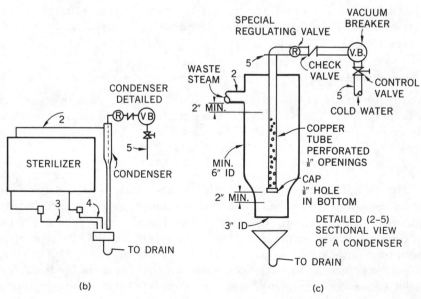

CONDENSER
DETAILED

STERILIZER

CONDENSER

TO DRAIN

(b)

SPECIAL
REGULATING VALVE

VACUUM
BREAKER

WASTE
STEAM

CHECK
VALVE

CONTROL
VALVE

COLD WATER

2" MIN.

MIN.
6" ID

2" MIN.

3" ID

COPPER
TUBE
PERFORATED
$\frac{1}{8}$" OPENINGS

CAP
$\frac{1}{8}$" HOLE
IN BOTTOM

DETAILED (2–5)
SECTIONAL VIEW
OF A CONDENSER

TO DRAIN

(c)

Figure 2-25 Autoclaves and other steam sterilizers.

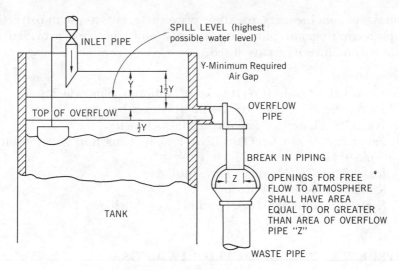

Figure 2-26

discharged to an indirect waste receptacle with a beehive or domed strainer.

2-10-5　General Duties of Survey Personnel

Nearly all codes indicate that all discharge to drains shall pass through a water sealed trap. All cleanouts on drain waste or vent piping shall be in place and air tight. All drains shall be pitched in the direction of flow; all vents shall be pitched back to the waste or drains they serve, and if water piping is trapped; that is, dipped or sloping down in the normal direction of flow, some means shall be installed so that the water supply piping can be completely drained. A stop and waste valve, a tee-nipple and cap, or a plugged tee are common means of draining such trapped water supplies.

If any fixture, appliance, apparatus or equipment has traps which siphon, aspirate or evaporate so the water seal barrier is reduced to less than one inch in depth, steps must be taken to eliminate this potential hazard of drain air (sewer gas) from entering the used areas of the building.

In conclusion, survey crews should be prepared to offer any helpful suggestions which are requested by the representative of the building owner or superintendent of maintenance.

A partial list of manufacturers who have developed acceptable valves, fittings, vacuum breakers, backflow preventers, etc., to use in correcting or protecting against plumbing hazards, and who have provided the author with illustrations are listed.

Manufacturers:

Sloan Valve Co. 4300 West Lake St., Chicago, Illinois 60624

Hersey-Sparling "Beeco," Dedham, Massachusetts

Watts Regulator Co., Lawrence, Massachusetts

Febco Inc., 9121 Glen Oaks Blvd, P.O. Box 368, Sun Valley, California 91352

Josam Mfg. Co., Michigan City, Indiana

Kohler Co., Kohler, Wisconsin

Nydell Vacuum Breakers, Grand Haven, Michigan

REFERENCES AND SELECTED READINGS

Dawson, F. M. Plumbing Cross-Connection and Back-Siphonage Research, National Association of Plumbing, Heating, Cooling, and Air Conditioning Contractors, Technical Bulletin #1, Washington, D.C.

Official Plumbing Code, City of Detroit, City-County Bldg., Dept. Building and Safety Engineering, Detroit, Mich., 1956 Edition.

Reinecke, E. *Handbook of Cross-Connection Control.* Los Angeles, Calif.: Rebco Inc., 1954.

Year Books of the American Society of Sanitary Engineering, (1951–1954), Cleveland, Ohio.

1950 Proceedings of Inservice Training Course in Plumbing Problems, University of Michigan, School of Public Health, Ann Arbor, Mich.

1962 Plumbing Problems, University of Michigan, School of Public Health, Ann Arbor, Mich.

2-11 SOUND AND NOISE

2-11-1 Introduction

Noise or unwanted sound is a major source of annoyance to patients and staff. It can adversely effect them physiologically and psychologically. It may cause temporary or permanent hearing loss; disruption of vital communications, such as the public address system used to summon physicians or indicate emergencies; irritability; and fatigue.

The increased use of therapeutic, operational, maintenance, electrical and mechanical equipment, and lighter weight construction materials tend to increase the problem of noise control. The activities of personnel, patients, and visitors further increase the noise level. Whereas certain noise levels, frequency and intensity are annoying or detrimental to health, low levels of sound are desirable because they mask unwanted sound, help patients especially older ones orient themselves at night and tend to reduce the depressing institutional feeling.

2-11-2   Nature of Sound

Sound is a pressure wave in air. It originates as a result of an oscillatory motion imparted to air molecules which cause a vibratory chain reaction. The sound wave is reflected if it strikes a hard surface. It is absorbed if it strikes a thick soft surface. A sound is considered to be loud or soft depending on whether its pressure intensity is great or small.

Noise Problems

Quantity and quality of noise is a function of site location; exterior noise; arrangement of areas; traffic patterns within the institution; construction materials (accoustical or nonaccoustical) used; mechanical equipment (boilers, pumps, fans, air conditioners, piping, bedpan washers, vacuum cleaners, etc.); talking; walking; radio and television sets; the condition of the patient; and individual idiosyncrasies. Special noise problems are created by moaning and crying of patients, especially those who are terminal cancer or comotose.

2-11-3   Noise Measurement Techniques

Noise may be measured by the use of sound level meters, sound survey meters, noise analyzers (such as an octave band analyzer), magnetic tape recorders and noise dosimeters. It may be further analyzed by using patient questionnaires, interviews with head and supervising nurses and on site studies.

Discussion

Although much is known about noise, noise measuring techniques and the effect of noise on people, little has been applied to the hospital environment. An excellent presentation of this subject is available in the Public Health Service Publication, *Noise in Hospitals*. It would be well for architects, engineers, administrators and manufacturers to review, use or expand this data when designing or redesigning hospital facilities and equipment.

2-11-4   Summary

The function of the institution is to provide a wholesome environment in order that the patient may recover from his illness or live his remaining days as comfortably as possible. Since noise can cause loss of sleep and rest, and can cause nervous strain, it interferes with the full development of this wholesome environment.

REFERENCES AND SELECTED READINGS

Accident Prevention Manual for Industrial Operations. Frank E. McElroy (Ed.), Chicago: National Safety Council, 5th ed., pp. 38-48, 43-9-12, 1964.

Noise in Hospitals. U.S. Dept. HEW, PHS, Pub. #930-D-11, U.S. Government Printing Office, Washington 25, D.C., 1963.

The Industrial Environment: Its Evaluation and Control. U.S. Dept. HEW, PHS, Pub. #614, Washington, D.C., 1965.

2-12   WASTE DISPOSAL

2-12-1   Introduction

The old-fashioned, unsanitary, open dumps were the depository for all types of waste including waste from hospitals. The dumps looked bad, smelled bad, and acted as a breeding ground for rats, flies, mosquitoes, and roaches. The opportunity for spreading disease was imminent. The dumps were odoriferous and constantly shrouded with a layer of smoke. Where incinerators were present on the grounds of the hospital, many were run inefficiently, and therefore created a disease hazard to the institution as well as contributing to community air pollution.

Although we have advanced in our scientific technology, our prospects for the future look as dim as the past. By the year 2000 the population of the United States is expected to double. This growth, coupled with the per capita rate of refuse production is drastically increasing the volume of waste to be stored, transported, and destroyed. Ground and surface water supplies, plus air are being increasingly polluted by the methods used to dispose of the waste.

This tragic picture is further complicated by the addition of contaminated and hazardous hospital waste.

2-12-2   Problem

Hospital wastes are useless, discarded materials resulting from the normal hospital activities. Refuse includes all putrescible and nonputrescible solid waste such as garbage, rubbish, ashes, and biological waste. Garbage is the putrescible animal and vegetable waste generated by the handling, preparation, and consumption of food. Rubbish is all non-putrescible solid waste except ashes. Biological waste results directly from patient activities. This includes diagnostic, medical, surgical, autopsy, and wound dressing. Some of the specific items are dressings, bandages, tissues, sputum, placenta, organs and amputated limbs.

A series of studies conducted in hospitals in 1959, indicated that the average garbage production equals 1.86 pounds per day per patient, noncombustibles 0.83 pounds per day per patient, and combustibles 1.67 pounds per day per patient. By 1967, the average total quantity has risen to between 7 and 8½ pounds per patient per day or 0.7 cubic foot per patient. This is due to the increased use of inexpensive disposable equipment. Over 170 disposable items are available. They range from paper bedding to cardboard bedpans.

2-12-3 Garbage

The collection, storage, and disposal of garbage is complicated by the liquid which it contains, by the variation and quantity during different seasons of the year. The increased quantity closely parallels the incredible number of fly larvae present. Thousands may be traced to a single unclean can. During the hot months odors are created very quickly, and therefore, a nuisance problem is created.

The garbage is generated in the main kitchen at the time of food preparation and in the wards when the food remnants are scraped from trays into garbage cans. In either case, they are usually collected in 20-gallon cans and then transported to a garbage collection room. The garbage storage room and cans, if not cleaned daily, emit nauseating odors.

Garbage from the communicable or infection units are collected in plastic bags, and placed directly into Dempster dumpers or incinerators. The garbage in the plastic bags in the dumpers decomposes and forms gases which expand the bag until it ruptures and spews its contents all over the dumper. Garbage should be stored in plastic lined metal cans with tight fitting lids in the kitchen or garbage storage areas. The cans should be washed well each day after emptying, and should be scrubbed out at least twice a week with a good detergent-disinfectant and hot water. The garbage room should be kept clean and free of odors. Floors should be washed thoroughly each day with the same floor washing procedure used in the O.R. Walls should be washed down each day. All such cleaning activities may be partially automated by various spray cleaning devices which inject detergent-disinfectants precisely into hose lines and/or can washers.

Garbage Disposal

Garbage can be removed by incinerating, burying, hog feeding, and garbage grinding. Placentas may be sold to pharmaceutical companies for extracting of materials. Proper incineration is the best method. Burying creates problems if the landfill is not properly operated. Flies and rodents will breed on the potentially infected garbage and may spread the hospital flora to the community, or reinfect the hospital.

Hog feeding is potentially a very dangerous means of disposing of hospital garbage for, certain ethnic groups in metropolitan areas eat food containing raw or partially cooked pork. If 400,000 swine had to be slaughtered during an outbreak of trichinosis during 1953–1955, think of the potential spread of many pathogenic organisms found in the hospital environment. Despite state and federal regulations prohibiting the feeding of raw garbage to swine, approximately 40,000 swine are still being fed this way each year.

Garbage grinding does not destroy the organisms but rather gives them a better chance to grow. If sewage treatment is adequate, the chance of spreading infection is quite minimal. However, if treatment is poor or lacking, the water supply could become contaminated with virulent organisms.

Dead experimental animals create a problem unless proper procedures are observed. They should be placed in a double polyethylene bag containing formalin and kept refrigerated until removal would lead to immediate incineration. If placed in a dumpster or warm storage area, decomposition would create gases which would rupture the bag.

2-12-4   Rubbish

Rubbish is generated from all departments of a hospital, and by all of the people who enter or live within the hospital or its associated buildings. It includes combustible and noncombustible material such as paper, tin cans, glass, wood, metal, plastics, bedding, rags, crockery, grass, bush clippings, and cardboard. Its quantity varies with the activity of the department, the number of people present, and the time of the year.

Rubbish from patient sources is placed in paper or plastic bags in the patient area trash cans (which should be washed daily) and removed to trash storage rooms, Dempster dumpers, or the hospital incinerator by means of trash chutes. Rubbish generated in other parts of the hospital may be kept in holding rooms, dumped in Dempster dumpers, or removed to the incinerator. Storage in trash cans creates problems when the cans are without plastic linings, or when they are overloaded. Removal of the material to the dumper or incinerator necessitates the use of some sort of vehicle which then may become a reservoir of infection or insect breeding.

Dempster dumpers tend to overflow and are difficult to clean. The overhead doors of the dumper are left open by employees since they are very heavy. This is equivalent to open storage of trash. Trash storage rooms when not properly insect and rodent proofed, cleaned, and ventilated are a source of insect and rodent breeding and odors. When the trash is dropped through the chute a piston action is produced. Air-laden organisms are forced back into the corridors and patient rooms. Immediate closing of the door prevents this phenomenon from occurring. Since trash chutes are difficult to clean, they should be sprayed with detergent-disinfectant and hot water under pressure twice a week using special chute cleaning devices which are available on the market. The area around the chute entrance may require special scrubbing after the cleaning procedure.

2-12-5   Contaminated Waste

Contaminated waste includes soiled dressings, bandages, disposable underpads, disposable diapers, catheters, tissues, soap, body secretion, sputum cups, masks, swabs, sanitary napkins, plastic casts, needles and syringes, animal fecal material, dead animals, surgical waste, autopsy waste, and placentas. It is generated in patient areas, operating rooms, delivery rooms, animal research facilities, and the morgue. It is usually placed in plastic bags which in turn are placed in metal cans.

The contaminated waste may either be dropped down the trash chute, into a rubbish holding room, directly into the incinerator, or may be removed to Dempster dumpers for storage until removed. The trash cans become contaminated by the waste if the plastic bags are not handled properly. The plastic bag that encloses the waste dropped down the trash chute may spew infectious materials along the chute, or into the trash holding room. Plastic bags placed in Dempster dumpers may generate the organisms present in the bag and thereby contaminate the Dempster dumpers. Disposal in city incinerator or private incinerator may be inadequate, and the infectious material may then be removed to a dump for landfill. Incineration should be carried out at a temperature of 1400°F. Burial is permissible, if four feet of hard packed earth covers the material. Placentas should be kept in a deep freezer, if they are to be used later by pharmaceutical companies. Disposable needles should be placed in used I.V. bottles, or in a box with a slot in it. This prevents the needles from acting as a source of infection to maintenance people who would otherwise be stuck when emptying the trash. It also prevents illegal reuse of needles and syringes.

Parts of the body such as amputated arms and legs may be found in the disposal area and may cause a serious public relations problem, if incineration is incomplete or burial improper. Throughout the procedure of collection, storage, and disposal all employees of the hospital, municipality and private contractors may become infected from the waste. This creates a serious occupational hazard. Maintenance people who usually handle infected material should be thoroughly trained in aseptic techniques involved in the collection and disposal of these materials.

The handling of human wastes in hospitals is one of the serious areas of breaks in technique. As long as a patient can go to a bathroom, the problem is somewhat similar to any institution. But where a bedpan has to be used, unusual procedures are needed to avoid contamination of the patient, the nurse, or the nurses' aides, other patients, and the environment. Frequently you see the nurse's aide carrying the bedpan incorrectly with the hands in the pan or grasping the rim. The waste materials may be dumped into toilets, hoppers, and sinks without real concern of the inordinate number of organisms present. Even in cases of enteric disease, insufficient care is given to this matter. The following bedpan cleaning procedure will apply to the various ways in which bedpans are cleaned and sanitized.

Procedure
1. Remove bedpan from bed by holding bottom of pan and grasping side.
2. Empty gross material into toilet.
3. Use cold water from bedpan washer to rinse top and inside of pan. Empty into toilet.
4. Use a disposable toilet swab to wash outside of pan and then inside. (Spray on detergent-disinfectant.)
5. Rinse out thoroughly in bedpan washer or with spray attachment.
6. Steam sanitize for three minutes or soak in 200 ppm chlorine for five minutes.
7. Use disposable bedpans in enteric infection areas. After use, place in plastic bags and incinerate.

Incinerator compacting or pulping of refuse—improved methods of waste destruction. It would appear that the best means of destroying hospital waste which in all cases has to be considered to be contaminated, and in special cases highly contaminated, is by incinerator at the hospital. Heavy duty, high temperature multi-chamber incinerators with drying shelves for wet waste and auxiliary heating units to insure temperatures of 1400–1800°F is highly desirable for destruction of hospital wastes. Particles in the emitted gases have to be trapped or settled out, and obnoxious, odorous gases have to be passed back through the burning chamber to destroy potential air pollution. Air pollution control-air devices include settlement chambers, liquid scrubbers or washers, and wet equipment water sprays. The heavy duty incinerator can be equipped with a heat exchange coil to provide hot water or steam to sanitize waste cans. Heat recovery could result in a savings to the institution. It is essential that the hospital engineer understand the operation of the incinerator and periodically as required remove residues from melted glass, cans, etc.

Compacting and Pulping

In institutions where it is difficult or impractical to build incinerators another waste destruction technique may be to shred paper and cardboard, wet it down in a special machine, grind, and then introduce into the sewage system. Another approach would be to compact, shred, remove water, and package into units which can be placed in trucks and removed to sanitary landfills. The disadvantages of these systems is that large cans and such things as heavy casts cannot be readily broken up. Therefore, it may cause a problem to the grinding and shredding machines. Glass also tends to become a problem. It would be undesirable to introduce septic waste into the grinding or pulping operation. This would be best used for cardboard boxes, other trash and garbage.

Experimental animals are difficult to dispose of in the routine trash disposal manner. The best means is to place the deceased animal in a plastic bag with formulin, double bag, and box. Then remove to sanitary landfills for proper burial.

2-12-6   Flammable, Toxic, and Corrosive Waste

Flammable, toxic, and corrosive waste includes solvents such as acetone, carbon tetrachloride, chloroform, diethyl ether, petroleum, benzene, alcohol, ethyl ether, toluene, ethyl acetate, dichloromethane, paints and paint solvents. Flammable, toxic and corrosive waste also includes corrosive acids such as sulfuric acid, hydrochloric acid, nitric acid, acetic acid and phosphoric acid. The collection, storage, and disposal of these materials can constitute a serious hazard unless handled properly. It could lead to fires, serious burns, or toxic effects to employees or individuals removing the materials. If the materials are poured down the drain, they can corrode and eat away piping and lead to further hazards. Flammable liquids should be stored in special steel safety cans which are so constructed that they substantially reduce the possibility of explosions and fires.

Disposing of Flammable Waste Liquids

Disposing of flammable waste liquids often presents a troublesome problem. Most regulations strictly prohibit the pouring of hazardous liquids into sink or floor drains or the burning of liquids in burners. In many cities, however, there are firms that make a specialty of collecting waste liquids. In other instances, the original supplier will pick up used liquids for reclaiming and resale. Another method of disposal is to burn waste liquids at a safe location outside the institution. The storage and transfer of waste liquids within the institution also presents a problem.

Disposing of Flammable Waste Solids

The careless, improper disposal of oily rags, solvent-soaked swabs, paint wipers, shavings and other flammable rubbish frequently cause fires. Although the fire loss from a small rubbish fire may not be serious, substantial water damage from an automatic sprinkling system is likely and can involve work in process, supplies, finished goods, machinery and other equipment. Approved safety receptacles are used for the disposal of flammable waste solids. These receptacles should be removed and emptied at frequent intervals.

Radioactive Waste

Radioactive waste includes all radioactive material used in treatment of patients or experiments within the institution. It has to be collected, stored, and disposed of in such a way that will not have a detrimental effect on employees, patients, or the public at large. All contaminated materials such as glassware, instruments, paper towels, liquid waste, and radioactively contaminated urine can create a hazardous situation. It is essential that this disposal be supervised by competent environmental personnel. Waste cannot be discharged into municipal sewage systems until it is no longer radioactive. If municipal sewage systems would receive radioactive waste, the waste would create a hazard for the sewage plant employees and contaminate the body of water receiving the effluent from the plant. Waste cans should be provided for liquid wastes, radioactively contaminated, such as urine from patients treated with large doses of iodine 131. Waste cans should be properly labeled and should contain the name of the enclosed contaminant. When the cans are full they should be removed to a secluded waste disposal area, locked up and kept there until they are no longer dangerous (this is based on half life of the substance). They should be emptied into either the municipal sewage system, buried in a sanitary landfill or burned in the incinerator at a minimum of 1400°F.

2-12-7   Storage and Removal Capacity

To determine the storage capacity and removal capacity, keep a record of the usage and of capacity used of the trash storage room, and the number of trash removals over a period of two weeks in the summer and two weeks in the winter. It is best to judge all trash needs by summer levels. Anticipate expansion of hospital facilities. Various efforts should be considered, and sufficient capacity should be allowed for an increase over a five year period. Additional consideration must be given to increased janitorial services, as well as storage and removal capacity when disposal programs are anticipated within the institution.

Other Waste Disposal Methods

Other waste disposal methods include: composting, which is not good for hospital waste; and compaction by grinding, crushing or shredding. These procedures increase available volume of trash storage and removal but also increase the airborne bacteria problem.

Discussion

Considerable research efforts are needed for the proper handling, storage, removal and disposal of hospital wastes. Research projects currently being carried out by various universities should include, or separately develop, the various needs of the institution and reasonable recommendations.

2-12-8   Summary

The ultimate reason for good waste disposal is the fast safe handling, transportation, and disposal of waste at a reasonable cost. Different techniques must be used, depending on the type of waste. Generally, infectious waste should be incinerated whereas toxic and corrosive chemicals and radioactive waste should be buried.

REFERENCES AND SELECTED READINGS

Anderson, J. R. (Ed.), *Community Sanitation Surveys.* Virginia Health Bulletin 16:2:2, June 1963.

Black, R. J., Bogue, M. DeVon, Mallison, Geo. F., and Wiley, John S. *Recommended Standards for Sanitary Landfill Operations.* (draft), U.S. Dept. HEW, PHS, September 1961.

Bond, R. G. *Bacterial Contamination from Hospital Solid Waste.* Univ. of Minnesota School of Public Health Project EF 00007-04, 1963.

Disposing of flammable waste, *Catalog of Protectorial Safety Equipment,* Chicago, p. 60, 1963.

Hughes, H. G. Chute in hospitals, *Journal of the Canadian Hospital Assoc.,* Vol. 44, No. 9, September 1964.

Koppenhauer, O. E. Incinerator of hospital waste, *Hospitals,* 35:91, May 1, 1961.

Magy, H. I. and Black, R. J. An evaluation of the migration of fly larvae from garbage cans in Pasadena, California, *California Vector Views,* 9:11:55, November 1962.

National Status on Control of Garbage Feeding. U.S. Dept. of Agriculture, January–June, 1963.

Philadelphia insists on closed refuse vehicles, *Refuse Removal Journal,* 6:12:20, December 1963.

Refuse Collection and Disposal—An Annotated Bibliography 1962–1963. Black, R. J., Wheeler, J. B., and Henderson, W. C. U.S. Dept. HEW, PHS, U.S. Gov. Printing Office, Washington, D.C. 20402, 1966.

Selected Materials on Environmental Aspects of Staphyloccoccal Disease. Atlanta, U.S. Dept. HEW, PHS, p. 43, January 1959.

Solid Waste Handling in Metropolital Areas. U.S. Dept. HEW, PHS, December 1966.

Stone, R. and Merz, R. C. Scientific Analysis of Sanitary Landfills, *A.M. Public Works Association Yearbook, 1961.* Am. Public Works Assoc., 1961.

Infection
Control

3-1 INTRODUCTION

You are about to learn an effective team approach technique to solving hospital-infection problems.

Hospital acquired infections may cause loss of work time, loss of effectiveness, discomfort, strain on family economic resources, emotional drain, permanent disability and hospital and professional liability.

Skilled physician, nursing, and environmental health specialists working as a team can systematically examine hospital conditions and write a definite report. Recommendations contained in the report can show the way to significantly decrease hospital acquired infections. This team should include the physician in charge of the service being studied, his supervising nurse and the Environmental Health Specialist. The tool this team can use is the Programmed Approach to Hospital Infection Control found at the end of this section.

This functional programmed approach developed as a result of the combined efforts of noted physicians, nurses, hospital administrators and environmental health specialists, using a critical review of the world literature on hospital acquired infection from January 1960 to June 1967, as a measure of completeness. This approach was tested, modified, and retested, over a ten year period.

3-2 PROGRAMMED APPROACH

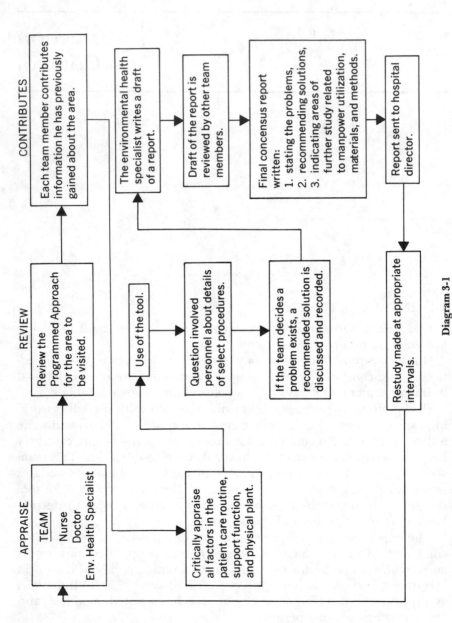

CONTRIBUTES

Each team member contributes information he has previously gained about the area.

The environmental health specialist writes a draft of a report.

Draft of the report is reviewed by other team members.

Final concensus report written:
1. stating the problems,
2. recommending solutions,
3. indicating areas of further study related to manpower utilization, materials, and methods.

Report sent to hospital director.

REVIEW

Review the Programmed Approach for the area to be visited.

Use of the tool.

Question involved personnel about details of select procedures.

If the team decides a problem exists, a recommended solution is discussed and recorded.

Restudy made at appropriate intervals.

APPRAISE

TEAM
Nurse
Doctor
Env. Health Specialist

Critically appraise all factors in the patient care routine, support function, and physical plant.

Diagram 3-1

3-3 PROBLEM AREAS

The hospital environment presents a special risk of infection to employees, patients, visitors, and the community.

The emergency room, admission section and outpatient clinics are potential foci of infection. In addition to patients, visitors and employees, even supplies and equipment may contribute pathogenic organisms.

The organisms are distributed by faulty patient-care techniques, mishandling contaminated material and equipment, poor housekeeping and inadequate physical facilities.

I. *Hospital-wide Problems*
1. Lack of training and inadequate supervision are often principal factors in spread of infection.
2. Unnecessary movement of personnel and supplies contribute to dissemination of infection.
3. Failure to appropriately mark the chart of each infectious case can lead to contamination of unaware personnel.
4. Improper transportation and storage of sterile supplies can cause contamination.
5. Failure to properly segregate clean and dirty linen and failure to properly clean and disinfect bedding can increase the risk of infection.
6. Careless handling of waste may introduce pathogenic organisms into the environment.
7. Because hospital food is often ground, creamed, and prepared in large quantities, the opportunity for contamination through improper handling and storage is considerably increased.
8. Unless bedpans and bed urinals are promptly removed from the bedside, properly handled and stored, thoroughly washed and heat or chemically disinfected, cross-infection may occur.
9. Any supplies, instruments or equipment that directly or indirectly contacts the patient can transmit infection.
10. Failure in any detail of isolation technique creates a risk of infection to employees, visitors, and other patients.
11. Failure in any detail of proper catheterization technique or follow-up care can cause urinary tract infection.
12. Other procedures that require special observation for infection control include inhalation therapy, tracheotomy and intravenous cut-down.

II. *Area Problems*
1. Surgical Department
   A. Flow of traffic in and out of the operating room.
   B. Flow of traffic between operating rooms.

    C. Handling of septic cases.

    D. Ventilation systems and air recirculation.

    E. Cleanliness of surgical scrub area.

    F. Lack of uniform technique during surgical scrub.

    G. Handling and storage of surgical instruments and equipment.

    H. In the surgical dressing room, street clothing and soiled scrub suits may contaminate surgical personnel and fresh surgical clothing.

    I. The wearing of surgical clothing outside of the surgery suite.

    J. Inadequate skin preparation.

    K. Suction apparatus inadequately disinfected.

    L. Contaminated bed entering operating area.

    M. Inadequate room preparation between cases.

2. Recovery Room

    A. Potential drop in level of aseptic technique.

    B. Intermingling of septic and nonseptic cases.

3. Surgical Ward

    A. Lack of standard procedure for wound dressing.

    B. Failure to teach proper technique of wound dressing.

    C. Improper disposal of contaminated dressings.

    D. Sterile dressing carts are moved in and out of contaminated areas.

4. Obstetrics and Gynecology

    A. Opportunity for urine and fecal contamination of mother, infant, and delivery area.

    B. Infected cases not handled with same precautions as in other surgical areas.

5. Nursery

    A. Improper cleaning of isolettes.

    B. Inadequate isolation of infected infants.

6. Pediatrics

    A. Mixture of medical and surgical patients.

    B. Entering patients may be in incubation period of childhood diseases.

    C. Enteric infection spread may occur due to lack of close supervision or child's failure to understand need for personal hygiene.

7. Medical Ward

    A. The age group in a medical ward is more likely to be infected and is more susceptible to infection.

8. Outpatient Clinics

    A. In the waiting room, sick and well patients intermingle.

    B. Noninfected patients may be seen in the same examining room as infected patients without the same precautions and cleanup procedures used for inpatients.

9. Emergency Room

    A. Sick and essentially well patients may intermingle.

B. Noninfected cases may follow infected cases without appropriate cleanup between cases.

C. Inadequate skin preparation prior to surgical procedures may lead to infection.

10. Autopsy Area

A. Strict aseptic technique is not always carried out in autopsy of infected cases.

11. Animal Laboratories

A. Research personnel may go from animal quarters to clinical area without proper clothing change.

REFERENCES AND SELECTED READINGS

Colbeck, J. C. *Control of Infections in Hospitals.* Chicago, Ill.: Hospital Monograph Series #12—American Hospital Association, 1962.

Dubos. R. J. and Hirch. J. G. *Bacterial and Mycotic Infections of Man.* Philadelphia, Pa.: Lippincott Co., 1965.

Environmental Aspects of the Hospital—Infection Control. Public Health Service Pub. #930-C-15. Vol. I, December 1966.

Reiman, H. A. Infectious diseases—Annual review of significant publications, *Postgraduate Medical Journal,* Vol. 40, October 1964.

Top. F. H. *Control of Infectious Diseases in General Hospitals.* New York: American Public Health Association. 1967.

Williams. R. E. O. and Shooter, R. A. *Infection in Hospitals.* Philadelphia, Pa.: F. A. Davis, 1963.

3-4 STUDY FORMS

_____ Hospital

PROGRAMMED APPROACH TO HOSPITAL INFECTION CONTROL

S = Satisfactory   I = Improvement Needed   U = Unsatisfactory

Building Name and No. _____ Floor _____ Date _____ Time_____

Names of Study Team _____

ADMINISTRATIVE PROCEDURES

_____ 1. Does any employee have a patient history of being a carrier of pyogenic infections?
_____ 2. Do all employees report pyogenic infections?
_____ 3. Is the employee who reports an infection immediately removed from patient care?
_____ 4. Is there a restriction of traffic within the given patient area?
_____ 5. Is there routine daily recording of infections on charts?
_____ 6. Is indiscriminate antibiotic use discouraged?
_____ 7. Are the interns given instruction in hospital infection control?
_____ 8. Are the residents given instruction in hospital infection control?
_____ 9. Are the nurses given instruction in hospital infection control?
_____10. Are nonprofessional employees given instruction in hospital infection control?
_____11. Are visitors restricted in time and number?
_____12. Do visitors observe special isolation procedures when indicated?

STERILIZATION PROCEDURES

_____ 1. Is each autoclave tested monthly for its ability to destroy bacterial spores?
_____ 2. Are autoclave indicators or dates used?
_____ 3. Are routine cultures made of utensils, trays, packs, instruments, catheters, gloves, sutures and parenteal solutions?
_____ 4. Are records kept of all isolations of significant bacteria such as "staph"?
_____ 5. Are all autoclaved items distinctly marked as sterile?
_____ 6. Are autoclaved items stored separately from nonsterile items?
_____ 7. Are autoclaved items protected from contamination while in storage?

LAUNDRY AND LINEN PROCEDURES

_____ 1. Are linens washed in such a manner that all pathogenic bacteria are destroyed?
_____ 2. Are bacteriological samples taken of the clean linen to insure that all pathogenic bacteria are destroyed?
_____ 3. Are the clean, ironed linens exposed to the dirty linens in such a way that there may be a transfer of pathogenic bacteria?

_____ 4. Are clean linens protected during transportation to ward areas?

_____ 5. Are clean linens transported on the same truck as dirty linens?

_____ 6. Are all linens, blankets, and other bed covers gently removed from beds to prevent air dispersion of bacteria?

_____ 7. Are all linens from infected patients placed in a specially marked laundry bag and closed at once?

_____ 8. Do all linens from infected patients receive special handling?

_____ 9. Are laundry bags from isolation placed in clean outer bags?

_____10. Are all blankets sterilized before reuse?

_____11. Are mattresses washed with a germicide between patients?

_____12. Are pillows washed with a germicide between patients?

_____13. Are beds washed with a germicide between patients?

_____14. Are nonporous covers used for mattresses and pillows?

_____15. Are the laundry trucks and carts cleaned daily?

_____16. When not in use, are the trucks stored in an area which is free of gross contamination?

TRASH AND SEPTIC WASTE REMOVAL PROCEDURES

_____ 1. Are infectious materials either autoclaved or placed in sealed plastic bags before being discarded?

_____ 2. Is food waste from infected patients placed in sealed plastic bags?

_____ 3. Are paper bags used in isolation rooms for discarded tissues, dressings, tongue blades, and other disposable items?

_____ 4. Are they immediately closed and placed in a sealed plastic bag?

_____ 5. Are bags containing infectious materials marked "Danger, Infectious Materials Within"?

_____ 6. Do employees who remove infectious materials discard their gowns at the completion of the waste disposal and then follow proper hand washing procedures?

_____ 7. Do employees who remove infectious materials wear gowns?

FOOD HANDLING PROCEDURES FOR INFECTED PATIENTS

_____ 1. Are all clean dishes, trays, and eating utensils protected against contamination during transportation or storage?

_____ 2. Are disposable single service paper units discarded after each use?

_____ 3. Are all remnants of meals scrapped into a plastic bag in the isolation room?

_____ 4. Are nondisposable utensils thoroughly and immediately disinfected after each use by infected patients?

_____ 5. Are all dishes, trays, and eating utensils washed and sanitized before reuse?

_____ 6. Is ice making equipment and ice storage equipment kept clean and sanitary?

_____ 7. Are there individual water containers and glasses for each patient?

_____ 8. Are these containers and glasses thoroughly washed and sanitized before reuse?

_____ 9. Are utensils for medications thoroughly washed and sanitized before reuse?

BEDPAN HANDLING

_____ 1. Are all bedpans, urinals, enema containers and other equipment for collection of excreta sterilized before reuse by other patients?

_____ 2. Are all such contaminated utensils handled in an aseptic manner after use by patients?

_____ 3. Are bedpans stored off the floor in a cabinet?

_____ 4. Is toilet paper stored off the floor in a sanitary manner?

EQUIPMENT HANDLING AND SANITIZATION PROCEDURES

_____ 1. Is there an individual thermometer for each patient?

_____ 2. Are thermometers stored in an adequate concentration of germicide to kill all bacteria?

_____ 3. When equipment such as portable X-ray units, flashlights, otoscopes, ophthalmoscopes, stethoscopes, ice bags, etc., are used for infectious cases are they cleansed thoroughly with a germicide solution before reuse?

_____ 4. Is there a Graduate Nurse assigned to the use of the dressing cart?

ISOLATION PROCEDURES

_____ 1. Are all patients with draining wounds isolated?

_____ 2. Is reverse isolation strictly enforced when indicated?

_____ 3. Are patients isolated in such a way and in such areas that proper procedure can be carried out?

_____ 4. Are isolated patients properly identified?

_____ 5. Is a suspected infected case reported the day it is noted?

_____ 6. Are clean gowns put on before entering isolation rooms?

_____ 7. Are the gowns discarded in containers in the isolation area?

_____ 8. Are hands washed with an acceptable technique before and after handling any contaminated material or patients?

_____ 9. Are all areas in which infectious cases have been treated thoroughly cleaned and sanitized before reuse?

CATHETERIZATION PROCEDURES

_____ 1. Are the genitalia thoroughly cleaned with an appropriate soap in preparation for the catheter?

_____ 2. Does the catheter come from a sterile package?

_____ 3. Does the syringe used for irrigation of the catheter come from a sterile package?

_____ 4. Are hands washed before donning sterile gloves?

_____ 5. Do the gloves used for sterilization come from a sterile package?

_____ 6. Does the urine drainage bottle overflow?

_____ 7. Is the urine bottle suspended above the floor?

_____ 8. Is the urine bottle autoclaved?

_____ 9. Is there a cotton plug in the air vent of the catheter?

_____10. Is an antiseptic present in the urine bottle?

DRESSING OF WOUNDS

_____ 1. Are dressings put on with gloved hands?

_____ 2. Are hands washed before and after dressing patients' wounds?

_____ 3. Are dressing trays and carts arranged to prevent contamination of sterile and clean equipment?

_____ 4. Are dirty drapes or dirty dressings kept on dressing cart?

_____ 5. Does cold sterilization take place on the dressing cart?

_____ 6. Are wounds dressed at specifically scheduled times?

SURGICAL FACILITIES

_____ 1. Are the operating suites separate from each other and other patient areas?

_____ 2. Is cross traffic through these units from other hospital areas eliminated?

_____ 3. Are the dressing rooms for physicians and nurses accessible directly from the rest of the hospital and do they open directly into the operating suites?

_____ 4. Is there adequate separation between utility areas used for clean and those used for contaminated equipment, supplies, or waste?

_____ 5. Are all surgical wastes placed in plastic bags for disposal?

_____ 6. Are sub-sterilizers (rapid instrument sterilizers) accessible to operating rooms?

_____ 7. Are facilities for scrubbing directly accessible to each operating room?

_____ 8. Are these facilities kept clean at all times?

_____ 9. Are locker rooms kept clean at all times?

_____10. Is there adequate space in clean areas for storage of sterilized items?

_____11. Are there facilities in the recovery room for isolation of infected cases?

_____12. Are there closed containers for all contaminated and soiled dressings and other contaminated material?

_____13. Are there adequate closed containers for disposal of gowns, masks, and booties in the locker room?

ANESTHESIA AND INHALATION THERAPY

_____ 1. Inhalation
   a. Is the equipment cleaned and sterilized after use by patients?

_____ 2. Intravenous
   a. Do the needles and syringes come in a sterile package?
   b. Does the plastic tubing come in a sterile package?

_____ 3. Spinal
   a. Is detergent used in cleaning needles?
   b. Is all equipment sterilized?
   c. Are solutions sterilized?
   d. Are contents of ampoules sterile?

_____ 4. Conduction Anesthesia (local)
   a. Are gowns, masks, gloves, worn when anesthesiologist does conduction anesthesia?

_____ 5. Is the anesthesia table stored outside of the O.R. within a traffic area?

_____ 6. Are endotraceal tubes cleaned and then sanitized in 70% alcohol plus Formalin? (1 part Formalin to 250 parts alcohol.)

_____ 7. Is the endotraceal tube then placed in a boiling sterilizer to boil off the Formalin?

_____ 8. Is humidification maintained during inhalation therapy?
_____ 9. Is the equipment cleaned properly?
_____ 10. Are the nasal catheters sterilized?
_____ 11. Is the humidifying solution sterile?

SURGICAL PROCEDURES

_____ 1. Do all personnel change from street clothes before entering surgical suites?
_____ 2. Are booties put on at the O.R.?
_____ 3. Are surgical room clothing and shoes worn outside of the operating room suite?
_____ 4. Are surgical gowns put on and discarded properly?
_____ 5. Are adequate surgical gowns provided for the surgeons?
_____ 6. Are surgical masks discarded after each procedure?
_____ 7. Are surgical masks discarded when wet?
_____ 8. Are hands washed before donning surgical suit, mask, and cap?
_____ 9. Are patients brought to the O.R. on beds?
_____ 10. Are they returned on their beds?
_____ 11. Does the operating table leave the O.R. suite?
_____ 12. Does the operating team scrub its hands thoroughly in an acceptable manner with soap or liquid hexachlorophene detergent prior to an operation?
_____ 13. Is the patient "prepped" in an acceptable manner immediately prior to the operation and before the surgeon gowns?
_____ 14. Are the razors and razor blades used for preoperative shaving cleaned and sterilized after each use?
_____ 15. Are disposable razors or razor blades used for preoperative shaving?
_____ 16. Is the nurse responsible for sterility of surgical procedures? (In unusual cases the surgeon makes this determination.)
_____ 17. Does the surgeon inform the nurse about a contaminated case?
_____ 18. Are precaution gowns provided for the circulating nurse and anesthesiologist?
_____ 19. Are contaminated patients scheduled for a separate operating room?
_____ 20. Are the contaminated cases scheduled last?
_____ 21. Are special precautions taken for T.B. cases in the O.R.?
_____ 22. Is the questionably contaminated case treated as a contaminated case?
_____ 23. On contaminated cases, are the gowns removed before the gloves?
_____ 24. Do personnel wash hands after a contaminated case and before going to the dressing room?
_____ 25. Is dropped equipment resterilized before reuse?
_____ 26. Is talking kept to a minimum during an operation?
_____ 27. Is the number of people in the O.R. kept to a minimum?
_____ 28. Is the suture package opened in an aseptic manner?
_____ 29. Is the adhesive tape stored in a satisfactory manner?
_____ 30. When operating in two different sites (grafting procedure) are separate instruments used?
_____ 31. When operating in two different sites, are different personnel used?
_____ 32. When operating in two different sites, do the personnel rescrub and regown:

_____33. Are special precautions taken during an intestinal anastomosis? (Is a sub-set of instruments used?)

_____34. Are the proper types of drapes used?

_____35. Is the proper thickness of drapes used?

_____36. Are dry drapes used?

_____37. Do they get wet during the procedure?

_____38. Are instruments retrieved from below the patient level and used?

_____39. Is sheet wadding sterilized when used on open procedures?

_____40. Are gloves changed when needle punctures them?

_____41. Are personnel with significant respiratory illnesses or with overt lesions excluded from the operating and delivery suites?

_____42. Are Kelly pads being used on the O.R. table?

_____43. Is the O.R. table cleaned properly between operations?

_____44. Is the operating room equipment cleaned properly?

_____45. Is the recovery room clean?

_____46. Is the recovery room maintained with the same basic technique as the operating room?

_____47. Is the operating room thoroughly scrubbed and washed with a germicide solution and allowed to sit for at least 24 hours after an infected case?

_____48. Are the walls spot cleaned between all operations?

_____49. Are the floors and other horizontal surfaces cleaned between all operations?

_____50. Is a germicide solution used in the above mentioned procedures?

_____51. Is there routine bacteriological surveillance of aseptic techniques and sterilization in the O.R.?

_____52. Do surgeons wash their hands, put on masks, and don sterile gloves before performing intravenous cutdowns?

_____53. Are intravenous catheters inserted in an aseptic manner?

_____54. Are intravenous catheters removed promptly when not needed?

HOUSEKEEPING

See self-inspection sheet for Housekeeping Program in Housekeeping section.

COMMENTS:

3-5   THE HOSPITAL INFECTION CONTROL COMMITTEE

3-5-1   Introduction

The Infection Control Committee was established in many hospitals in 1956, when it became obvious to members of the staff that there had been a marked increase in staphylococcal infections in both surgical and medical patients. Concomitantly multiple reports of epidemic staphylococcal disease within hospitals were appearing from both the United States and abroad. Staff members notified the administration of their desire to initiate an active infection committee to deal with the problem.

3-5-2   Meetings and Membership

During the first six months of its existence the committee met two or three times a week. This was necessitated by the fact that there were a substantial number of staphylococcal infections occurring within the hospital. Many questions concerning changes in technique throughout the institution were considered and action taken. Subsequently, the committee met regularly once per week throughout the calendar year.

The membership of the committee consists of representatives from the Departments of Medicine, Surgery, Administration, Housekeeping, Nursing,* and Environmental Health.

3-5-3   Method of Reporting Infections

It is a firm institutional rule that all infections or suspect infections of either medical or surgical variety must be cultured. At the weekly meeting of the infection committee, the Department of Microbiology presents a list of all patients with positive cultures for the past week. These patients are then distributed to the various members of the committee who survey their charts and fill out an infection form. At the next meeting, the cases are discussed and classified. In this hospital, where the committee has been in existence for $11\frac{1}{2}$ years, its members have surveyed and classified some 6000 patients. They have found that this method of reporting infections is most effective.

Publications

During the past 11 years, the membership of that committee has published 24 scientific articles in the medical journals of this country.

---

*Includes the infection control nurse and the nurse in charge of the dressing cart.

The number of papers presented by committee members and talks given, number well over 100. A scientific exhibit on staphylococcal disease was created by the committee and was shown at every major medical convention in the United States and also at a number abroad. A pamphlet summarizing this exhibit and its principles was reprinted numerous times, and over 70,000 copies were distributed throughout the world.

3-5-4 Functions and Activities of an Infection Control Committee

Perhaps the most important achievement of the Infection Control Committee is to effectively combine and utilize the efforts of many professional people who are interested and knowledgeable about the problems of infection. Because they are active in patient care, both on a professional and administrative level, they are conscious of problems relating to infection throughout the institution. Likewise they are readily available for consultation and discussion.

The following is a partial list of the activities of a committee on infection.

1. Publication of a handbook on the management of patients with infection.
2. Lecture on hospital infections and techniques of prevention to residents, interns, medical students, and nurses.
3. Conduct bacteriological surveys of hospital personnel, areas where infection appears to have increased in incidence in the institution, and of multiple institutional fomites when other techniques fail, or a specific emergency exists. The operating room ventilating system is surveyed bacteriologically at regular intervals. Efficacy of germicides is established and recommendations made as to the type of solutions to be used in the institution.
4. Surveys techniques of sterilization and usage of equipment.
5. The committee is constantly available for consultation and decision-making related to patient isolation and type of room, or admission to the intensive care unit.
6. Early in its existence members of the committee should establish a clinic for the treatment of hospital employees who develop infection. This clinic, or a delegated member of the committee, should examine all employees who have infections. The physician decides whether the employee may continue to work in some area of nonpatient contact or be relieved of all duties until the infection has cleared.
7. Surgical techniques and preparation of patients for surgery is recommended to the various surgical services when warranted. Members of the committee representing the department involved have the responsibility of seeing that these changes are carried out.

REFERENCES AND SELECTED READINGS

Caswell, H. T. How to maintain an infection control program, *Modern Hospital*, Vol. 97, September 1961.

Hayt, E. *Legal Considerations in Control of Hospital Infections*. U.S. Dept. HEW, PHS, CDC, Atlanta, Ga.

Himmlesbach, C. *Role of the Hospital Infection Committee*. U.S. Dept. HEW, PHS, CDC Course #1050-G, Atlanta. Ga.

Linden, Rosemary, *Organization and Functions of the Hospital Infection Control Committee*. U.S. Dept. HEW, PHS, CDC, Atlanta, Ga.

Weinzettel, R. J. *The Effective Infections Control Committee: Administrative Aspects*. U.S. Dept. HEW, PHS. Atlanta, Ga.

4

Fire
Safety

4-1 INTRODUCTION

Morally and legally every hospital is generally responsible for the safety of its employees, patients, visitors and others on hospital property or affected by hospital operations.

Further, every hospital is obligated to protect its buildings, equipment, and other resources, and even adjoining properties from destruction or damage due to a related fire.

The importance of fire safety is greatly magnified in hospitals due to the general helplessness and dependency of its patients plus the numerous inherent fire hazards associated with medical care and its facilities. Such fire hazards include the presence of: fuels, boilers and pressure vessels; refrigeration and air conditioning; electrical systems and electrical equipment; work shops and maintenance operations; kitchen stoves, fryers, and exhaust ducts; linen chutes, dryers and other laundry equipment; unusual amounts of combustible linens, mattresses and dressings; extensive use of flammable gases, liquids and oxygen; the storage of a great variety of necessary dry stores and other supplies.

Fire incidents may also be complicated by the presence of radioactive materials, acids and caustics, and conditions involving operating rooms, research laboratories, hyperbaric chambers, and other special units.

4-2 FIRE PREVENTION

Fire prevention is simply the elimination of unsafe conditions and unsafe actions that could cause a fire. This is accomplished through the basic "E's of Safety" — Engineering, Education and Enforcement (plus Enthusiasm).

Fire prevention is a definite hospital responsibility and function that should be carried out strenuously and systematically with complete management support, and by every person connected with the hospital operation, along with the best professional aids and assistance obtainable.

4-3 FIRE FIGHTING

Fire fighting is not the sole or prime responsibility of the hospital, where an established municipal fire department is in the immediate area. It is however, the hospital's responsibility to establish, train and equip a hospital fire brigade, and to train all employees in the method of reporting fire, emergency rescue techniques, extinguishment of fire, and other emergency functions.

It should be clearly understood that the fire department should be notified immediately upon the discovery or suspicion of a fire.

Hospital personnel should render emergency service that may extinguish the fire or hold it in check until the fire department arrives and assumes control.

It should be clearly understood that the hospital's primary responsibility related to fire is the saving of lives.

In areas with minimal, remote or nonprofessional level fire departments, it may then be the hospital's responsibility to organize, train, and equip a fire brigade or private fire department that could handle extensive fire fighting and evacuation operations.

4-4 HOSPITAL FIRES—SOURCES AND CONTROL

An extensive study in the New York City area revealed that 52% of hospital fires occurred in "service rooms" (storerooms, maintenance and utility rooms), 15% were due to fires originating outside the hospital buildings, 14% involved heating plants, 11% were in patient rooms, 5% in nurses' quarters, and 3% were in operating rooms.

In most cases, "service rooms" were closed or otherwise not occupied at the time fire was discovered, which indicates need for automatic fire protection as afforded by sprinkler systems.

Matches and smoking was the alleged media for one of five hospital fires, indicating need for proper smoking areas, education and enforcement of smoking regulations.

The misuse of electricity and/or the unsafe condition of electrical equipment was the next leading fire cause factor, indicating the need for inspection, proper installation, and maintenance.

Fires involving heating plants were attributed to the normal type hazards associated with improper cleaning, maintenance, insulation, etc.

It was notable that the severity of fire damage was greatest where hospital staff attempted to put out the incipient fire without first calling for fire department aid.

4-5 FUNDAMENTALS OF FIRE

To understand fire prevention and fire fighting, it is necessary to know that three elements are required to have a fire. These are:

1. *Combustible Material (Fuel).* May be in a solid, liquid or vapor-gas state.
2. *Oxygen (Air).* Oxygen supports and accelerates combustion. Found principally in surrounding air (21%), it is also prevalent in most chemicals bearing the suffix "ates" such as chlorates and nitrates.
3. *Ignition Point (Heat).* This is the amount of temperature a material must be raised by application of heat to maintain combustion.

4-6 THE BASIC PRINCIPLE OF FIRE PREVENTION AND FIRE EXTINGUISHMENT

Since three elements are required to have a fire, the elimination of any one of these elements will prevent a fire or extinguish it.

1. *Combustible Material (Fuel).* The substitution of combustible materials with noncombustibles, the minimum use of combustibles, proper storage and good housekeeping practices will help prevent fires. In the event of fire, removal and/or diversion or shutting off the liquid, gas, or solid fuel supply will extinguish the related fire.
2. *Oxygen (Air).* Oxygen may be eliminated by use of an inert gas. Air may be excluded with a cover, and also by use of a chemical that will dilute the oxygen in air to a point below that required to support combustion (fire will burn in 16% of air).

     This method of fire prevention and extinguishment is commonly known as the "blanketing-smothering" technique.
3. *Ignition Point (Heat).* Fire may be prevented or extinguished by maintaining temperatures below the ignition point. In extinguishment, "quenching-cooling" is accomplished with water or chemicals, and also by the introduction of cooler materials through agitation.

This latter method is now common in the prevention and extinguishment of fires in tanks or containers with fuel or other flammable liquids.

METHOD: Although more than one method of fire extinguishment may be utilized, efforts should be made to concentrate on the most effective method for the particular class of fire.

4-7   CLASSES OF FIRE AND EXTINGUISHERS

Portable fire extinguishers are classified according to their fire extinguishing potential which is indicated by a numeral and letter designation. The letter designates the general class of fire for which the extinguisher is suitable, and the numeral indicates the approximate relative extinguishing potential of the device.

Class A Fires. Fires in ordinary combustible materials such as wood, cloth, and paper where the "quenching-cooling" effect of water or solutions containing large percentages of water is most effective and of first importance in reducing the temperature of the burning material below the ignition temperature.

Class B Fires. Fires in flammable petroleum products or other similar flammable liquids, greases, etc., where the "blanketing-smothering" effect of oxygen—excluding extinguishing agents is most effective.

Class C Fires. Fires involving electrical equipment where the electrical nonconductivity of the extinguishing agent is of first importance.

Class D Fires. Those in combustible metals, such as magnesium, titanium, zirconium, sodium, and potassium. In this class of fire, special extinguishing agents and techniques are required, and the extinguishing media, usually a special dry chemical, must be specifically designed for the particular metal and quantity involved.

Class D fire exposures are not common in hospitals, but they may occur in laboratory and experimental operations. This points up the necessity of knowing what chemicals are brought into the hospital, where they are kept, the provision of any necessary special type fire extinguishers, and the education of personnel (and the local fire department) concerning their presence and methods necessary for extinguishing a related fire.

4-8   FIRE EXTINGUISHER SELECTION

Prospective users should first ascertain from authorities, having jurisdiction, as to their minimum requirements regarding type, quantity, and placement of fire extinguishers.

To insure standards of quality and performance, it is recommended that all fire extinguishers purchased meet with Underwriters' Laboratories, Inc., and/or Factory Mutual Approval. As minimal requirements for proper installation, the nationally recognized standards of the National Fire Protection Association should be followed, as outlined in their Standard #10 *Installation, Portable Fire Extinguishers,* and Standard #10A *Maintenance and Use of Portable Fire Extinguishers.* It is recommended that general hospital areas be classified as "ordinary type of hazard," which according to N.F.P.A. Standards requires at least one fire extinguisher rated as 2-A* for every 3000 square feet to be protected, with a maximum travel distance of 75 feet to the extinguisher. (New York City requires 2500 square feet with a 75 foot travel distance for hospital class occupancy.)

In more hazardous areas such as carpentry shops, warehouses, etc., where there is a higher Class A Fire potential, the area should be considered in the "Extra Hazard Class" for which the N.F.P.A. recommends 3-A extinguisher protection for 3000 square feet with a 75 foot maximum travel distance.

Where flammable liquid and/or grease fires can be anticipated such as in boiler rooms, kitchens, laboratories, paint shops and operating rooms, Class B extinguishers should be installed in locations that will require not more than 50 feet travel distance.

"Light" hazard areas require Class B extinguishers with a 4-B rating, "Ordinary" hazard areas—8-B, and "Extra" hazard areas 12-B.

Extinguishers with Class C ratings are required where there may be energized electrical equipment and a nonconductive extinguishing media is necessary, such as in electrical switch gear, generator rooms, computer and X-ray departments, etc. Since the fire itself would be a Class A or Class B hazard (with the added electrical danger), this nonconductive extinguisher should be of a size and in a location based on the anticipated Class A or B hazard.

With the exception of Foam and Loaded Stream Extinguishers, those extinguishers bearing a Class B rating will also be of Class C (i.e., CO_2, Dry Chemical, Vaporizing Liquid, and Multi-purpose).

Selection Tips

Class A. In areas not subjected to freezing, the $2\frac{1}{2}$ gallon Pressurized Water Fire Extinguisher is one of the best for Class A Fires. Compara-

---

*2 indicates units of fire extinguishing potential, and A indicates type of fire designed for—i.e., ordinary combustible materials. Usually $2\frac{1}{2}$ gallon water type extinguishers have a 2-A Rating.

Class and Types of Fire Extinguishers

Class A	Class B	Class C
Water types	Foam	Carbon dioxide
Soda action	Loaded stream	Dry chemical
Loaded stream	Carbon dioxide	Vaporizing liquid
Foam	Dry chemical	Multi-purpose
Multi-purpose	Vaporizing liquid	
	Multi-purpose	

NOTE: For Class D (Metallic Fire) check with established fire extinguisher supplier.

tively light; it may be recharged from a gas station type air compressor; has a readily visible gauge to indicate a state of charge; contains no harmful acids, although use of an anti-rust solvent is recommended; has a good carrying handle; has controlled on and off discharge by merely squeezing the handle; does not need to be inverted; contents are not messy; and it usually requires no annual recharging.

Where exposed to freezing, special Anti-freeze Pressurized Water or Anti-freeze Cartridge Operated Fire Extinguishers are recommended.

Class B-C

a. In areas containing food-stuff, delicate electrical equipment, and other areas where cleanliness of extinguishing agent is necessary, the Carbon Dioxide Fire Extinguisher is considered best.

b. In areas containing large quantities of oil, or other flammable liquids, the ammonium phosphate or sodium bicarbonate base Dry Chemical Fire Extinguisher is considered superior.

Other Types

a. Vaporizing Liquid Fire Extinguishers (carbon tetrachloride or chlorobromomethane), may be dangerous due to the toxicity of its liquid and vapors, also the liquid may corrode the container and components. Use of this type extinguisher is not recommended.

b. Foam Extinguishers are not generally recommended since they lead to confusion and possible dangerous misuse of the similar looking soda-acid (Class A) extinguisher on Class B fires. Further, this Class B extinguisher requires special knowledge in handling; it cannot be used on alcohol or other (polar) solvent fires; it cannot be used on Class C (electrical) fires; is subject to freezing; is messy, and harder to handle and maintain than CO_2 or Dry Chemical Fire Extinguishers of similar capacity.

c. Multi-purpose Extinguishers (also known as "All-purpose" and "A-B-C" Fire Extinguishers), are a comparatively new type of fire extinguisher which can be safely and effectively used on A, B, and C Class Fires. Exclusive use of such extinguishers will help prevent confusion or error concerning which type extinguisher is to be used.

However, the extinguishing media is quite messy and may leave a corrosive residue, which can cause costly damage to metal, particularly components of delicate and valuable equipment that may be found in labs, computer rooms, etc.

Before purchasing Multi-purpose units, it would also be prudent to check with local regulatory authorities for acceptance in the particular region involved.

Installation

Extinguishers should be mounted on the wall, column or other stationary member in a safe accessible location.

Unless local law otherwise indicates, extinguishers should be mounted so that the extinguisher bottom is not less than two feet or more than four and one-half feet above floor level

In rooms it is recommended to install extinguishers near the entrance door. Standard location placement is advantageous, such as at a fire alarm box and/or fire exit on each floor. Where applicable, signs indicating the presence of fire extinguishers should be installed.

4-9   ENGINEERING FIRE SAFETY

Prevention of hospital fires should start well before construction, and with assistance from professional fire protection engineers in cooperation with planners, architects, construction engineers, and municipal authorities.

4-9-1   Types of Building Construction

There are five standard types of building construction in use today that are defined and recognized by the National Fire Protection Association. They are classified as:

1. Fire-resistive
2. Heavy timber
3. Noncombustible
4. Ordinary
5. Wood frame

The term "fireproof" has been officially discontinued by most authorities for its use is misleading since no material is immune to the effects of fire of sufficient intensity and duration.

Fire-resistive construction may be simply defined as that in which structural members, including walls, partitions, columns, floors and roofs, are of noncombustible materials having minimal fire resistance ratings for specific components ranging from 2 to 4 hours for buildings having an overall 3 hour fire-resistive classification, and 1½ to 3 hours for a fire-resistive building of a 2 hour classification.

Heavy Timber construction may be simply defined as that which utilizes noncombustible two hour rated bearing walls, noncombustible exterior walls, and where columns, beams, and girders may be of heavy timber, with wood floors and roofs installed to meet certain specifications.

Noncombustible construction is merely that type of construction in which structural components are noncombustible, but do not qualify as "Fire-resistive Construction."

Ordinary construction refers to buildings with two hour rated noncombustible exterior bearing walls, but with roofs, floors, and interior framing of wood, or partly of wood (or other combustible material), of smaller dimensions than are required for "Heavy Timber Construction."

Wood frame construction is where exterior walls, bearing walls and partitions, floors and roofs and their supports are of wood or other combustible materials.

Although "fire-resistive construction" is extremely desirous and mandatory in most areas for new hospital construction, the use of fire-resistive building materials does not necessarily assure safety to life and freedom from fire damage.

Proper attention must be given to all features including proper fire exits; enclosure of vertical floor openings to prevent fire and smoke spread (stairs, elevator shafts, ducts, dumbwaiters, chutes); limitation of combustible interior finish material; and the subdivision of floor areas to prevent horizontal spread of fire and smoke, and to provide same level places of safe refuge for the horizontal evacuation of patients.

Depending upon area, other architectural safeguards may be necessary to protect against earthquake, tornado, floods, etc.

In some areas lesser construction may be permitted, particularly in one-story structures and/or if additional means of fire prevention and protection are afforded, such as automatic sprinkler systems.

Isolating the Hazard. Where possible and practical, operations which normally present an unusual fire and explosion potential should be located in structures separate from those housing patients, or otherwise isolated from these regions. This would include the hospital's power plant, laboratories, laundry, warehouse, and the like.

4-9-2 Fire Protection Equipment—Automatic Sprinklers

Automatic sprinklers are the #1 fire protection device which has constantly given unparalleled performance in the saving of life and property.

Sprinklers are normally incorporated to sound an alarm in the building serviced, at a monitoring service office and in some areas directly to the local fire department. They provide an almost immediate and continuous flow of extinguishing water to areas not often readily accessible to fire fighter hose streams. They will also extinguish or at least hold down an incipient fire to allow precious time for safe evacuation.

Two basic types of automatic sprinkler systems are generally utilized in hospitals, with adaptations for special situations and exposures.

Wet System. Water supply under pressure is in the sprinkler piping being retained by the sprinkler head. At a predetermined temperature (usually 135°F) a bulb, fusible pellet or metal link will disintegrate allowing water spray to emit and extinguish the fire by "quenching and cooling." Due to the presence of water in its pipes, wet systems are not installed in areas subjected to freezing temperatures, unless special conditions allow use of an anti-freeze solution.

Dry Pipe System. This special type system is designed for use where sprinkler pipes would be exposed to freezing temperatures. Somewhat similar in construction as the "wet pipe system," this system contains air under pressure in its pipes which when released by the sprinkler head will allow a valve to open and thus supply water through the pipes and onto the fire.

Comment. Contrary to common belief by many laymen, correctly designed automatic sprinkler systems will function in an excellent manner on grease and flammable liquid fires, such as in kitchen grease hoods and ducts, and in flammable liquids storage vaults and laboratories.

Most fire protection authorities also recommend use of automatic sprinklers in computer rooms and other areas containing similar electrical equipment, supplemented with an automatic carbon dioxide fire extinguishing system designed to reach the interior of equipment which may be shielded from sprinkler water.

The principal reason for automatic sprinkler protection preference over CO_2, Dry Chemical, and Steam Smothering Fire Extinguishing Systems, is the practically inexhaustible supply of extinguishing media (water) and the least likely chance of mechanical failure.

Sprinkler Economics. Generally speaking, fire insurance premiums can be reduced to about one-third when automatic sprinklers are installed in non-fire-resistive buildings. Thus, in many instances, sprinkler installation costs can be amortized out of insurance savings within four to ten years, while providing dependable protection for life and property.

Although insurance premium reductions may not apply to sprinklers in fire-resistive buildings, losses may be prevented through complete or partial sprinklering. Of particular need would be high hazard occupancies such as workshops, storage rooms, chutes, shaftways, ducts, and certain laboratory areas. Sprinkler installations are also needed where dead-end corridors exist and where additional protection may be needed to safely reach exits.

In most fire insurance policies, the fire insurance carrier will pay for any water damage resulting from accidental discharge of sprinkler systems, or breaks in the sprinkler system water supply lines.

Sprinkler Safeguards. It is imperative that sprinkler supply valves be open at all times, that sprinkler heads are protected against damage. Also, sprinklers must be kept unobstructed to allow designed water flow pattern. Generally, a minimum clearance of 18 inches should be maintained between sprinkler heads and stored items.

Water supply valves should be sealed in the open position with metal wire and lead seals. Some authorities advocate use of padlocks and chains.

Each sprinkler control valve should be identified by a sign indicating "sprinkler control valve" and each valve should be given an identity number. A weekly inspection should be made to ascertain that all valves are open, and written records of each inspection maintained. Also, the system should be tested by use of a drain valve which will create a water flow, and also flush out the line. Since this will usually set off the alarm system, notification should be given before testing, or the alarm bypassed.

If any valve must be closed for repairs, etc., the local fire department and the institution's fire insurance carrier should be notified. Until sprinkler protection is resumed, special fire prevention and protection methods should be followed. This may include the stretching of fire hose for instant use in the area, posting of special watchmen to be alert for fires and who may reopen the water supply where applicable in event of fire, the prohibition of smoking and use of open flame in the area, and the removal of dangerous materials and/or operations.

Sprinklers in Chutes. It is imperative that automatic sprinklers be installed in linen and trash chutes. Aside from the normal installation of sprinklers at top and bottom of the chute, it is advisable to also install recessed protected sprinkler heads interspaced along the vertical length of the chute, generally at each floor level. This will prevent items which may create a stoppage in the chute from blocking the flow of water to extinguish a fire below, which was one of the significant factors in the 1961 Hartford Hospital Fire.

4-9-3   Fire and Smoke Detection Alarm Systems

Fire detection alarm systems may be grouped into three basic types— fixed temperature, rate of rise, and a combination of both.

Fixed Temperature Systems. These respond when the temperature of an immediate area reaches a fixed point such as 135°F or higher. Such units may use detector heads so spaced and located to cover specific areas, or a heat sensitive miniature cable run along a specific pattern to cover the area desired to be protected.

Rate-of-Rise Systems. A more sensitive type, this system responds to a sudden rise in surrounding area temperature, usually in the range of a 5°F increase in 20 seconds.

Combination Rate-of-Rise and Fixed Temperature Systems. This system is generally preferable to the single type systems since it provides a dual response. A gradual build-up of heat as would develop from a slow, smoldering fire would be detected by the fixed temperature element. On the other hand, the rate-of-rise system would respond much more rapidly to a blazing fire even in its early stages.

Other Fire Detection Alarm Devices

Some units are on the market which can give a false sense of security. These devices are generally self-contained units, usually consisting of a small battery, a buzzer, and a heat sensing element. Claims for their reliability can often be misleading. The main deficiencies are that the alarm will sound only in the area where the fire occurs and may not be heard in other parts of the building. Also, most of these devices cannot be tested.

Smoke Detection Alarm Systems

There are several types of smoke (and gas) detection alarm systems which utilize various principals designed to detect fire (smoke and gas) at an early stage.

The ionization chamber combination gas and smoke detector utilizes a detection head containing one sealed and one open ionization chamber in which the entrance of invisible gases of combustion will create decreased electrical conductivity in the exposed chamber and thus an unbalance between the two chambers which then triggers an alarm. This is perhaps the most sensitive and fastest type of automatic alarm system.

The photoelectric smoke detector operates to sound an alarm when smoke interferes with the light beam and interrupts the electrical circuit. In some types an indirect light would be reflected or deflected by smoke particles to focus on the photoconductive cell, changing resistance and operating an alarm.

The ultraviolet flame, smoke, and combustible vapor detector utilizes a tube which adds up the impulses of electrical energy generated by the tube as it counts ultraviolet rays, and which sets off an alarm at a predetermined amount.

The flame radiation photoelectric detector system operates on the principle of modulated radiation by flame, and is beneficial only where un-obstructed scanning of an area is possible.

Installation and Costs. The best detection systems are generally one-quarter to one-half the cost of an automatic sprinkler system. However, in most instances, fire insurance premium rates will not be reduced for detection systems, as for automatic sprinklers.

When using detection systems, they should meet Underwriters' Laboratories, Inc. Approval. As minimal requirements for proper in-stallation, the National Fire Protection Association's Standards #72, A, B, C, and D (as applicable to type of system) should be followed.

Limitations. It should be clearly understood that smoke and fire detec-tion alarm systems merely warn that a fire may be in progress. Such systems cannot extinguish a fire. However, they can be adapted and utilized to close dampers and doors, and to shut down equipment.

In consideration of detection alarm systems, important factors that must be reviewed are: building construction, exits, staffing at all hours, mental and physical condition of patients, response and type of local fire department—all of which may indicate that a detection alarm system may or may not allow sufficient time for safe evacuation and/or fire extinguishment. Also to be considered is the extreme sensitivity of some smoke (and gas) detection systems which could lead to repeated false alarms and possible disregarding of a "true alarm."

4-9-4 Manual Evacuation Alarm Systems

Every hospital should have some type of an audible signaling system that can be activated by anyone discovering a fire or similar emergency.

Such alarm boxes should be accessibly located on each floor and in every area. As a minimal standard, at least one alarm box should be installed for every 10,000 square feet on any floor, and sufficient boxes should be installed to allow a maximum horizontal travel distance of 200 feet to the nearest box utilizing the normal paths of exit from the area.

It is generally recommended, and required in many municipalities, that the evacuation alarm ring throughout every area of an individual building. The usual system will sound a coded signal which indicates the location and/or floor where the alarm box was pulled or otherwise activated. Such signals being repeated at least three times. A chart, indicating the code signals should be installed at each alarm box, and also in other key areas such as administrative and other key personnel offices, nursing stations, and elevators.

4-9-5 Monitoring of Fire, Smoke and Evacuation Alarms, and Sprinkler Systems

For all alarm systems the need for prompt response is paramount. In general, there are five methods in common use:

1. *Central Station Alarm.* This system transmits an alarm to a constantly supervised monitoring company's office, where the alarm is recorded and the fire department automatically and almost instantaneously notified.
2. *Proprietary Alarm.* This system transmits the alarm to a supervised location on the protected property, where the alarm is recorded and monitoring personnel will call the fire department and/or take other necessary action.
3. *Local Alarm.* This is a common and least expensive system where an audible alarm sounds only on the premises to warn occupants.
4. *Auxiliary Alarm.* This system or hook-up utilizes a municipal fire alarm system to a fire station or to fire alarm headquarters.
5. *Direct Fire Department Connection.* This system uses a direct line connection to sound an alarm at the municipal fire department's location.

Comment. To insure prompt response by the fire department and to eliminate delayed alarms, it is advisable to utilize a system that will automatically notify the fire department if the detection system, sprinkler system, or manual fire alarm system is activated.

In most large cities, this must be done through commercial central station alarm companies which specialize and charge for this service. In some cities and smaller locations, it may be possible to tie the hospital's system into the municipal fire alarm system or utilize wires directly to the fire department.

Proprietary alarm systems are usually installed where the institutional complex is large and/or the location is remote from a good municipal fire department. It is also necessary that institutional personnel constantly monitor the alarm system, and staff or the institution's private fire department is present, equipped and capable of handling any fire emergency.

Where only local alarm systems are used, all concerned should fully realize that the municipal fire department must be summoned immediately, via phone, municipal alarm box, or other approved means.

Pre-Signal Alarms. In some locations, local alarm systems may be allowed which will first ring only in prearranged locations, such as administrative offices, engineering office, etc., rather than throughout the entire building. Then, upon evaluation by an administrator, the alarm system can be activated to sound the alarm throughout the building.

The reasoning given for such systems is to avoid disturbing the patients or other staff unnecessarily.

With the mobility and possible shortage of key staff, particularly during evening hours, such a system could dangerously delay response, and lead to other serious errors. It is therefore recommended by most fire authorities that pre-signal alarm systems be not generally used in buildings or areas that house patients, or where a source of personnel to cope with an emergency could be summoned, such as a nurses' or staff residence building.

4-9-6   Fire and Smoke Barriers

Stair Doors. To prevent spread of smoke and fire, all stairs should be equipped with Underwriters' Laboratories Approved Class B fire doors which, depending on material and type, give a one to one and one-half hour fire rating. Such doors should be automatically self-closing and kept closed at all times except during actual momentary use. They should not be wedged or otherwise held open.

In some areas, authorities will allow wire inserted glass vision panels in certain Class B fire doors. Generally, the maximum allowable opening for glass is 100 square inches with a maximum dimension of 12 inches, using two thicknesses of one-quarter inch wired glass with a maximum mesh of seven-eighths of an inch, and of at least #25 steel wire gauge or its equivalent, with wire glass set at least five-eighths of an inch into the frame.

Corridor Doors—Smoke-fire Barriers. Doors, barriers, and partitions are utilized to subdivide floor areas into fire zones or places of refuge. In forming these subdivisions, it is imperative that noncombustible materials be utilized having at least a one hour fire rating, and that the barrier extend from the lower floor to the upper floor. This should include extending through hung ceilings and other concealed spaces where fire and smoke could spread.

It is generally recommended that the maximum number of patients kept in any one fire zone be limited to 30, with an ideal census of 16.

Corridor and other fire zone doors should be at least U.L. Approved Class C fire doors (three-quarter hour rated), and all such doors should be self-closing. There should be no more than 150 feet of corridor length without a fire barrier or horizontal exit.

Since traffic flow problems may arise with some of these doors, wire inserted glass vision panels up to 1296 square inches are generally allowed in most areas.

Some municipal authorities are now allowing corridor and other smoke-fire barrier doors (not fire stair doors) to be held open by a magnetic door holder which will automatically release (close) the door when activated by a fire-smoke detection device, if the hospital's manual fire alarm is pulled, or if the automatic sprinkler system functions. Of course, with such devices, it is necessary to ascertain that the areas surrounding the door are never blocked by wheelchairs, stretchers, etc., and that doors are visually checked during time of emergency.

Fusible Links. In general these links, which are attached to a door, etc., and to a wall or other stationary member, contain a soft metal center which melts and separates at a predetermined temperature (125°F and up), allowing the door, lid or cover held to automatically close. Usually, untenable smoke can exist before heat is sufficient to melt a fusible link and allow the door to close. Therefore, the use of fusible links to hold open corridor or smoke-fire barrier doors is not recommended.

4-9-7 Watchmen Stations

The use of watchmen and watchmen stations serves the dual purpose of systematically checking for fire and other safety hazards, plus conditions related to security such as burglary and thefts, unauthorized visitors, disturbances and other unusual occurrences.

The usual method in most hospitals is to equip a watchman with a portable clock which is activated by a key located at watchmen stations and thus records the station visited and time. Stations are spaced and located so that the watchman should traverse all parts of the hospital.

Local regulations may vary concerning the use of watchman and watchclock rounds. Some areas may even waive the use of watchmen making rounds, if the premises is equipped with automatic fire-smoke detection alarm systems. However, such practice may be unwise since an automatic system cannot check for blocked fire exits, accumulated trash, inoperable exit lights, etc.

In general, rounds each hour are advocated in patient areas commencing at a time when evening visitors have left, and/or when patients are prepared for the night, but not later than 10:00 p.m. and continuing until the day shift arrives.

In addition, areas that may be unused, vacant or unstaffed — such as construction sites, storage and workshop areas, auditoriums and business offices — should be visited during the untenated hours (evenings, weekends, holidays, etc.).

4-9-8   Standpipes and Hoses

Standpipe and hose systems provide accessible means for application of water to fires. They are of great value where automatic sprinklers are not installed, but never take the place of sprinkler protection. Standpipe and hose systems are needed, and in most areas mandatory, for multistory buildings and where areas of a building may not be readily available to hose lines stretched from outside hydrants.

In most areas, it is advisable to have a standpipe outlet that will accommodate a two and one-half inch hose as generally used by the fire department. However, as this larger hose line is difficult to handle by nonprofessional fire fighters and may cause injury and water damage, it is advisable, if local law allows, to install a $2\frac{1}{2}-1\frac{1}{2}$ inch removable reducer, and install $1\frac{1}{2}$ inch hose at each standpoint outlet.

Hose lengths should be kept to 50 or 75 feet lengths as longer initial runs are unwieldy and may result in kinks. It is imperative that all threads be the same as those utilized by the municipal fire department to allow interchange and hooking up additional hose lines.

Building height, structural conditions, weather, area, local law, and water supply are determining factors in standpipe installations. Usually an exterior connection is required so fire department apparatus may pump water into the standpipe lines. Automatic fire pumps and good secondary sources of water supply are also advisable.

Aside from interior use, roof outlets can be valuable to fight roof fires, fires in cooling towers, to wet down buildings, and to fight or control fires involving immediately adjoining buildings or grounds. Where exposed to freezing conditions, standpipes should be of the dry-pipe type or if circumstance allows, anti-freeze can be added to the exposed lines.

Hose lines vary and usually a U.L. Approved unlined linen hose or light-weight cotton rubber-lined hose is adequate if kept clean and dry.

Hose nozzles also vary and it is prudent and economical to equip standpipe hose with the simple nozzle generally known as the "open nozzle," "straight tip nozzle," or "open hose nozzle." Where unusual exposures or circumstances prevail, other type nozzles may be considered such as the more expensive "controlling nozzle" which allows flow or shut off of water at the nozzle, "fog nozzles" for use on flammable liquid fires or "combination nozzles" which can be adjusted to straight stream or fog spray.

Inspection. It is imperative that standpipe systems be periodically tested and all components, including hose lines, be inspected frequently.

4-9-9   Fire Exits

The general safety rule of, at least two remote means of safe exit from each floor or fire zone, of which one leads directly to the exterior or to a fire tower or fire stair should prevail.

Local law may also dictate the maximum distance to exits (usually 100 feet in non-sprinklered and 150 feet in sprinklered institutions), the size of corridors (eight feet), exit doors (usually 40 inches minimum width and swinging out in direction of exit travel), use of panic hardware, exit signs and emergency illumination.

Where local laws allow, it is advisable to use as minimal specifications the standards set forth in the National Fire Protection Association's Standard #101 *Life Safety Code* (formerly *Building Exits Code*), which contains specific sections for hospitals and nursing homes.

When planning fire exits, it is recommended to have room doors of sufficient width to allow passage of a patient bed (plus side rails and any other attachments). Although evacuation via bed is generally not recommended, there are times when it may be advantageous to move patients to safety via bed. One such example occurred in 1963 at New York's Montefiore Hospital when a great number of exploding propane gas tanks from an adjoining construction site fire threatened patients in rooms facing the fire scene. In this instance, patients while in their beds were merely moved into corridors and room doors closed to prevent injury from flying glass and debris.

4-9-10   Storage and Service Areas

Hospital design should provide for sufficient areas to contain lockers, desks, stretchers, wheelchairs and other items which commonly block corridors or otherwise create a hazard. All corridors and other exit routes, exit doors and stairways should be kept clear at all times.

4-9-11   Door and Window Locks

Under normal circumstances, toilet doors and room doors, utilized by patients or residents and which they can lock, should be equipped with locks that can be quickly opened in an emergency from the exterior side.

Also, window detention screens or similar window guards should be of a type that can be removed by the fire department from the exterior to rescue and to gain entry.

In penal institutions or in certain psychiatric patient areas where doors must be locked, reliable means should be provided for rapid release, such as remote control locks. Attendants should also be equipped with master keys to allow opening of windows and doors in an emergency.

4-9-12   Revolving Doors

Revolving doors should not be considered as legitimate fire exits, and also due to an accident potential, their use is not recommended. Where installed, revolving doors should be equipped with a panic pressure release which will allow collapse of the leaf doors and help prevent a jamb up. Such a safety device should be tested frequently. In addition, the normal speed of a revolving door should not exceed 12 revolutions per minute.

4-9-13   Elevators

Elevators should not be considered legitimate means of emergency egress, such as fire stairs.

Elevators should be equipped with an emergency power source to allow freeing of trapped patients and/or others in the event of power loss, and to afford other emergency use. Elevator cabs and doors should be of solid noncombustible material and shaftway walls should be of brick, concrete or concrete block construction.

Elevator cabs should be equipped with an emergency stop and an emergency alarm. It is also advantageous to equip elevators, particularly those utilized for patient transportation, with telephones.

The use of elevators during a fire, particularly automatic elevators, can be extremely dangerous since the elevator could malfunction and accidentally stop and open its doors at the immediate fire scene, or the elevator could stall in the shaft exposing occupants to fire and smoke.

4-9-14   Roof Areas

Lightning protection should be afforded as building and local conditions may require including the common grounding of electric and telephone service, radio and television masts, and piping systems such as water and gas.

Chimney and stacks should be provided with spark arrestors.

Cooling towers utilizing wood baffles or other combustible components should be equipped with automatic sprinklers, even though water generally flows through such units.

Roof covering should be noncombustible and of a Class A type as defined by the National Fire Protection Association and the Underwriters' Laboratories, Inc.

4-9-15   Furnishings

To eliminate potential fuel for a fire, extensive use of metal furniture is advocated, such as tables, desks, cabinets, chests, bookcases, shelves, etc. Overstuffed furniture should be avoided and coverings on upholstered articles should be flame resistant or fire retarded.

Drapes, cubicle curtains and similar items should be of noncombustible material or flameproof.

Ceiling tile, wall covering and other exposed relevant interior finishes should be noncombustible, fire-retarded or otherwise be a U.L. Class A Interior Finish, with flame spread of 0–25 maximum.

Although standards may exempt floor coverings, it is advisable to also utilize Class A materials to prevent possible smoke and fire spread, particularly where flammable liquid fires may occur.

The use of fire-retarding paint is also advantageous, particularly in high hazard areas.

Trash containers should be of nonburnable material, preferably with self-closing covers.

Mattresses should be fire retarded and equipped with handles which will allow emergency transportation of the patient.

Canvas type stretchers placed in a centrally accessible location on each floor are valuable for emergency evacuation. Such stretchers take little storage space and can be moved with ease. However, they must be of a good type, protected from deterioration and inspected frequently.

Visible alarms, plus audible alarms may be required where occupants may be deaf (such as institutions for deaf and dumb), or where there may be a high noise level.

Refrigerators. Only U.L. Approved Explosion-proof refrigerators should be utilized for the placement of flammable liquids, gases, or solids. All refrigerators in laboratories, medical care locations or other areas where improper use is possible, should bear a clearly visible sign stating in effect

> *Warning—This is not an explosion-proof refrigerator. Storage of flammable liquids, gases or solids is prohibited.*

Bed lights should be of a type that will not allow them to come into close proximity to bedding.

Safety showers (and emergency eye wash fountains) should be installed in laboratory and other exposure areas. Access to such units should be kept clear and they should be periodically tested. In addition, fire blankets in containers should be mounted in similar areas for use on burning clothing or to snuff out other fires.

Exhaust hoods, with self-closing doors, should be installed and utilized in areas involving flammable or toxic liquid or gas, and exhaust systems installed in working or teaching laboratories to remove any dangerous fumes. It should be kept in mind that flammable vapors are heavier than air and will settle to floor level, thus requiring exhaust outlets at floor level.

4-9-16   Emergency Cut-Offs

Provisions should be made for master valves or switches to be utilized in emergency for shutting off fuel, water, electricity, gas, and other items which could influence or be influenced by a fire emergency. Such controls should be located in safe accessible locations away from any equipment or operation which may produce fire or explosion.

Controls should be clearly identified, a listing, or diagram of control locations should be posted in key locations, and involved responsible personnel on each shift should be trained in these locations and usage.

4-9-17   Engineering for Fire Safety

Engineering for fire safety involves many other facets dependent upon type of structure, locale, and related operations. In certain areas the physical structure may require explosion and smoke venting; safeguards to eliminate static electricity; water-tight floors with raised door sills and special drains to retain and safely drain spilled flammable liquids; automatic and/or remote control safety devices to shut off boilers and other equipment; special yard mains and hydrants; explosive-proof lighting and electrical systems; emergency generators; and many other items.

In engineering for fire safety, the goal is to eliminate all possible fire hazards of a structural and operational nature and thus minimize the potential of human failure.

4-10   EDUCATION FOR FIRE SAFETY

After engineering the best possible fire-safe facilities and operations, personnel must be trained to prevent fires, and to take positive action in event of a fire emergency.

Fire Emergency Plans

The Chief Executive Officer of every hospital should be responsible for and ascertain that a written fire emergency plan is developed and maintained which outlines authority, responsibilities, supervision, rules, procedures, and training. Such a plan should include emergency instruction charts which outline duties consistent with the needs of the institution to be performed on specific floors or areas and should be kept up to date.

The applicable chart(s) should be posted in a conspicuous place on each floor or area and should contain the name or job title of persons for each shift and their function or duty in the event of an emergency. This should include: Person in Charge, Alarm and Communication Operator, Area Controls, Searchers, Evacuation Team and Fire Brigade.

Basic instructions in the event of fire discovery can be taught and remembered by the key word RACE.

Remove anyone in immediate danger from fire or smoke.
Alert by sounding the alarm.
Confine the fire and smoke by closing doors and any openings.
Extinguish the fire if possible.

4-10-1   Initial Training

Before a new employee starts work, he or she should be briefed on simple fire emergency procedures. This should include: smoking regulations, method of sounding the fire alarm, and where to report in the event of a fire alarm. In addition, any employee manual should contain basic fire emergency information and the employee should be given a copy and requested to read it.

How and by whom this initial training is given may vary at different institutions, but it should be spelled out in the master emergency plan.

In some hospitals, this initial training is done by the personnel department; others utilize their security department, where new employees are fingerprinted; in many locations it is done by the department head or supervisor.

Orientation. Many hospitals, particularly the larger ones, have a formal orientation program which reviews the institution's layout and organization, benefits, rules and regulations, etc. At this time some hospitals may include a portion of fire prevention and fire emergencies.

Often subject matter is too much and too varied, and it can be anticipated that a new and inexperienced employee will retain only the simplest of instructions. Therefore, special training classes should be held which are solely devoted to fire.

Fire Training Session #1. This session is generally held at a frequency of one a month, depending upon size of institution and labor turnover. It should be no more than two hours in duration and should set the mood, give elementary knowledge and lay the groundwork for future advanced fire training sessions.

Where on staff, such training sessions are conducted by the institution's fire marshal, safety officer or other person in charge of the fire program, or one with related knowledge and ability.

a. Explain the hospital's policy concerning fire prevention and fire emergencies.
b. Explain fire prevention rules and regulations (i.e., smoking and use of open flame, use of equipment, etc.).
c. Review basic steps to be taken in case of fire (RACE).
d. Review methods of sounding an alarm. (In this case, use of dummy fire alarm boxes and telephone hooked into a loudspeaker will help demonstrate methods.) Allow personnel to activate alarm and simulate phoning in an emergency.
e. Explain the basics of fire chemistry (Fuel, Air, Heat) and demonstrate briefly the type and usage of fire extinguishers in the hospital, and other methods of extinguishment.
f. Explain the necessity for keeping fire exits clear and doors closed.
g. Show a film which will visually and dramatically show major points covered. One such film that will have a dramatic and education impact is *They Called It Fireproof*, 16 mm 28 minutes color sound. This film, if unobtainable locally, may be rented and/or purchased from Contemporary Films, Inc., 267 West 25th St., New York, N.Y. 10001 and it may be purchased (only)

from the National Film Board of Canada, 680 Fifth Ave., New York, N.Y. 10019, or 150 Kent Street, Ottawa, Ontario, or 3255 Cote deLiessa Road, Montreal 3, Quebec.

Fire Training Session #2. This session should be limited to two hours maximum and designed to include those who have had Session #1. It should be scheduled to follow Session #1 within one months time.

a. Review highlights of Session #1.
b. Show film *Fire and Your Hospital.* This 16 mm 20 minute black and white sound film is one of the best all-round training films which outlines basic hospital hazards, emergency planning, and use of fire fighting techniques. If unobtainable locally, it may be purchased or rented from Association Films, Inc., 600 Madison Ave., New York, N.Y. 10022. This organization also has offices in Ridgefield, New Jersey; Oakmont, Pennsylvania; La Grange, Illinois; Hayward, California; and Dallas, Texas.
c. Demonstrate and allow persons present to use fire extinguishers, hose lines and other apparatus and techniques for fire extinguishment. If possible and practical, this session should move out of doors where actual controlled fires may be extinguished.*

   Wire baskets can be utilized to contain wood and paper for Class A Fires; U.L. Approved safety cans should be utilized for any flammable liquids to be used in demonstration; fires should be lit with long handle torches; back-up fire extinguishers, hose, and fire blankets should be available for any emergency.

   Class B Fires can be demonstrated by floating and igniting gasoline in a large metal container partially filled with water. Another method is to hang a metal bucket containing several drip holes in its bottom from a metal stand and have a metal trough (about 6–8 feet long) run below the pail and downward to the ground.

   A small quantity of gasoline is poured into the bucket, allowed to drip and run down the inclined trough and ignited. Utilizing a Class B Fire Extinguisher, the employee must start at the bottom of the incline to extinguish the fire, working up to and into the bucket. This demonstration vividly simulates a fire from a leaking drum or a spill.

   Other demonstrations and drills can be used to show how to extinguish fires by cutting off oxygen with covers, blankets, and other available materials, utilizing fire contained in a metal trash can and also using a hospital bed with ignited bedding.

   Warning: In demonstrations, the use of live persons in a bed which is set on fire, regardless of safeguards taken, is extremely dangerous and is absolutely not recommended.

*It is imperative that the trainer is experienced and that activities do not present a danger to persons or property. If possible, municipal fire department representatives and apparatus should be present.

Fire Training Session #3. This should be an advanced session of two hour maximum duration for all staff or at least those who could be involved in rescue of patients or injured. Although it is advantageous for personnel to complete Sessions #1 and #2, it is not absolutely necessary as these sessions could be completed at a later date.

a. As a guide and/or text, it is advantageous to use the (60 page) booklet *Emergency Removal of Patients and First-Aid Fire Fighting In Hospitals.* This booklet by Lt. Robert McGrath may be purchased from the National Safety Council, 425 North Michigan Avenue, Chicago, Illinois 60611. However, some institutions have developed their own material on this subject.

   If possible, some written and pictorial material should be given to those attending this session and briefly reviewed.

b. Show film *Emergency Removal of Patients* which is the companion to Lt. McGrath's booklet on this subject. This 16 mm 25 minute color sound film, if unobtainable locally, may be obtained on a free loan from Abbott Laboratories, Inc., Medical Film Dept., North Chicago, Illinois 60064 or may be purchased or rented from Mervin W. Larue, Inc., 159 East Chicago Avenue, Chicago, 11, Illinois.

c. The hospital's evacuation plans should be reviewed and methods of evacuation explained (i.e., horizontal and vertical evacuation, leading ambulatory patients to safe areas, transportation by wheelchair and stretchers, etc.).

d. To avoid confusion and to standardize training in emergency lifting and carrying, it is best to preselect only a few methods for actual practice, and expand the repertoire at subsequent sessions.

   Initially, it would be advantageous to concentrate on the one man "Pack Strap Carry," and "Hip Carry," "Cradle Drop," and "Blanket Pull," the two man "Swing Carry," and "Extremity Carry." If applicable, this session should also review methods for evacuating babies.

e. It is prudent to ascertain that all persons involved have no physical conditions that would prohibit them from engaging in this strenuous activity.

f. It is advantageous to have trained "team captains" to assist and give individual attention to the trainees.

g. Actual physical conditions should be simulated with use of beds, dummies and dolls, stretchers, wheelchairs, blankets, etc. Fellow employees may be utilized to simulate patients, but extreme care must be taken to see that they are in good physical condition and are not endangered.

Fire Training Session #3 Follow-up. Additional sessions should be scheduled soon after Session #3 until necessary basic evacuation techniques are learned.

Annual Review. To insure that previously trained employees have retained their knowledge, it is beneficial to schedule an annual "hospital-wide" demonstration, preferably out of doors where apparatus and techniques can be put into effect. Some hospitals find it timely to hold such demonstrations during "Fire Prevention Week" in October and/or "Clean-up Week" in the Spring.

Special Training Sessions

(a) *Fire Brigade*. Special training sessions, in addition to Sessions #1, #2, and #3, should be held for those staff members who will compose the hospital's fire brigade or fire department. Depending upon circumstance, it would be advantageous to hold these sessions or drills on a weekly basis until a level of skill has been developed.

Session duration should be kept short, one to two hours at the most, with handout material that could be studied on off hours. Where necessary, it would be helpful to utilize the services of a professional fire department training officer. In some locations it may be possible to utilize the local fire department's training school and instructors to teach your fire brigade special skills.

Sessions should ultimately cover such subjects as: use and care of fire fighting apparatus and equipment (hose, couplings and nozzles, fire extinguishers, and fixed systems); the correct use of forcible entry tools (axe, claw tools, wire cutters, pole (plaster) hook, etc.); hose line evolutions, as may be required; use of self-contained gas masks or similar apparatus; artificial mouth-to-mouth resuscitation, cardiac massage and other related first aid; use of emergency cut-off, special fire dangers of properties, operations and departments; plus other skills which may be required in event of a fire emergency, including protection of property and salvage.

(b) *Laboratory*. Special periodic training sessions should be held with laboratory personnel to review normal hazards, check for any new hazards, and to review methods to be used in various specialized situations, including those involving radioactive materials

Some available films on laboratory fire safety are:

Safety in the Chemical Laboratory, 16 mm 19½ minutes color and sound, utilized in schools to emphasize general safety, handling of flammable liquids, and preparation of sodium amide. This film may be purchased or rented from the Manufacturing Chemists Association, 1825 Connecticut Avenue, N.W., Washington, D.C. 20009.

Radiation Protection in Nuclear Medicine, 16 mm 45 minutes color and sound, demonstrates procedures and equipment used by hospital staff to protect against radiation hazards. This film may be borrowed from the U.S. Navy Department, Bureau of Medicine and Surgery, Washington, D.C. 20250.

(c) *Operating Room*. O.R. personnel should receive special training regarding inherent dangers in their department, preventative measures, and emergency actions in event of fire and/or explosions.

One film on this subject which can be used for part of the O.R. staff training is *Fire and Explosion Hazards From Flammable Anesthetics*, 16 mm 30 minutes color and sound. This film may be borrowed without charge, or purchased from Abbott Laboratories, Inc., Medical Film Library, North Chicago, Illinois 60064.

(d) *Fire Training Records*. To avoid duplication and to insure that each employee receives the proper training, proper records should be kept. Usually such records are maintained by the Personnel Department utilizing an index card filed by employee's name and other identity needed and which indicates the Training Session Number and Date attended. This may be also cross-indexed by a file card containing employee's name data and date of attending the particular session, and this card is filed alphabetically in a file for the particular session (i.e., Fire Training Session #1). Thus, by running through these cards, it can be quickly determined who requires additional training. It should be hospital policy that an employee must attend designated fire training session, unless unusual circumstance warrant written administrative approval to waiver or postpone training.

4-10-2   Fire Inspections

Fire inspections provide an excellent method to detect and correct unsafe fire conditions and activities. They also serve to educate the employee inspector and others concerned with the area or operation inspected. Of course "continual inspection" should be practiced by every hospital employee who should report, and/or correct, unsafe fire and accident conditions.

Where a hospital does not employ a full time safety officer or fire marshal, a good practice is to assign an Inspection Committee Chairman and operate this Committee as a subcommittee of the hospital's Safety Committee.

To ease and expedite inspection tours, it may be beneficial to organize the hospital facilities into zones and assign inspection teams, consisting of two or three persons, to tour a specific zone within a specific time period and/or make periodic inspections in these assigned zones. This should include inspection teams assigned from and operating on each shift.

A written record of each inspection should be made, indicating date and time of inspection, hazards found, and corrective action taken. Such completed forms should be coordinated by the Inspection Committee Chairman who will follow-up on any conditions that remain uncorrected, and will report progress to the Safety Committee. In this plan, it is wise to use supervisory level personnel and/or persons with a knowledge of fire prevention. In addition, it is best to have the person in charge of a particular area accompany the inspection team so questions can be answered and any corrective action needed, be implemented without delay.

To assist inspectors and to gain uniform coverage, an inspection checklist form should be utilized. However, inspectors should be instructed and reminded to also report any unusual conditions that may not be specifically covered by the form.

Outside Inspectors. To supplement your own inspections, additional fire inspections should be routinely made by your municipal fire department, insurance carrier engineers, and various service or regulatory agencies.

In addition to fire department inspections and depending upon circumstances, it is advantageous to encourage drills where fire department apparatus is brought onto property. Knowledge gained may prevent errors and assist in the event of a real emergency. Such drills could check for vehicle clearances, positioning of vehicles and ladders, means of entry and stretching of hose lines, etc.

Fire and Evacuation Drills. Most regulatory authorities require that a hospital or similar type agency conduct fire and evacuation drills at a minimum frequency of 12 drills per year held at irregular intervals during day and night. Such drills should include the transmission of a fire alarm signal and simulation of emergency fire conditions except movement of infirm or bed-ridden patients. If possible and practical, it is suggested that 12 fire and evacuation drills be held each year—on each shift.

When fire and evacuation drills are held, all staff should participate unless such participation or deviation from routine would jeopardize a life, such as interruption of an operation, etc.

If a fire drill is considered merely as a routine exercise from which some persons may be excused, there is a grave danger that in an actual fire the drill will fail in its intended purpose.

The person conducting the fire drill should first notify the telephone operator and others who may receive or transmit a call for fire department action, and as a courtesy also advise the top administrator on duty.

Varied floors or areas should be selected for the simulated fire scene and the fire drill conductor should approach any available staff person, advise that a drill is to be held and request this person to sound the alarm.

When the hospital fire alarm is activated and/or other means of notification are made, every area of the hospital should participate. To help evaluate participation, some hospitals utilize members of their fire and/or safety committee who are posted on various floors or areas in advance, and, utilizing a "fire drill observer's checklist," records what occurs during the drill. Some "yes" or "no" questions to be answered on this checklist are: are all doors closed; all windows closed; all hallways cleared; all chutes closed; unnecessary appliances and utilities (except lights) turned off, exhaust and ventilating fans turned off; were patients and personnel properly informed and reassured; did alarm sound properly; was alarm audible; was public address audible; were records, valuables, narcotics, etc. secured; was a communication officer stationed at emergency telephone; telephones not used except in emergency; did assigned personnel search toilets, lounges, etc. and escort patients and visitors to rooms?

Also, on floor of simulated fire emergency, a record would be made regarding response of the fire brigade and evacuation teams.

Immediately following the drill or soon thereafter, it is beneficial to hold a critique to review findings and institute any procedures necessary to correct unsatisfactory conditions.

4-10-3   Other Educational Media

Education for fire safety should utilize all possible and effective methods including: films; posters; slogans; payroll inserts; contests; suggestion boxes; literature; departmental "stand-up" meetings; safety fairs and demonstrations; visits by selected groups to other hospitals, industries, and fire department facilities.

It has also been found beneficial to relate fire safety to the employee's home or off-the-job activities. Some institutions, through bulk purchase and reduced costs may sell fire alarms, fire extinguishers and other items at cost to employees to create interest in fire safety.

Helpful materials can be gained from established safety organizations such as: the National Fire Protection Association; the National Safety Council; various insurance carriers, service organizations and industries.

4-11   ENFORCEMENT

Unfortunately people will do things they should not do, and whether it is done unintentionally or intentionally, they may produce the same tragic results.

Hospital policy, rules and regulations regarding fire prevention should be clear, practical, and enforced.

4-11-1 Smoking

Smoking is one problem which usually requires enforcement techniques. Unless local law has more stringent regulations, smoking in hospitals and other medical care institutions should be prohibited, except in specially designated areas where signs indicating

Smoking permitted in this location — prohibited in other locations

are posted. In other areas and at entrances signs should be posted which stipulate

Smoking, or using a flame or fire producing device is prohibited in these premises except in designated locations.

Safe smoking locations should be selected in cooperation with advice from and approval of the municipal fire department and/or other regulatory agencies. Considered areas may include waiting rooms, lounges, toilets, solarium, cafeteria, certain meeting rooms and business offices. It is elementary that such locations should not contain combustibles, and if possible, should be sprinklered. Heavy duty noncombustible ashtrays and stands should be provided, waste receptacles should be metal with self-closing covers, and doors to areas should be self-closing where feasible.

It should be the general rule that no smoking is allowed in patients' rooms (by patients, visitors, or staff). Patients desiring to smoke should be removed to authorized smoking locations. Where this is impractical and/or medically unwise, controlled smoking by a patient may be allowed only when a staff member is present, and only if there are no hazards from oxygen, medical gases, etc.

Contractors. To insure that contractors and their employees will not create hazards that may jeopardize the institution, written contracts should, where applicable, include references to accident prevention, fire prevention, and fire protection. Basic, is the stipulation that contractors and their employees must conform to hospital safety regulations including those regarding smoking, use of open flames, and reporting fires.

Where new construction or alteration is involved, items as applicable should be included that will require contractors to provide fire-fighting equipment. Such equipment including the provision of fire extinguishers, fire buckets, etc.; watchmen; the daily or more frequent removal of combustible waste; notification to a designated hospital administrator and hospital approval before any utilities to the hospital are shut off. Similar notification and approval should be sought before welding, burning, or engagement in similar hazardous activities, and also the stipulation that hospital access and/or exits will not be blocked in such a way as to prevent access by emergency vehicles and emergency egress. In addition, it may be beneficial to further stipulate in the contract, depending upon particular circumstances, that water pressure should be maintained in any standpipe system being installed, up to each floor as constructed. Similarly, where automatic sprinklers are being installed, it is advantageous to have sprinklers put into service immediately, and to utilize sprinkler protected areas for storage of combustible materials and/or articles received that will go into the building (i.e., beds, furniture, etc.). It is also advantageous to prohibit the use of combustible "shanties" within buildings under construction and to limit the amount of flammable liquids and gases that may be brought into buildings or onto hospital property.

Local laws, building and fire department inspectors, insurance and legal stipulations regarding the liability of contractors may in some cases legally relieve a hospital of some or all responsibilities concerning the actions of contractors. However, in most cases, hospitals (and hospital occupants) will suffer in the event of a fire or similar catastrophe and the hospital will bear or share legal and financial responsibility. It is imperative therefore, that enforcement techniques be utilized to ascertain that contractors or others follow good fire prevention practices while on hospital property.

Other Areas of Enforcement. A number of items relative to contractors may also be applicable to hospital staff, particularly where the hospital's maintenance department may engage in construction and alteration work which may require welding, use of combustibles, etc.

Many institutions will utilize their security department to enforce many of their fire prevention regulations and to otherwise check for usual fire-producing situations. In lieu and/or in addition to a security department, persons or committees may be utilized. Some areas that may require enforcement action include: blocking or chocking fire exit and fire-smoke cut-off doors; failure to secure and protect medical gas cylinders; accumulation of trash; storage or placement of items in corridors; blocking or tampering with fire extinguishers and other emergency equipment; unauthorized use of equipment (i.e., hot plates, heaters, fans, etc.); unauthorized repairs (repairs to electrical equipment, use of heavy fuses); the bringing of dangerous materials into the hospital (i.e., flammable or sparking toys); use of flammable decorations;

the failure to shut off equipment (i.e., stoves, electrical appliances and machines, gas jets, etc.); the failure to lock doors to unoccupied laboratories, store rooms, motor rooms, etc.; unsafe operation and parking of motor vehicles; improper handling and storage of combustible and volatile materials, liquids or gases; failure to use conductive shoes and follow other safe practices in O.R.'s; improper disposal of aerosol cans; and overcrowding rooms or areas beyond safe capacity.

4-12   DISASTER PROGRAMS

In most cases, regulatory authorities require hospitals to have a disaster program with plans to cope with both off-premises and on-premises disasters.

Potential off-premises disasters may include: aircraft, train and motor vehicle accidents; floods; tornadoes; earthquakes; fire; explosion; radiation; bombing and other acts of war.

On-premises disasters may also involve most items that may occur to the community, plus the individual problems of loss of water, electricity and gas; destruction of areas of the hospital due to fire, explosion or flood; radiation contamination of areas, etc.

A major portion of a disaster plan pertains to the handling and medical treatment of victims. In many cases portions of the plan will involve circumstances similar to those involving fire emergencies. In fact, some on-premises disasters may start off as fire emergencies.

It is imperative therefore, that an institution's disaster program and plan be coordinated with the fire plan. For example, if the fire plan calls for a central labor pool to group in a specific room or area, the disaster plan should be consistent and also utilize the same area for its labor pool. Similarly, the same fire plan organizational structure should be utilized as far as possible in the disaster plan utilizing those who are trained or otherwise responsible in evacuation, area controls, communications, etc.

A comparatively new facet of disaster planning for hospitals involves that related to riots and other civil disorders. This requires additional protection of physical facilities, staff and patients, including victims — who may be hostile. In addition, hospital staff and supplies may be seriously curtailed during such emergencies, and police and fire department services at a minimum due to their vital need at the areas of violence.

Above all, disaster programs should strive to cover all possible circumstances, they should utilize established organizational structures, and they should be kept as simple and flexible as possible. In addition, such plans should be tested, evaluated and revised as necessary.

4-13 REFERENCE LIBRARY

To do a job you must have proper tools. Reference books and knowledge of where to get technical assistance is imperative for any Fire
Safety Program.

Listed are basic publications that can form a nucleus for a good
reference library. This library should be supplemented with specialized
books pertaining to operations and other situations relative to your
particular location and institution.

NATIONAL FIRE PROTECTION PUBLICATIONS

National Fire Protection Association
60 Batterymarch Street, Boston, Massachusetts 02110

N.F.P.A. Handbook of Fire Protection (13th edition). This handbook of about 2128 pages is a
most widely used reference covering in detail practically every phase of fire protection.
($22.50 approx.)

National Fire Codes
Vol. 1 Flammable Liquids, Ovens, Boiler-Furnaces
Vol. 2 Gases
Vol. 3 Combustible Solids, Dusts and Explosives
Vol. 4 Building Construction and Facilities
Vol. 5 Electrical
Vol. 6 Sprinklers, Fire Pumps and Water Tanks
Vol. 7 Alarms and Special Extinguishing Systems
Vol. 8 Portable and Manual Fire Control Equipment
Vol. 9 Occupancy Standards and Process Hazards
Vol. 10 Transportation

These volumes are published annually and contain most of the N.F.P.A. Standards,
Codes and Recommended Practices.
($5.00 per volume — $40.00 per set approx.)

N.F.P.A. Standards (Pamphlets). Although found in related volumes of the National Fire
Codes, separate pamphlets are printed to cover individual subjects. As follows are
pamphlets that may be most pertinent to a hospital's fire protection program:

N.F.P.A. No.	Title	Approx. Price
3M	Hospital Emergency Preparedness	$1.00
56A	Inhalation Anesthetics	$1.50
56B	Inhalation Therapy	$0.75
56C	Hospital Laboratories	$0.75
56D	Hyperbaric Facilities	$1.00
56F	Nonflammable Medical Gas	$0.75
76A	Essential Electrical Systems for Hospitals	$0.75
76CM	High-Frequency Electrical Equipment in Hospitals	$1.00

N.F.P.A. Inspection Manual. This is a pocket manual that is particularly valuable in reference and training for inspectors and fire-brigade members.

($4.00 approx.)

Fire Protection for Chemicals. This book gives basic data concerning the prevention, detection, control and extinguishment of chemical fires.

($3.00 approx.)

N.F.P.A. Membership. It is advantageous for a hospital to take out an Associate Membership in the National Fire Protection Association. Annual dues are $30.00 which includes subscription to *Fire Journal*, a monthly Fire News, one free volume of a National Fire Code, plus samples of various fire-safety materials.

Handbook of Industrial Loss Prevention by the Factory Mutual Engineering Corp. Published by McGraw-Hill Book Company, 330 West 42nd St., New York, N.Y. 10036.

This 864-page handbook contains detailed, highly technical, recommended practices for the protection of property and operations against damage by fire, explosion, lightning, wind, and earthquake.

($20.00 approx.)

Accident Prevention Manual for Industrial Operations. Published by the National Safety Council, 425 North Michigan Avenue, Chicago, Illinois 60611.

This is the standard general handbook most widely used in the field of "safety engineering" which covers a wide scope of safety matters, including fire-safety. Although a number of sections deal with industrial operations, a great percentage of contents can be utilized by hospitals.

($16.00 approx.)

Dangerous Properties of Industrial Materials by N. Irving Sax. Published by Reinhold Publishing Corporation, 430 Park Avenue, New York, N.Y. 10022.

This is a most complete handbook containing every type of information regarding fire and safety concerning chemicals and materials.

($25.00 approx.)

Best's Safety Maintenance Directory. Published by Alfred M. Best Company, Inc., Park Avenue and Columbia Road, Morristown, New Jersey 07960.

This 772-page bi-annual publication contains an extensive directory of safety and fire equipment plus a manual of modern safety techniques.

($11.50 approx.)

Hospital Safety Manual. A joint publication of the American Hospital Association and the National Safety Council, published by the National Safety Council.

This 128-page book is a general guide for hospital safety.

($2.55 approx.)

Emergency Removal of Patients and First-Aid Fire Fighting in Hospitals. Published by the National Safety Council.

Sixty pages concerning carrying and general evacuation techniques, plus fire fighting.

($1.80 approx.)

N.S.C. Membership. For about $30.00 per year a hospital can subscribe to the National Safety Council's Hospital Safety Service. With this membership, the hospital will receive a free copy of the N.S.C. *Hospital Safety Manual* and the book *Emergency Removal of Patients and First-Aid Fire Fighting in Hospitals*, the monthly *Hospital Safety Newsletter*, samples of hospital related safety posters, and special technical papers and other materials as released.

5

Patient and Employee Safety

5-1 INTRODUCTION

> It may seem a strange principle to enunciate as the very first requirement in a hospital that it should do the sick no harm.
>
> FLORENCE NIGHTINGALE

Hospitals are established in a community to provide care for the sick of that community. Employees are hired by the hospital to help provide that care. The general public looks to the hospital as an institution of healing. However, providing the best surgical team for a patient becomes quite inconsequential if that patient dies from an overdose of a drug. Providing cordial working conditions for an employee becomes insignificant when he must spend several months out of work, because he was severely injured while performing his job. The visitor who trips over the doormat and breaks his leg while entering the hospital soon forgets the humanitarian aspect of a hospital's functions.

Not very many years ago these accidents to patients and visitors were a moral problem only, since the doctrine of charitable immunity applied to most hospitals. Before 1910 even injured workers' recoveries were few. However, due to the Workmen's Compensation Laws which have been enacted in all states, and the hospitals' loss of charitable immunity in most states, the cost of these accidents is upwards of $100,000,000 a year. Not only are the number of lawsuits against the hospital increasing but the amount of the judgments are also increasing. Hospitals and their equipment are becoming more complex, and the scope of their responsibility has broadened tremendously. Where once the hospital was "the doctor's workshop," now, under certain conditions, hospitals are being held liable for the professional negligence of their attending staff.

Hospital administration can no longer ignore the need for an overall and effective safety program, which must include:

182

Patient Safety
Employee Safety
Visitor Safety
Fire Protection
Evacuation Plan

The following accident prevention program and organization is flexible and can be adapted to fit almost any size hospital with only minor modifications.

5-2 ORGANIZATION

Accident control must start at the top. Both the hospital administrator and the medical director must actively support a strong accident prevention program, which recognizes the hospital's *total responsibility* for the welfare of the patient, and its obligation to employees and visitors. It is mandatory that hospitals recognize the full extent of their responsibility before any effective program of accident prevention can be established.

For the purposes of this test the responsibility for maintaining effective safety programs in the specific areas of Patient Safety, Employee-Visitor Safety, and Fire Safety is delegated to three separate committees whose composition and duties will be outlined individually. It is recognized that for various size hospitals these committees may be combined into a general safety committee, encompassing all three. In still other institutions, these committees, and possibly others like laboratory safety committee, building safety committee, etc., would report to a central steering committee. The specific organization depends on the hospital's size, and function (i.e., general or specialty). The one aspect which is common to all, however, is active support by the administrative and medical staffs.

Since fire safety is of such obvious importance a separate chapter was devoted to it.

5-3 PATIENT SAFETY

5-3-1 The Patient Safety Committee

The Patient Safety Committee's membership should include the Administrator, who would act as chairman; the Medical Director, or Chief of Medicine and Chief of Surgery; the Director of Medical Education; the Director of Nursing; and the Hospital Safety Director.

The committee's functions would be:

1. Periodically review the hospital's administrative, medical, and nursing procedures to insure the maximum safety of the patient.
2. It should oversee all of the activities in the hospital which include patient contact except those areas for which control has already been established such as the tissue committee, infection committee, etc.
3. It should insure complete and unobstructed communications among administration, and the medical and nursing staffs.
4. It should periodically appraise the house and attending staffs as to the nature, seriousness and cost of incidents occurring to patients in the hospital and solicit their cooperation in any safety activities deemed necessary. This is extremely important.
5. It should coordinate all nursing and medical staff safety activities.
6. It should make studies of patient falls, mandatory consultation procedures, emergency room procedures, etc.
7. It should also review all patient incidents and either institute the necessary corrective action, or if major medical policies are involved, make the necessary recommendations, studies, etc., for presentation to the medical staff for their review.

Overall, this committee should coordinate all of the activities which are being carried on in the hospital for the patients' safety and should make sure that there are no gaps left in this picture of *total patient responsibility*.

5-3-2   Patient Incidents

The Doctrine of Charitable Immunity. While there is a great diversity among states regarding the extent to which a charitable organization (i.e., a voluntary nonprofit hospital) is liable for torts committed by its servants, the general trend is to hold charities liable to the same extent as other organizations.

For ease in identification, incidents involving patients can fall into three categories — Medical, Quasi-Medical, and General.

Medical incidents would be those involving the practice of medicine and subject to negligence or malpractice, litigations due to errors of omission or commission. Such incidents involve incorrect diagnosis and treatment, surgical errors, patient abandonment, and other medical situations which may be judged on a doctrine of ordinary care, regulations, standards and law, and the degree of care which prevails in similar institutions or in the community.

Quasi-medical incidents involve those which may involve nonprofessional persons or routine hospital care. In this grouping would fall: defective hospital type apparatus and equipment; improper consent for operations and other procedures; improper dispatchment and handling of emergency room cases; exposure to infections; improper drug administration; incorrect blood procedures; and the general area of patient falls related to the patient's condition.

General incidents would be those associated with hazards normal to accidents which could affect hospital employees, visitors, and others. These may include the foreign body in food, slip and fall on wet floors, etc.

Consent. In general the performance of an operation or other event without the patient's consent or that of his relative or other legal representative can result in a liability claim against the hospital. Such consent forms involve: authorization to perform an operation, use anesthetics and perform other medical services; the agreement for blood or blood plasma transfusions; the refusal to permit blood transfusions; permission to use radioactive therapy, shock therapy, radioisotopes, experimental procedures, treatments or drugs under clinical investigation; authorization to allow observers to witness an operation, delivery or other procedure; consent to taking and publication of photos, motion pictures, and televising an operation or other procedure, authorization for an autopsy or to retain and dispose of a body, parts or organs; authorization for use of eyes by donor and next of kin; consent to operate for cosmetic purposes; consent to operate for grafting and/or removal of tissue; consent for transplants; authorization for abortions or treatment of a recent or partial abortion; authorization for sterilization; release for ritual circumcision, consent for diagnostic procedures, acknowledgment of emergency treatment; consent or refusal to submit to treatment; authorization for use of birth control pills or devices; consent by all parties involved in artificial insemination.

In all cases, consent or authorization must be "informed", meaning that where applicable, the patient or others involved are fully aware of and understand the dangers that may be involved.

In combating medical incidents, it is beneficial to have a separate medical committee composed of representative specialists in their particular field who will set up safeguards to prevent medical type incidents and who will review, evaluate and recommend any necessary corrective action to prevent the reoccurrence of a medical incident.

Such a committee could report directly to a top administrator or may be a subcommittee of the hospital's general Safety Committee and could briefly report on applicable trends, problems and actions.

Quasi-Medical Incidents

Patient Falls. Most patient accidents occur in a patient's room and about half of these accidents occur in the immediate area of the patient's bed. Some measures to prevent patient falls include the zoning of patients into areas dependent upon their need for supervision (i.e., intensive care units; medical care units; and ambulatory care units).

The use of vari-height beds kept in the low position except during actual treatment, the incorporation and use of safety rail (side rails) on each bed, and the use of safety vests which restrict but allow movement are also helpful in curbing falls.

Proper indoctrination of patients, a good communication system, and proper staffing also influence fall prevention. To prevent falls from bedpans, a bedside commode can be used if medically advisable.

Room and furniture design, plus other environmental features, including illumination and use of night-lights, installation of handrails and grab bars, the removal of sharp or protruding portions of furniture, designed storage areas to eliminate cluttering of rooms, the use of properly based overbed tables and bedside chairs, and the use of walkers, tripod canes and other aids may aid in prevention of falls. In addition, side reactions to drugs and medications, particular ailments or infirmities, and age and alertness of patients will also influence the fall pattern. Above all, supervision and attention by nurses, auxiliary personnel and volunteers is a paramount requirement to patient fall prevention. In conjunction with prevention of patient falls, the use of safety belts on wheelchairs and stretchers should be a standard practice.

Toilets, Baths and Shower Facilities. Where local regulations do not conflict, the following safeguards are recommended:

a. Shower stalls should be equipped with a rust-proof sturdy chair with openings for bathing a patient's rectal and back areas.
b. Shower floors should be flush and without a curb, although slightly sloped for drainage, and the floor surface should be of a nonslip material.
c. All tubs, showers and toilet enclosures should be equipped with grab bars at least of one inch outside diameter, mounted with at least five inches of clearance between bar and wall. The use of towel racks or similar apparatus that will not safely serve as a grab bar should be prohibited.
d. Each water closet should have grab bars on each side approximately one inch to one and one-half inches outside diameter by twenty-four inches long, mounted approximately thirty-two inches above and parallel to the floor.
e. Each tub should have a grab bar at one end approximately thirty-two inches above and parallel to the floor.
f. Each shower should have one grab bar approximately thirty-two inches above the floor, easily accessible to patients while stepping into the shower. Each shower should also have one grab bar fourteen inches long and mounted approximately thirty-two inches above and parallel to the floor on the wall with the shower controls.

g. All exposed heating pipes, hot water pipes, and drain pipes should be covered or insulated.

h. All hot water outlets should be provided with water thermostatically controlled to provide a maximum temperature of 110°F at the fixture, and such controls should be locked.

Footstools. Where necessary, footstools should be not less than ten inches by fourteen inches wide and eight inches high; tip-proof and equipped with floor gripping rubber feet and with rubber tread cemented to the top of the step. To help patients see footstools if color is not obvious, it is advisable to paint the perimeter of the step with a fluorescent or other obvious paint.

Radiators. Should be protected with guard covers to prevent body contact, and beds and chairs should be kept at least two feet from any radiator.

Ramps. Should have a maximum slope of 5%, surface should be of nonslip material, and firmly anchored handrails should be provided on both sides which will not project more than three and one-half inches and which are thirty to thirty-six inches above the floor surface. Where incline is greater than 5%, patients should not be allowed to use such ramps without attendant.

Illumination. Electric lighting should be provided in accordance with the latest recommended levels of the Illuminating Engineering Society. The use of candles, kerosene oil lanterns, or other open flame for illumination should be prohibited.

Night-lights in corridor, toilets and similar areas should be not less than five footcandles; and night-lights in patient rooms not less than one footcandle. All light switches should be accessible with the ceiling light switch located at the entrance door.

Communication System. An electrical call system should be installed which will register above the door to the patient's room and at the nurse's station, utility room, and floor pantry. In addition, there should be an emergency call system for each toilet, bath and shower, utilizing a signal distinctly different than that used in patients' rooms.

Miscellaneous Environmental Safeguards

All lockers, bookcases and other similar upright fixtures should be secured to the wall, floor or other stationary member to prevent them from being pulled or otherwise knocked over causing injury to patients and others.

Beds should be approachable from one end and both sides; they should be equipped with wheel locks and retractable gatch handles;

should be kept at least three feet from a window, and at least three feet six inches from any lateral wall. An unobstructed passageway of at least five feet should be maintained between bed ends.

Only flameproof cubicle curtains should be used which are so secured that they will not give way if a patient should grab them for support.

Doors to patient rooms should bear an identifying number.

Outlets for electrical apparatus should be provided at each patient's bed, and all electrical equipment should be properly grounded.

Trash cans should be of washable metal or other noncombustible material.

5-4   EMPLOYEE-VISITOR SAFETY

5-4-1   Employee-Visitor Safety Committee

The employee-visitor safety committee's responsibility should be the establishment and maintenance of a dynamic employee-visitor safety program. Membership should include the Assistant Administrator — Chairman, Safety Director (Personnel Director) — Secretary, the Assistant Nursing Director and department heads of all major departments. These departments should include engineering and maintenance, housekeeping, dietary, lab, X-ray, and O.R. The health service nurse, a rector, in-service and several nursing supervisors should also be included.

The functions of this committee would be:

1. The establishment and following up on the employee orientation program. This orientation should include those aspects of safety which are common to all departments, i.e., accident reporting, turning in fire alarms, lifting problems, attitude, etc. (*See* Employees Safety Education, p. 192.)
2. The supervision and establishment of departmental safety educational programs. These individualized programs would include the specific hazards, operations, and safe practices found and utilized within the respective departments. (*See* Employees Safety Education, p. 192.)
3. The maintenance of a procedure manual of the standard safe practices utilized for all frequent procedures in each department.
4. Department heads will report to this committee on the safety activities conducted during the month. The committee will periodically review the safety rules and safe practices set up by each department and make necessary corrections or changes.
5. The committee will delegate supervisory personnel in each department to make inspections of their own areas on a periodic and frequent basis.

6. A general inspection team should be appointed which would make periodic inspections of the entire hospital. This inspection team should consist of the Assistant Administrator, chief engineer, housekeeping supervisor and nursing supervisor. The entire hospital should be inspected at least twice annually. This usually requires that only certain portions of the hospital be inspected each month.

The committee should meet at least monthly to review the employee education programs in each department and review and follow-up on the general inspection team. This committee should also review all employee and visitor incidents as reported on the incident report forms and assign the necessary corrective action, where applicable. (*See* Accident Investigation and Reporting, p. 197.)

5-4-2 Supervisors' Safety Education

One of the greatest hindrances to an effective safety program is the lack of fundamental knowledge of safety techniques by the supervisory staff. These people, who are the key to the program, often have misunderstood the basic theory of accident prevention. They must have a working knowledge of the following:

A. Definition of an accident.
B. Causes of an accident.
    1. Unsafe acts
    2. Unsafe condition
C. Investigation of accidents.

Definition of an Accident

An accident is an unexpected happening, caused by an unsafe act(s) and/or unsafe condition(s) that interrupts the normal routine. It is important here to notice that the definition does not include the word injury. An accident which *results* in a near miss or minor contusion is just as much an accident as one which results in a death. Theoretically, what transpires the instant after the accident has occurred (the result) should not be taken into consideration when analyzing the cause of the accident.

Causes of an Accident

Accidents are caused—they do not just happen. The way to prevent accidents is to eliminate that which causes them. Once these two simple statements are accepted it becomes apparent how important a role the supervisor plays in accident prevention. Who else in the hospital's structure better knows the possible contributing factors (causes) of an accident?

Virtually all accidents are caused by either an unsafe act (by a person), or by an unsafe condition (the environment), or a combination of the two. A recent study showed that unsafe acts were a contributing factor in 85% of the accidents and that environmental conditions contributed in some degree to 15% of the accidents. Obviously, in a number of the accidents *both* an unsafe act and an environmental condition combined to produce the accident.

Unsafe Acts. There are many ways in which men commit unsafe acts. Some typical ones are:

1. Operating equipment without authority.
2. Failure to secure against unexpected movement.
3. Operating/working at an unsafe speed.
4. Failure to warn or signal.
5. Removing or making safety devices inoperative.
6. Using defective tools or equipment.
7. Using tools or equipment unsafely.
8. Taking an unsafe position or posture.
9. Servicing moving, energized, or otherwise hazardous equipment.
10. Riding hazardous moving equipment.
11. Horseplay, distracting, startling, etc.
12. Failure to wear personal protective equipment or wearing improper garments, jewelry, etc.

Investigation of Accidents

More important than the actual unsafe act itself is the reason the unsafe act was committed. The reasons why employees commit unsafe acts can be grouped into three broad categories:

1. Lack of knowledge or skill.
2. Conflicting motivations and attitudes.
3. Physical or mental inadequacies.

In order to eliminate the cause of the unsafe act, it is imperative that the reason the employee committed the act be recognized. It is apparent that the remedy for one who committed an unsafe act due to a lack of knowledge, would be different from that if the act was due to a mental inadequacy. Therefore, let us examine the above categories more closely.

Lack of Knowledge or Skill

Lack of Hazard Awareness. Employees often commit unsafe acts because they do not realize the dangers (hazards) associated with a specific job.

Lack of Job Knowledge. Many unsafe acts are committed because employees do not know the safe job procedure. Although they may realize a procedure is hazardous, they do not know the safe way to complete the task.

Lack of Job Skill. Skill differs from knowledge in that it takes physical coordination and practice as well as the knowledge of a job. A person may be an automotive engineer and realize the dangers of driving a car but obviously this does not guarantee that he is a good driver. This takes skill, i.e., a certain amount of physical coordination and practice.

Conflicting Motivations and Attitudes

Although a person may have both the skill and knowledge to work safely, this does not mean the employee will do what the safe job procedure calls for. Employees will often deliberately risk unsafe alternatives to:

Save Time. Whenever the safe way requires more time than an unsafe alternative some employees will choose the unsafe alternative to save time. (Does the employee go for a ladder or step on that convenient box?)

Save Effort. Whenever the safe way requires more physical exertion than the unsafe alternative, some employees will choose the unsafe alternative to save effort. (Same example as above.)

Avoid Discomfort. When the safe way involves more physical discomfort than an unsafe alternative some employees will choose the unsafe alternative to avoid even minor physical discomfort.

Attract Attention. Unable to satisfy their needs for recognition and attention in normal ways, some employees resort to exhibitionism and showing off. This takes the form of working unsafely in the most flagrant and daring ways.

Assert Their Independence. Some employees resent close supervision and when they are away from supervision will often act contrary to instructions for no other reason than to assert their independence.

Gain Group Approval. Most employees will go along with the example set by the oldtimers, even if this example is a bad one. (If the oldtimers do not wear goggles while grinding, do you think the new man will?)

Express Resentment. Many employees express resentment by committing unsafe acts. This they think defies supervision.

It is important to remember that anyone who commits an unsafe act, for one of the reasons outlined above, believes that he can do it, without an accident. It is this conviction plus the conflicting motives discussed that influence an employee to deliberately take chances. A worker would not commit the unsafe act if convinced of the hazardous nature of the practice.

Physical or Mental Inadequacies

A person's mental and physical condition determines the way he or she acts. When either of these conditions is impaired it may cause a person to act unsafely. This impairment may be temporary or permanent, easily correctable or not correctable at all.

Physical Impairments
    Temporary   intoxication, fatigue, sprained ankle, etc.
    Permanent   poor sight, poor hearing, poor coordination, chronic illness
Mental Impairments
    Temporary   worry, day dreaming, hostility, etc.
    Permanent   low mental aptitude

Unsafe Condition. Unsafe conditions can occur for a variety of reasons. They may be due to:

1. Deterioration or corrosion.
2. Arrangement or layout.
3. Storage.
4. Misuse or excessive use.
5. Construction.
6. Design.

5-4-3 Employees' Safety Education

General Orientation

All new employees should be given an initial safety orientation by either personnel or the safety department. This should include general safety rules and procedures common to all departments The hospital's accident prevention policy should be outlined, stressing the administration's active support. Fire drill procedures, the accident (or incident) reporting system, critical safety rules, personal protective equipment policies, etc. should all be discussed with the new employee. This general orientation should be given on the employee's first day, and then repeated periodically.

Department and Job Orientation

When an employee moves into a new position he should be told of the specific hazards and safety rules of his department and in particular the safe and proper way to do his specific job. It is imperative that this departmental and job orientation take place within the first day or two. To let an employee work at a job for a week and then show the worker the correct way to perform it, will undermine all future safety efforts. Once a job orientation has been given, the supervisor should follow up, to make sure the new employee has not deviated from the safe procedure. The supervisor should watch the employee carry out the entire job cycle, and then discuss the more hazardous aspects of this work.

Safety Contacts and Talks

In order to maintain a safety awareness in each department, supervisors should frequently talk about safety to their staff. This is best done individually or in small groups of two or three, but definitely not in larger groups or it takes on the atmosphere of a lecture. A supervisor should attempt to talk to all of his personnel at least once or twice a month in this manner. If an employee is contacted individually the supervisor can reemphasize the hazards and precautions of the particular job. This is without a doubt the most effective safety education technique known.

The supervisor can personalize what he says and how he says it. The employee will pay more attention if it is his job and his alone, which is being discussed. It appears that the supervisor is *personally* interested in the safety of the individual and shows that the supervisor thinks working safely is important.

Lastly, it is usually easier to instruct or discuss a topic with one person than with a group. It is possible, however, to hold effective discussions with small groups. These are called "tool box talks." Here topics or hazards common to all must be discussed. This could include departmental safety rules, discussion of an accident which has occurred in the department, accident reporting, etc.

Standard Safe Practices

Each department should have a set of standard safe practices. These are rules governing each major operation in the department specifically detailing the procedure to be used for any hazardous operation. As part of maintaining safety awareness these rules should be reviewed periodically with the employees for revisions where necessary. Naturally any new job would require that a set of rules be formulated for it.

5-5   VISITORS, CONTRACTORS, AND VOLUNTEERS

5-5-1   Visitors

Visitors may be involved in accidents while on hospital property and they have been known to cause accidents. The control of visitor accidents should be a part of every hospital's safety program.

Aside from exposure to the same hazards that may cause accidents to hospital employees and patients, visitors may be in an emotional and/or physical condition that makes them susceptible to their own errors in judgment or prone to succumb to the slightest irregularity.

Frequent accidents to visitors include: falls on hospital paths, grounds and roadways; vehicle accidents on hospital roads and in parking fields; accidents involving entrance doors, and particularly revolving doors; slips and falls in corridors, lobbies, etc.; injuries by closing elevator doors or improperly leveled elevators; being struck by food and linen trucks, and other wheeled vehicles; falls in stairways and on steps; and injuries from unauthorized use of hospital equipment or facilities—such as cranking up a patient's bed and heating food or beverages in the pantry.

To prevent such accidents, physical conditions should be the best possible, properly inspected and maintained. Roads and parking areas should be adequately illuminated, marked, and controlled. It is found beneficial to paint curbing an obvious color such as traffic yellow to denote change in level, and to use designated marked cross-walks for pedestrian travel.

Doors should be easy to open and slow-closing, and glass panels should be shatterproof, clearly marked and if possible, protected by metal kick-plates and guard bars. The speed of revolving doors should be kept below 12 revolutions per minute and the use of mats or other floor covering which could cause tripping should be eliminated. If possible, floor surfaces should be of a nonslip material and where waxing is necessary, only an U.L. Approved Nonslip wax should be utilized.

Elevator starters and operators should guard against persons rushing into or out of elevators when doors are closing, and automatic elevators should be equipped with electric eyes and/or pressure sensitive door edges that will prevent anyone from being caught in a closing door. Of course, elevators should not be overloaded, and should be equipped with emergency stop and alarm buttons, and also telephones. Aside from proper leveling of elevators, one safeguard to help reduce tripping when an elevator is improperly leveled, is the painting of a strip in an obvious color such as traffic yellow immediately below the elevator cab door saddle and below each shaftway door saddle. Thus, if the elevator is not level, the warning color is exposed denoting the change in level.

The use of wheeled vehicles within a hospital should be controlled by training personnel in techniques of safe operation, the use of vision mirrors at intersections, and enforcement of safe speed and other regulations.

Falls on steps and stairways can be reduced through proper illumination, the painting of nosings an obvious color, and the use of contrasting color for handrails to make them stand out from walls. A helpful aid is the stenciling of signs on stairway walls stating "Go Slow—Use Handrail!"

In reference to visitor accidents sustained in pantries and other non-public areas, it is beneficial from a safety and legal aspect to install signs on entrance doors to such areas which state "Staff Only—Entrance By Others Prohibited." Of course, such regulations should be enforced.

Common accidents caused by visitors are the helpful acts of arranging a patient's bed, helping a patient in and out of bed or performing other services which the visitor, through lack of experience and training, is not capable of doing safely. Also visitors may bring in food, beverages, cigarettes, electrical and other equipment, and medicines that could be injurious to the patient. A frequent visitor related accident occurs in pediatrics where a parent or other visitor may lower crib rails and leave the child unattended, with a resulting fall.

Aside from good physical conditions, constant vigilance must be utilized by all hospital staff to prevent accidents to and by visitors.

5-5-2 Contractors

In most cases a hospital could be legally liable for damages or injuries caused by a hired independent contractor if: it interferes with the work being performed and such interference causes an accident; where the job contracted to be done is unlawful; where the acts performed create a public nuisance; where statute requires the hospital employee to do a thing efficiently, and an accident results from an inefficiency; where the hospital knowingly hires an incompetent contractor; where the work involved may be inherently dangerous; and where the hospital exercises any supervision over the work being done or over the employees of the contractor

In this context, an independent contractor may be simply defined as one employed to produce a given result, being free to select necessary means and methods which are not otherwise specified in advance.

From a legal aspect, proper contractual agreements and insurance coverages will help relieve a hospital of potential financial losses due to accidents caused by a contractor or his subcontractors. However, the hospital cannot be relieved of the many side effects that an accident can produce such as unfavorable publicity and public relations, losses in manpower and operations, reduced personnel morale, etc. Therefore, a hospital safety program must give recognition to accident hazards that may be produced by contractors.

For example, in the course of adding to an existing building, staff and patients must be protected from various fire and safety hazards due to building materials, use of open flame, blocking of exits, etc. Windows, paths and other areas should be protected from falling objects, by use of sidewalk bridges and/or safety screens. Precautions should be taken to prevent disruption of utilities and services (i.e., electricity, water, gas, medical gases). For safety and security reasons, it is generally a good practice to restrict construction employees from the occupied portions of the hospital, if possible. This may entail setting up separate lavatory facilities, rest, eating, locker and parking areas, etc. Above all, the lending of hospital equipment to contractors should be prohibited as in most cases the hospital could be held liable if the equipment was defective or otherwise contributed to an accident.

It should also be decided in advance as to the hospital's role in the treatment of a contractor's employees who may be injured during construction.

Key factors in the prevention of fires and accidents contributable to contractors are: good planning and contractual arrangements; an alert hospital administration; the establishment of proper channels to receive hospital complaints and rectify unsafe conditions expeditiously without detrimental legal involvement by the hospital; and the encouraged use of regulatory authorities such as fire, building and other departments.

5-5-3   Volunteers

Volunteer hospital workers are generally not considered hospital employees or covered under the hospital's workmen's compensation insurance policy. Thus many hospitals will carry a special policy to protect volunteers in the event they are injured on hospital property or through a hospital activity. In most areas, a hospital could be liable for accidents caused by a volunteer.

The use of volunteers is of great value in many hospitals as they provide much of the human relationship with patients and they perform functions that could not otherwise be done due to personnel shortages and budgetary limitations.

Proper selection, training and supervision of volunteer hospital workers is the key to the prevention of accidents to them and those they may be involved with. Volunteers should be of good character and in reasonably good physical condition with no ailments that may lead to accidents or other problems. They should receive thorough training in their duties and they should know what they may do and what they are not allowed to do. In some operations, it is helpful to print guidelines for the volunteer worker which describe the particular job operation and how to do it safely. Volunteers should always work under careful supervision and their functions periodically evaluated.

The safety aspect of volunteers should always be included in the hospital's safety program and the volunteer department represented on the hospital's Safety Committee.

Minors

The employment of underage persons or the use of such persons as volunteers may produce unusual legal and safety problems which may be more or less emphasized by state or local laws. In some states the unlawful employment or use of a minor who is subsequently injured may result in double indemnity or other penalties of which the excess cannot be covered by insurance and must be borne by the hospital.

In the use of persons who may be defined as minors, care must be taken to insure that they are legally used, capable and trained to perform assigned functions, properly supervised, and never put in positions of hazard to themselves or in which they may cause injury to others.

5-6 ACCIDENT INVESTIGATION AND REPORTING

The investigation of an accident (or incident) should be a systematic effort to establish all relevant facts regarding how and why an accident occurred. This is done in order that a conclusion may be drawn about what must be done to prevent a recurrence. Accidents should be investigated as soon as possible after their occurrence.

5-6-1 Employee Accidents

It is imperative that the first line supervisor investigates all accidents occurring under his or her supervision because:

1. The supervisor knows the job, personnel, and working conditions best.
2. Investigating the accident increases the supervisor's awareness of personnel responsibility for accident prevention.
3. The supervisor learns of unsafe procedures, unsafe acts and unsafe conditions in the area of assigned responsibility.
4. It is the supervisor who usually initiates the corrective action and unless the supervisor has done the investigating, many required remedies are not implemented.

In investigating accidents the supervisor should:

1. Interview the employee who had the accident and remind the worker of the investigation's purpose, i.e., to learn what occurred and how, in order to prevent a recurrence and not to "fix the blame."
2. Get the complete story of the accident and ask questions to make sure he fully understands how and why it happened.
3. Discuss with the employee how to prevent the accident from recurring.
4. Interview accident witnesses promptly and separately.
5. If necessary reenact the accident.

The following should be established:

1. *Who* was involved in the accident?
2. *When* did the accident occur?
3. *Where* did the accident occur?
4. *What* job was being done at the time?
5. *Why* did the accident occur (what unsafe act and/or unsafe condition caused the accident and why did the employee commit the unsafe act)?
6. *How* can a recurrence be prevented?

Remember, it is imperative to find out not only what unsafe act was committed, but also *why* it was committed, before proper corrective action can be taken. Was the employee's attitude the reason for committing the unsafe act? If so, you must determine what you can do to change this attitude. Did the employee lack sufficient training, sufficient skill, or sufficient mental capability? As you can see, the corrective action you must take as a supervisor depends on *what caused the employee to act unsafely.*

5-6-2 Patient and Visitor Incidents

Here again, answer the questions,

Who was involved . . .
What was he doing . . .
When did it occur . . .
Why did it occur . . .
Where did it occur . . .

and most importantly

How can a recurrence be prevented?

As previously outlined, all patient incidents are to be reviewed by the Patient Safety Committee. If corrective action has not already been taken, this committee should then do so

Only with an involved administration, active patient and employee-visitor safety committees, and interested medical and nursing staffs, can a hospital hope to be responsive to the safety needs of its patients, employees, and visitors.

6

The Hospital Occupational
Health Program

6-1 INTRODUCTION

This chapter is intended as a ready reference for the physician or nurse assigned responsibility for a hospital occupational health program. It should be valuable to hospital management needing to establish such a program and a guide for improving facilities already present. It can serve as a guide to provide continuity and stability to the program when personnel changes occur. It can also serve as basic information for the orientation of medical personnel and to answer the most frequently encountered questions; provide direction for the usual activities; indicate sources for additional aid; and thus lead to a more effective occupational health program.

6-2 OBJECTIVES AND FUNCTIONS OF THE OCCUPATIONAL HEALTH PROGRAM

Three of the greatest items of expense to a business or industry are absenteeism, personnel turnover, and compensation for occupational illness and injuries. In a broad sense, it may be said that the function of an occupational health program is to keep these three to a minimum. This may be accomplished through the following activities:

1. Providing healthy work environment
2. Physical examinations:
   a. Preplacement physical examination—to place an employee in work for which he is physically, mentally, and emotionally suited. He should be placed in a position in which his health is at a minimum risk and in which he does not constitute a risk to others.
   b. Periodic health evaluation to insure that the worker's health has not been compromised; that he is able to handle his job; and to encourage

him to care for his health and to seek early treatment for minor non-disabling conditions.
3. Provision of medical care for:
   a. Emergency occupational injuries and illness.
   b. Nonoccupational conditions — to keep the worker on the job, if possible, or to refer him to his own physician when further care is required.
   c. Emergency nonoccupational conditions to protect life and limb until the employee can be placed in the hands of his own physician.
4. Maintenance of health through:
   a Education.
   b. Immunizations.
   c. Surveys to reveal chronic conditions and promote early treatment.
   d. Counseling on health, social and family problems.

The modern manager usually recognizes the advantages of a complete and vigorous occupational health program because the work output is improved as well as the promotion of a constructive image of management to the employee. Occupational medicine should expand and utilize new techniques to promote the health and comfort of the worker in his total environment. His total environment affects his value and production as an employee. To accomplish this, all health and social services need to cooperate and the Occupational Physician can serve as the link between them. The Occupational Physician should review carefully the standing orders for nurses, make such changes as he feels are necessary for his special programs and then sign orders.

6-3   ORGANIZATION OF THE OCCUPATIONAL HEALTH PROGRAM*

6-3-1   Personnel

The individual factors involved in an occupational program require that any guideline for personnel be individually interpreted. Among the local factors to be considered are type of occupational hazard, availability of other medical facilities, number of shifts working, and experience of the employees. An experienced and dependable nurse is the key to the functioning occupational health program. A relief nurse should also be available. A reception and records clerk is essential. In a small hospital, this person may have additional duties.

Usually, it is recommended that for less than 300 employees, a full-time

*Felton, J. S. Organization and Operation of an Occupational Health Program, *Journal of Occ. Medicine.* Vol. 6, pp. 25–68, January 1964.

registered nurse and part-time physician is satisfactory. For 1000 employees, a full-time physician is desirable, and he may serve up to 4000 employees, unless there are many engaged in hazardous work. Additional nurses are recommended at one per 1000 employees. The figures are approximations and depend to a large extent upon the local needs.

In most hospitals, the laboratory and X-ray facilities available are adequate for all needs of the occupational health program.

6-3-2   Facilities and Equipment

Facilities

The facility should be attractive in appearance. There should be racks for outer clothing, magazines, and health educational material. Decorative touches, such as plants and flowers, help create a relaxing atmosphere. The flow of traffic should be arranged so that waiting patients are relatively undisturbed until called. It should be possible for acutely ill or injured patients to enter and leave without being seen from the waiting room. Privacy for patients being interviewed and examined is essential. Separate and adequate toilet facilities for women and men will be required. These should be located to facilitate handling of urine specimens. An adequate number of examining rooms should be available, containing diagnostic and hand-washing facilities. Even in the smallest hospital, one bed for limited rest and observation, and used for no other purpose, is suggested. An area for taking electrocardiograms and giving physiotherapy treatments is required. In small areas, it is important to have several dressing rooms. The total area required for the occupational health program should be not less than one square foot of area per employee, up to 1000 employees, and should be at a minimum, 300 square feet.

Medical Equipment

The usual diagnostic instruments will be determined by the physician's preference. In addition to these, the following should be provided:

1. Patient Transport—wheeled litters and wheelchairs.
2. X-ray view boxes.
3. Beam scale.
4. Vital capacity apparatus (timed).
5. Facilities for steam sterilizing.
6. Facilities for suturing and other minor surgery.

7. Ear irrigation equipment.
8. Material for application of casts.
9. Assortment of crutches for loan.
10. Special diagnostic instruments: audiometer; orthorater, etc.
11. Tonometer.

Emergency Equipment

1. Inflatable splints.
2. Resuscitator with oxygen.
3. Pressor agents and blood expanders.

Other Equipment

An electrocardiograph machine is important. (Appropriate records should be kept.)

Physiotherapy

This may include diathermy, ultrasonic, and hydrotherapy apparatus. Such treatment is given only on physician's orders. The nurse can usually be instructed to perform such treatments. A prescription form stating mode, intensity, area, duration, and frequency of treatment, is helpful.

Night Services

Most hospitals have a sizeable night shift. In many instances, the professional staff of the Emergency Room provides night coverage for the occupational health program. Special emphasis is necessary to provide for proper and complete records and reports of all occupational cases treated outside regular hours. A form for providing a record of circumstances, treatment, and instructions should be developed for this use.

Laboratory

The hospital clinical laboratory is usually equipped to handle routine urine and blood work and such special tests as may be required for periodic evaluations for hazardous occupations.

X-ray

Adequate X-ray facilities are usually available at all hospitals. Routine 14 × 17 inch chest films are preferable for prehire and periodic examinations. If films are loaned to private physicians or consultants, accurate records should be maintained on the whereabouts of the film. A radiologist should be available for consultation. A duplicate of the report should be placed with the X-ray film, and the original placed in the patient's medical record.

Industrial Hygienists

The Industrial Hygienist is a specialist in recognizing, evaluating, and recommending controls for hazardous environments. It is advisable to have a complete industrial hygiene survey of the hospital each year to insure that the employee's health is being properly protected.*

6-3-3   Records

Preplacement Physical Examination

A preplacement physical examination should include an occupational exposure history as well as the routine medical history. A brief description, including physical, mental, and emotional requirements of the job that the applicant is being considered for should be a part of the preplacement record. An appropriate examination to determine if the applicant meets these requirements should be performed and recorded.

Periodic Examination

Periodic physical examination is usually limited to determining the current health and status of the employee and the effect of the work environment on his health.

Record System

Suggestions on a complete record system for an occupational health program together with sample forms are contained in *Guide to Records for Health Services in Small Industries*, available from the Secretary-Treasurer, American Conference of Governmental Industrial-Hygienists, 1014 Broadway, Cincinnati, Ohio, 45202, for $1.00 per copy.

---

*Information on the availability of an Industrial Hygienist in your locality can be obtained from: The American Industrial Hygiene Association, 1425 Prevost, Detroit, Michigan 48227.

Medical Information

The utmost care must be exercised to prevent unauthorized or unnecessary access to confidential medical records.

6-4　ROUTINES AND PROCEDURES

6-4-1　Reception and Records Clerk

General Responsibilities

The reception and records clerk is responsible for maintaining the orderly process of handling employees and their records. This person should be able to deal with people courteously and effectively, as well as having the technical skills of typing and filing. Considerable warmth, tact, and patience is required. In addition, this person must also be capable of handling emergency situations.

One of the major responsibilities is to preserve the confidential nature of the medical information being handled. Diagnostic or other information must not be released to unofficial persons. Medical records are not to be removed or examined by nonmedical personnel. Moreover, medical information, including details of diagnosis or treatment, are not to be discussed outside the clinic. During the filing of records and preparing of reports, it is the clerk's job to see that the records are not exposed to public view and that at the close of each working day, all charts and medical records are properly filed. This clerk must also insure that a copy of all correspondence regarding a patient is filed in the patient's medical record.

Additional Responsibilities

Additional responsibilities may include:

a. Ordering and stocking forms and office supplies.
b. Under the direction of the nurse, scheduling examinations and visits.
c. Answering the telephone.
d. Preparing correspondence, reports, and forms.

Reception Desk

General. Receive the clinic visitors and route them to the waiting room, treatment room, or examining room, as appropriate.

Emergencies. Direct the patient to the nurse or doctor and then procure the patient's record.

Helping Patients. After the patient has been seen by the nurse or doctor, direct him to the Pharmacy if he has a prescription. Arrange for transportation of the patient if the patient is to be sent home, and notify his supervisor.

Daily Log

Each employee visiting the clinic will be entered in the daily log which provides information for preparing reports.

Preemployment Examinations

The clerk takes the forms from the applicants, directs them to the waiting area and prepares the routine requests for laboratory and X-rays. After the examination, the clerk types any necessary correspondence or records.

Health Record

Each new employee shall have a health record. This record is maintained in the active files of the Medical Department until employment is terminated.

6-4-2   Nursing Staff

General Responsibilities

The Occupational Health Nurse not only has the usual nursing responsibilities to the patient, but has, in addition, a public health responsibility to all the employees. When she sees a patient, she must not only consider his health problem but how his health problem affects the health and well-being of his fellow employees and management, and others with whom he may come in contact.

Supervision. The Chief Nurse should exercise general supervision over the other nurses, the clerk-receptionist, and the maintenance and janitorial staff for the clinic area.

Administration. She is responsible for scheduling examinations, preliminary laboratory and X-ray work, preserving the confidentiality and filing of medical records and reports.

General Nursing Duties. In all cases of injuries, illness, and return from sick absence, the nurse must be certain to record exactly what happened, where, when, and how.

In each visit, the vital signs—blood pressure, temperature, pulse, and respiration should be recorded. Even though these signs may not relate directly to this visit, they may reveal previously unnoticed conditions and serve to develop base-line values. The patient's weight recorded periodically over the years is valuable, and should always be recorded for diabetics and cardiacs. The temperature is important to detect early infection. Periodic recording of an employee's blood pressure is valuable for base-line studies, determining the effectiveness of hypotensive drugs, and determining how the working environment affects blood pressure regulation.

After the doctor sees the patient, the nurse completes any necessary treatment, makes the appropriate chart entry and checks to see that the patient fully understands the doctor's instructions. The patient is then returned to the clerk-receptionist for scheduling a revisit or making out an injury report, if necessary.

Referrals. The nurse should be familiar with the procedures for referring employees to private physicians. She may even arrange the appointment with the physician's office. She is also responsible for sending any necessary forms, X-rays, or medical reports which should accompany the patient.

It is convenient to have a list of all physicians in the area of the hospital with their specialties, office address, office telephone, and emergency telephone numbers.

Professional Development. The nurse's contribution to her occupational health program increases as she increases her knowledge and professional skills.

Membership in the American Association for Industrial Nurses, and the Industrial Nursing Section of the American Nurses Association provides stimulus for continuing self-education and provides information on the seminars and training courses in the field of occupational health.

To perform her responsibilities most effectively, the nurse should be encouraged to regularly visit all areas of the hospital to see, first-hand, what is going on, and the working conditions. She should work closely with the Environmental Health Specialist.

Health Promotion. The nurse has an excellent opportunity to promote health education and to advise employees about their diet, personal hygiene, and their general health. She should be familiar with the community services available and know where to refer a person for assistance. The local United Fund or other such agency may have a directory of these services.

Health Evaluation and Preplacement Examinations

a. The nurse and doctor should develop procedures for handling preplacement examinations. The following procedures are recommended as minimum for preplacement:

Weight and height
Blood pressure, pulse, respiration and temperature
Audiogram
Visual test
Urinalysis, including microscopic
Hematocrit, wbc and differential
Screening blood sugar
Serological test for syphilis
PA chest X-ray, 14 × 17 inches
Tonometry in all applicants over 35 years of age.

b. Periodic health evaluations.

Executive Health Examinations. The health of hospital executives is extremely important to hospital management in that the absence or replacement of personnel at this level tends to disrupt the administrative program. Consequently, a complete health appraisal by the Occupational Physician at least every two years is considered good business practice. Such examinations should include, as a minimum, complete physical examination, chest X-ray, electrocardiogram, audiometry, visual screening, complete blood count and urinalysis.

Hazardous Occupations. Employees working with specific health hazards should be examined periodically and appropriate observations made as required by the hazard.

Medical Follow-up. Employees with special medical conditions such as pregnancy, diabetes, heart conditions, and injuries should be examined periodically. A file card should be kept for each patient containing personal data, diagnosis, occupation, and the date of visit and revisit.

Return from Sick Leave. Any employee off work more than three days for illness should have a note from his doctor giving the reason for his absence. This is done to be certain that the individual is able to return to work; to determine whether he is able to return to the same job; to alert the occupational health personnel to a potential public health problem; and to determine whether the illness might be related to his occupation.

Injuries. The employer can be responsible for providing medical diagnosis and treatment of job related illness and injuries. The employee is not expected to be able to determine if his illness is related to his employment, so employees should be encouraged to visit the Occupational Health Clinic if they feel ill on the job. Sometimes, the nurse may be required to evaluate a patient's condition, and possibly render such emergency treatment as necessary until the patient can be placed in the hands of a doctor. For this reason, the physician should prepare and sign standing orders.

6-5   ENVIRONMENTAL TECHNICIAN

The hospital environment contains biological, chemical, and physical hazards. A list of many of the hazards will be found in the Study Forms in the appendices (*see* p. 215). Since the Occupational Physician and nurse have almost full-time responsibilities in the Occupational Health Clinic, an Environmental Technician is necessary in medium-sized or larger hospitals to routinely evaluate the entire hospital environment and report his observations to the Occupational Physician. The Environmental Technician's responsibilities should include observation of the general housekeeping, infection control procedures, food handling, radiation control, disposal of sanitary waste, physical hazards control, and ventilation.

6-6   THE PHYSICIAN

6-6-1   Responsibilities

The Occupational Health Physician is responsible for the entire occupational health program.

Occupational health is the application of medical, nursing and engineering practices and principles to conserve the health of employees. The quality of the employee health service must be maintained at a high level through high professional standards, and a sincere interest in and respect for the individual employee. The program must be consistent with the code of ethics of the medical and nursing professions and not interfere with the relationship between the employee and his personal physician.

An important responsibility of the physician is to maintain contacts with the medical profession in the hospital and the community. He is concerned, not only with the immediate working environment, but to a lesser degree, the water supply, sewage disposal, food sanitation, health practices of the hospital employees, and housekeeping. In many of these areas, other departments will be responsible for the details. In attaining these objectives, the physician will, of necessity, share or delegate certain functions and cooperate closely with other officials and departments. He should organize his own department so that routine matters are handled efficiently.

It is expected that the closest relationship will be with the Occupational Health Nurse or Chief Nurse, if there is more than one nurse on the staff. She must be familiar with operating procedures and sources of information. She should be provided with simple and concise standing orders to cover normal routine and medical emergencies. If the nurse is not prevention-oriented and trained, the Occupational Physician may discover that further instruction is required, with discussion and clarification of the details. It cannot be overemphasized that procedures for handling injuries and illnesses must be written by the physician and approved in advance so that the nurse will understand these completely.

6-6-2   Professional Liability

The Occupational Physician is advised to carry professional liability insurance.

6-6-3   Job Visitation

The physician should be familiar with the physical layout of the hospital and observe, personally, the various activities of the hospital. In this manner, he can appreciate the conditions which may cause injury or health risk. It is suggested that at least 10% of the Occupational Health Physician's time be spent visiting the various wards, surgical suites, medical laboratories, research laboratories, autopsy rooms, and maintenance and janitorial spaces.

The occupational hazards file should be readily available. An indexed hazardous materials and processes file, with the locations, precautions or methods of control for toxic materials, Threshold Limit Value, symptoms of exposure, and methods of treatment, should be included.

6-6-4   Treatment

Occupational Health Physician. He should be responsible for treatment of all minor occupational illness and injury and for overseeing that the employee with an occupational illness or injury beyond his training or experience, and for which facilities for treatment are not at hand, be appropriately referred.

Occupational Conditions. The aim in treatment of occupational injuries is to return the patient to work as soon as practicable. Often, he can be returned to light duty almost immediately but if the condition requires a patient to rest, the physician should not be influenced by the supervisor, the patient himself, or anyone else, to keep the worker on the job.

Non-occupational Conditions. Medical care may be provided for minor conditions for which the employee would not ordinarily visit his private physician.

Employees should be encouraged to seek the advice of the Occupational Health Physician on illness that they think might be related to their occupation. In this way, the physician has the opportunity to determine whether the condition is job related or not; to understand the employee's attitude toward his work environment; and to provide health counseling.

6-6-5 Examinations

Preplacement Examinations

The purpose of the preplacement examination is to place the employee in a job that is not beyond his physical or emotional capabilities, or hazardous to his health or the health of others. This allows the placement of the handicapped as well as the non-handicapped person. Sometimes, the decision as to whether the applicant is qualified is difficult. It may be necessary before the decision is made to obtain medical reports from a private physician, another hospital, or the Veterans Administration.

The applicant's previous work history is valuable to learn what occupational hazards he has already been exposed to and that may present a special health liability or determine his physical capability. A health defect in an applicant for heavy labor might not be disqualifying if the applicant had worked for years in a similar occupation without experiencing difficulty but, on the other hand, it might be disqualifying if his previous work had all been sedentary. Ideally, the decision should be based on the applicant's present condition. If the person has had a heart attack, or even cancer, he should not necessarily be disqualified, even if there is a possibility that he may be disabled some time in the future. However, these decisions are influenced by the State laws and compensation practices.

After the Examination

When the examination is completed, the applicant should be given a report of what tests he has received, any abnormal findings, and the doctor's recommendations. This is a good opportunity to explain the functions of the Occupational Health Clinic. This may be accomplished by providing a small brochure on the services of the clinic. The employees should also be advised to report any significant change in their health status to the Occupational Health Clinic. Particularly, mention should be made of the development of heart disease, hypertension, diabetes, or pregnancy.

Periodic Health Examinations

Employees with special health problems, such as diabetes, heart disease or hypertension should be called in periodically to determine their fitness to continue working and to evaluate their condition in terms of adequate medical care.

Hazardous Occupations

Workers exposed to radiation, heat or cold stress, bacteria, chemicals or other occupational hazards, as found in the Study Form in the Appendices, should be appropriately examined at the recommended intervals.

Executive Physicals

Key personnel should be examined at least every two years on a voluntary basis. A full report of this examination should be provided to the executive's personal physician. The extent of these examinations may vary, depending on the extent of time and facilities available. Detailed information on these examinations may be found in the Public Health Service Publication 1010, *Periodic Health Examinations*.

Fitness for Duty Examinations

Since the capabilities and health status of an employee may change, it is appropriate for his supervisor to ask the Occupational Health Clinic to evaluate an employee's fitness for duty.

In order to aid the physician performing this function for management, the requesting official should provide the following information:

1. Physical requirements and job description.

2. Description of the duties the employee is not satisfactorily performing, and the reason for considering that ill-health is the underlying factor.
3. Statement that the employee has the knowledge of the situation, and understands that his ability to perform the job is being questioned, and that the employee has consented to the examination.

6-6-6 Women Who Work

Placement

Women can perform as efficiently and as safely as men in most jobs. However, the average woman is shorter and lighter than is a man. She requires special consideration of her conditions. Most equipment and machinery is designed for men. Since there is no practical test for measuring strength or endurance, the best guide to placement may be consideration of the woman's previous work experience and, possibly, a trial period in the job.

Lifting

Individual variance in the ability to lift keeps employers or anyone from setting absolute limits for either sex. Therefore, the physician must make an individual judgment in each case.

Pregnancy

The woman should be encouraged to report her condition to the Occupational Health Clinic. The physician or nurse in the clinic should try to determine that she is receiving regular prenatal care, and that her condition progresses normally, and is not adversely affected by her employment. A pregnant woman should be allowed to work only during the day shift, and not more than 40 hours a week. Consideration should be given to possible toxic exposures, including those which may cause anemia, including aniline, benzol, toluol, lead, chlorinated hydrocarbons, mercury, and turpentine. If adjustment in the working conditions are deemed advisable, the Occupational Health Physician should consult with the patient's private physician. It is considered that the pregnant patient should be seen at the clinic at least monthly, and checked for weight, blood pressure, edema, and asked about such symptoms as nausea, vomiting, weakness, or edema. The length of time the patient may continue working depends on the type of work she is doing and the absence of symptoms. A maternity sick leave allowance of six weeks before and eight weeks after delivery is recommended.

Other Problems

If a woman develops menstrual disorders, she should be referred to her personal physician for the necessary care. Occasionally, a woman with dysmenorrhea may be able to complete her work shift if given medication for symptomatic relief.

6-7   SUPPLEMENTAL INFORMATION FOR PHYSICIANS

6-7-1   Occupational Diseases

The working environment should be carefully controlled to prevent the development of occupational illnesses or injury. There are hostile agents in the hospital environment and it is an obligation of Management to insure that these hostile agents do not injure the worker's health. One of the Occupational Physician's roles is to inform Management of the potential hazards to the worker's health. The types of hazards involved may be:

a. Airborne dusts, vapors, fumes, or mists.
b. Harmful chemicals.
c. Excessive noise.
d. Infections.
e. Radiant energy, ionizing and nonionizing radiation.
f. Vibration.
g. Abnormalities of air pressure, temperature and humidity.

The person assigned the responsibility for initially developing the occupational health program may wish to consult a specialist in the field of occupational medicine during the planning stages of the program, and periodically thereafter. A list of specialists in occupational medicine in any area of the United States may be requested from: The American Academy of Occupational Medicine, University of Michigan Medical Center, Ann Arbor, Michigan 48104.

6-7-2   Sight Conservation Program

This is a program to prevent eye injury by assuring that the employees have the necessary vision to meet job requirements; by providing protection against eye injury; by providing proper care of eye injuries; and by educating employees in health and safety. Persons with monocular vision should be required to wear safety eye-wear. Monocular vision may not disqualify a person for a particular job that has been performed safely in the past. Eye hazard areas should be determined by the Environmental Technician. Grinding or sandblasting operations or any machine operation which produces high impact particles or burns or splashes should be designated eye-hazardous areas. Anyone assigned such work should be assured appropriate eye protection and be required to wear it. Employees should not be permitted to wear contact lens in eye-hazardous areas, and should not be permitted to work around toxic chemicals in humid temperatures, or be exposed to infrared rays. In general, employees should be discouraged from wearing contact lens unless their work is inside and sedentary.

6-7-3 Hearing Conservation Program

The object of the hearing conservation program is to protect the employee from permanent impairment of hearing due to loud noise in his working environment. This program should include routine audiometric examination of new employees; periodic supervision of potentially high noise areas to determine if there is a noise hazard present; and periodic audiometric examinations of all workers exposed to noise levels greater than 90 decibels to determine if there has been a temporary threshold shift.

6-8 APPENDICES

6-8-1 Recommended References

Industrial Hygiene and Toxicology. Vol. II, Patty, F. A. (Ed.), New York: Interscience Publishers, 1963.
Occupational Diseases and Industrial Medicine. Johnstone & Miller, Saunders Co., 1961.
Occupational Diseases of the Skin. Schwartz, Tulipan, and Birmingham, 3rd ed., Lea & Febiger, 1957.
Clinical Laboratory Diagnosis. Levinson and MacFate, 6th ed., Lea & Febiger, 1962.
Threshold Limit Values (TLV). American Conference of Governmental Industrial Hygienists, 1014 Broadway, Cincinnati, Ohio 45202.

6-8-2 Study Forms

Each hospital will have a different set of occupational health problems. It is recommended that the Occupational Health Physician, the Occupational Health Nurse, the Environmental Technician, with consultants

STUDY FORM

BIOLOGICAL HAZARDS (EXAMPLES)

P = Physician
N = Nurse
ET = Environmental Technician
CIH = Consulting Industrial
Hygienist

Agent, Job Equipment or Process	Hazard	Location	MEDICAL CONTROL		ENVIRONMENTAL CONTROL		
			Procedure	Interval Months	Procedure	Interval Months	Professional
Contaminated dressings	Bacteria		Special handling procedures		Training and survey	3	N, ET
Food handling	Bacteria		Physical exams	6	Training and observation	3	ET
Garbage and refuse disposal	Bacteria		Physical exams	12	Training and observation	6	ET
Handling animals	Zoonoses		Physical exams	6	Observation	6	P, ET
Handling pathology specimens	Bacteria Fungi		Physical exams	6	Observation	6	P, ET

STUDY FORM

PHYSICAL HAZARDS (EXAMPLES)

P = Physician
N = Nurse
ET = Environmental Technician
CIH = Consulting Industrial Hygienist

Agent, Job Equipment or Process	Hazard	MEDICAL CONTROL			ENVIRONMENTAL CONTROL		
		Location	Procedure	Interval Months	Procedure	Interval Months	Professional
X-ray mach.	X-rays radiation		Physical exam. CBC	12	Industrial hygiene survey	12	ET, CIH
Radio isotopes	Alpha, beta gamma, radiation		Physical exam. CBC	12	Industrial hygiene survey	12	ET, CIH
Ultra sound and diathermy	Microwave radiation		Slit-Lamp exam.	12	Industrial hygiene survey	12	ET, CIH

STUDY FORM

CHEMICAL HAZARDS (EXAMPLES)

P = Physician
N = Nurse
ET = Environmental Technician
CIH = Consulting Industrial Hygienist

Agent, Job Equipment or Process	Hazard	Location	MEDICAL CONTROL		ENVIRONMENTAL CONTROL		
			Procedure	Interval Months	Procedure	Interval Months	Professional
Drug handling	Toxicity		Physical exam.	12	Observation	12	P
Laboratory chemicals	Toxicity		Physical exam.	12	Observation	12	ET, CIH
Solvent handling	Toxicity		Physical exam.	12	Observation	12	CT, CIH
Mercury handling	Toxicity		Urine mercury	6	Observation	6	ET, CIH

in industrial hygiene and occupational medicine, prepare a set of Study Forms for the Environmental Technician to use in a routine surveillance program. The Environmental Technician should completely survey the hospital and write down each agent, job, equipment, or process that is thought to be a health hazard, and then develop recommended medical and environmental control procedures for each potential hazard with the help of the nurse, doctor, and consulting industrial hygienist and specialist in occupational medicine. Simple Study Forms for biological hazards, physical hazards, and chemical hazards, with a few examples, are provided.

6-8-3 Consultants

A list of consulting Industrial Hygienists in any area may be obtained from: The American Industrial Hygiene Association, 1425 Prevost, Detroit, Michigan 48227.

A list of consulting Occupational Medicine Specialists can be obtained from: The American Academy of Occupational Medicine, University of Michigan Medical Center, Ann Arbor, Michigan 48104.

7

Special
Techniques

7-1 DETERGENTS AND DISINFECTANTS – EVALUATION AND USE IN HOSPITAL ENVIRONMENTAL SANITATION PRACTICE

7-1-1 Detergents in Hospital Practice

In recent years, significant improvements in sanitation techniques have come about as the result of advances in chemistry, application devices, design facilities, and newly developed products. The phenomenon of detergency has been the object of many millions of dollars of scientific inquiry, taking advantage of sophisticated instrumentation, radioactive tracer techniques, and other modern research tools. The basic chemical industry, too, has made important contributions with respect to the raw materials involved. The advances made in related scientific disciplines have importantly broadened the scope of the chemistry of cleaning.

The hospital environment, immense, complex and critical, presents detergent science with some of its most challenging problems. Every type of cleaning used is present in a hospital and thus, the need for virtually every cleaning technique. The hospital Environmental Health Specialist, whose duties encompass all departments and who therefore encounters the full variety of cleaning problems, obviously benefits from a fundamental knowledge of cleaning principles and detergent chemistry.

It is the purpose of this chapter to draw together in summary form the basic principles with which the environmentalist can approach these problems.

7-1-2 Basic Detergent Mechanisms

Any cleaning process involves a variety of detergent or cleaning mechanisms, although all available mechanisms are obviously not involved in any single cleaning operation. These mechanisms can be described briefly as follows:

Emulsification

Emulsification is the action of breaking up fats and oils into very small particles, which are uniformly mixed with the water used. In a stable emulsion, fat and oil particles are held apart and kept suspended uniformly for long periods of time. This action may be purely mechanical, as it is in the homogenization of milk, or it may be largely chemical, using an emulsifying ingredient, which actually reacts with oil and fat to enable one literally to "mix oil and water." Emulsification is one of the most important basic cleaning mechanisms and is accomplished by many chemicals. Synthetic detergents such as those found in most general purpose cleaners or dishwashing detergents and also natural soap are among the most common materials which can assist emulsification.

Saponification

Saponification is the chemical reaction between an alkali and an animal or vegetable fat or oil resulting in production of a soap. In oversimplified terms, the alkali makes the fat or oil partially soluble in water. The advantage of this action in cleaning is obvious; fatty or oily soils that are normally insoluble in water are made somewhat soluble and removal is thus greatly aided.

Wetting

Wetting is the action of a water solution in contacting all soil or surfaces. Water does not freely wet many surfaces because of its surface tension — that property of water which makes it form into droplets on a surface rather than spread out and penetrate evenly. Reduce the surface tension and water will spread out and penetrate, i.e., "wet." Chemicals that reduce surface tension substantially are therefore commonly called wetting agents. The synthetic detergents are the most common wetting agents.

Penetration

Penetration is the action of a liquid entering into porous materials, through cracks, pinholes, etc. This action may be considered a part of wetting and certainly in order to have good penetration, good wetting action is necessary.

Suspension

Suspension is the action which holds up insoluble particles in a solution. Ingredients which have a strong suspending action are valuable in a detergent because they prevent insoluble soil from settling back on to the surface (soil redeposition).

Rinsibility

Rinsibility is the condition of a solution which enables it to be flushed from a surface easily and completely. There are some detergents or detergent ingredients which may tend to cling to certain surfaces and resist normal efforts to rinse them off. This property of poor rinsibility may be a disadvantage in some circumstances, though by no means all.

Water Softening

Softening is defined as the removal or inactivation of water hardness. Many of the common minerals in tap water in many parts of the country may seriously interfere with cleaning action by a variety of chemical means. Thus, some types of detergents for specific purposes require chemical ingredients which soften the water. This type of chemical softening of the water is accomplished by means of ingredients which sequester the water hardness minerals. The process of sequestration is that in which the magnesium and calcium hardness minerals are, figuratively speaking, "surrounded" or "tied up" by these sequestering agents. In the sequestered condition, the water hardness minerals are effectively neutralized or rendered harmless in solution. A term which is closely related to sequestration is chelation. While the terms are fairly synonymous, sequestration is a word usually used in connection with the polyphosphate types of softening ingredients, and chelation is used in connection with the organic softening ingredients such as EDTA (Ethylenediaminetetraacetic acid).

At the time of this writing, controversy over the ecological role of phosphates in detergents rages hotly in the news media, and in political circles. Phosphates are accused of being a major cause of excessive growth of algae in lakes, a problem which potentially effects about 15% of the population of the United States. However, most scientists and informed environmental health specialists, after careful review of current evidence, conclude that detergent phosphates have a very limited, if not nonexistent, part in the eutrophication of lakes and stagnant waterways. They conclude that even if all phosphates in detergents were totally removed, there would still be sufficient phosphorus from natural sources plus animal and human waste to supply the needs of even the most vigorous of algae growths.

Furthermore, it is generally felt that carbon, i.e., typical organic sewage, is the critical limiting nutrient in the algae growth cycle. Thus, proper sewage treatment through new and improved sewage plants is thought to be the only means of controlling excessive algal growth where it is a problem.

Despite these facts, hospitals in some locales may be faced with local regulations and controversy on detergents. For the hospital, such issues may be easily resolved because the overall safety and effectiveness of detergents in the hospital environment must be the only consideration due to their important role in patient care.

Although the phosphate issue is controversial, a major control of hospital acquired infection is through the proper use of detergents in the cleaning process. Detergent phosphates have an enviable record of safety and efficacy which is unmatched by any substitute offered to date and in a health care facility, those considerations must take precedence over any ecological issues.

Dissolving

Dissolving is a chemical action in detergents which liquifies water soluble materials or soils. This is a very important cleaning mechanism, because many soils, such as alkaline deposits (lime), are not readily soluble in plain water or in alkaline cleaning solutions. However, certain acids will dissolve such resistant soils.

pH

pH is a term often used by people in the cleaning field, and often misused. pH is only *one* measure of acidity or alkalinity. The pH scale ranges from 1 to 14 with 1 being very acid and 14 being very alkaline and the number 7 representing the neutral point. You can get a neutral solution by adding the right amount of acid to a quantity of alkaline solution.

A measure of acidity or alkalinity which is even more important than pH is a factor which we might term "total acidity" or "total alkalinity." The more correct term is the buffering capacity of an alkali or an acid. Thus it is possible to have two different detergents, both of pH 10 or moderately alkaline, and have one of these detergents require only two ounces of a standard acid to neutralize it while the other would require

10 ounces. Obviously, the detergent that requires 10 ounces is a much more strongly alkaline product than the other—yet the pH's are the same.

Both alkaline and acid cleaners are needed in hospital environmental sanitation.

One frequently hears about so-called neutral general purpose cleaners. Actually there are very few truly neutral cleaners, and those that are neutral are usually not very good cleaners. A certain amount of alkalinity is highly desirable in a general purpose cleaner and does not necessarily mean that it will attack waxes and floor finishes or hurt the skin.

7-1-3 Detergent Formulation

It can be readily understood that detergent ingredients have many important functions and that a good balanced cleaner will contain ingredients which perform all functions well according to the nature of the soil present. Unfortunately, no single ingredient will perform all functions properly. It is, therefore, necessary to combine available materials in such a way that all of the functions receive due consideration. Particular combinations of ingredients may also produce highly desirable synergistic effects. Thus, careful formulation is essential and the possible combinations for particular effectiveness against certain soils and problems is literally endless, while the development of hundreds of new chemicals synthesized each year presents the continuing possibility of new and improved products to the detergent research laboratory, and fully justifies the millions of dollars spent in such research each year.

Thus, nothing could be further from the truth than the often heard statement "Detergent products are all more or less the same." Equally untrue are the occasional claims that a particular detergent is suitable for all purposes. No such detergent exists and it is highly unlikely that one will ever be developed. It is necessary for the environmentalist to be able to recognize the cleaning problems and soils involved and thus to recommend the appropriate type of detergent for the particular condition. Occasionally, problems may present themselves which are beyond the scope of the environmentalist's knowledge and at such time he should call upon the research facilities of one of the larger and more reputable detergent manufacturers.

7-1-4 Types of Hospital Detergents

Most hospitals use at least 50 or more cleaning and disinfecting products from 25 or more companies. This is because it is difficult for various department heads to distinguish between the many brands and recognize differences or similarities. The opportunity, therefore, exists for the hospital environmental health specialist to assist all department heads, and the purchasing department in particular, to simplify, consolidate, and standardize the types of products used in the hospital. It is perfectly reasonable to have only 15 or 20 products from four or five different companies serving virtually all needs in even the most complex institution.

Referring only to detergents as opposed to disinfectants, it is generally possible to classify all brands into a relatively few number of categories. Likewise, it is almost always possible to classify cleaning problems and functions so that a very wide variety of objects or surfaces can be cleaned with the same product.

Manual Immersion Cleaning

This refers to cleaning which is done by immersing objects beneath the solution, where they are brushed, agitated, or otherwise manipulated by hand to remove soil. A period of soaking is usually recommended to permit the detergent solution to act in the many chemical ways described previously, thus reducing the amount of hand labor involved.

Products for this purpose can be either powder or liquid. The powdered products usually contain ingredients to provide controlled alkalinity and water softening. However, the main ingredient would be either a natural soap or, more commonly, one or more synthetic organic detergents. There may also be special additives for corrosion inhibition and skin protection.

There are a wide variety of such products found in the hospital, many of which could be consolidated. Products which are used to wash dishes in the dietary department by hand may also be perfectly suitable for cleaning surgical instruments and laboratory glassware, though it is common to find these items being cleaned by products with exotic names and labels and claiming to be "the only thing suitable for surgical instruments." Chemically, the two types of products could well be identical, despite wide differences in selling price.

Liquid cleaners in the category are also very widely used and effective. Chemically, they are usually blends of anionic and nonionic synthetic organic detergents. Well formulated liquid products may perform just as well as the powders, and have the additional advantages of being far easier to dispense and control. The liquids also permit a far wider variety of chemical ingredients in their formulation, because most of the synthetic detergents, of which there are literally thousands available, are by nature liquid.

Here again, as in the powders, a large variety may be found in the hospital with wide differences of price and function. Simplification and consolidation is again possible with a high quality liquid detergent such as might be used in the dietary department—possibly just as effective as the more expensive product used for surgical instruments and laboratory glassware.

Housekeeping Cleaners

Within this category would be a wide variety of cleaners, both powder and liquid, for cleaning various surfaces, both by hand and by machine.

Liquid All-Purpose Cleaners

All-purpose cleaners would be the most common type of cleaner, for the most part composed of anionic and nonionic synthetic detergents, similar to the liquid cleaners described under immersion cleaners. The major difference would be that the all-purpose housekeeping cleaner would be lower sudsing and specifically formulated not to damage or dull the synthetic or wax floor finishes used on floors.

All-purpose cleaners of this type are generally suitable for most light to medium duty cleaning on virtually any hard surface throughout the hospital but would be most appropriate on floors, walls, furniture, and equipment. However, in most hospitals many of these needs, formerly served by an all-purpose cleaner such as this, are being met by use of the combination detergent-disinfectant which serves the function of both the cleaner and a disinfectant.

Heavy Duty Cleaners or Wax Strippers

These are liquid products, formulated specifically to emulsify and soften waxes and synthetic floor finishes so that they may be easily removed prior to refinishing. Such a stripper is more highly alkaline than the all-purpose cleaner type product and has many uses as a heavy duty cleaner as well as a stripper.

Used as a heavy duty cleaner, this type of product is generally not suitable for floors unless such floors are not treated with a wax or floor finish. Obviously such a product will damage the finish. They are most suitable for situations in which heavy fat or grease is encountered or for wall washing.

Low Sudsing Cleaners

In the modern hospital, large uncluttered floor areas are best cleaned by the use of battery operated automatic machines which both scrub and vacuum the floor in one pass. Such machines require a liquid detergent which has very fast cleaning action and is also very low sudsing. The low sudsing characteristic is necessary because the vacuum part of the machine naturally agitates the cleaning solution as it picks it up off the floor, and as a result the pick-up tank of the machine would rapidly become filled with suds instead of soil-laden cleaning solution. Some all-purpose cleaners may be satisfactory for this purpose.

Wall Cleaners

While both the all-purpose cleaner and the heavy duty cleaner – wax stripper – can be used for the cleaning of walls, it is occasionally desirable to use a special powdered product specifically designed for wall cleaning. This would be especially true for painted surfaces, which are the most difficult to clean. The powdered wall cleaner would include among its many ingredients tri-sodium phosphate, which has the specific ability to dissolve and remove deteriorated paint residues, a necessary part of soil removal on any painted surface.

Wall washing is also done with special wall washing machines which pump hot detergent solution to turkish towels wrapped around special trowels. These machines generally work best with the liquid all-purpose cleaner or heavy duty cleaner type of product rather than the powders.

Concrete Cleaners

This would be a powdered type of product similar in general chemical nature to the powdered wall cleaner, but would be even more highly alkaline and specifically formulated for cleaning soiled concrete surfaces.

Machine Products

These types of products could be either powdered or liquid and are carefully designed for use in dish, utensil, or laboratory glassware washing machines. These products are the most highly alkaline of all and would present skin irritation hazards if used manually. There is a very wide variety of these to suit highly specific conditions of soil, water hardness, and the objects to be washed.

In every case, the hospital is strongly advised to consult the larger, more reputable detergent manufacturers specializing in this type of product for recommendations in this area. Consolidation is generally possible but not without skilled help.

Automatic electronic dispensing and control of these products is often essential. However, it is beyond the scope of this chapter to go into detail on this subject.

Specialty Products

Included under this category would be products which do not seem to fit elsewhere. The most notable of these would be acid detergents, of which there are two basic types. One of these is the acid toilet bowl cleaner composed of synthetic detergents and hydrochloric acid, plus, in some, a disinfectant. These strong acid bowl cleaners, while dangerous, are extremely effective on rust and other mineral stains encountered in toilet bowls. They should be used only on vitreous china bowls and not on bathtubs and sinks, which are generally porcelain. Hydrochloric acid presents, of course, a safety problem in that it corrodes most metals, damages concrete, eats holes in many synthetic fabrics such as nylon and can produce severe injury to the skin. However, with care, such hazards can be minimized and the results usually justify the use of such products.

The other, milder type of acid detergent is based on organic acids or phosphoric acid and nonionic detergents. These products are very useful for removing mineral films from stainless steel surfaces such as water baths and kitchen equipment, removing urine scale from patient urinals, and dissolving soap and mineral films from tile walls, shower stalls, and other bathroom fixtures. Where an alkaline detergent fails, an acid detergent may be effective.

Another specialty detergent is the carpet shampoo. This type of product is a liquid, very high sudsing detergent, which dries to a powdery residue that can be removed by vacuuming the carpet or rug. While suds contribute nothing to cleaning, directly, high suds in a carpet shampoo are necessary in order to prevent the solution from overly wetting the carpet and thus producing problems of shrinkage, slow drying, and deterioration of the carpet backing.

There are many other specialty products available, but they need not be described. Probably better than 99% of all cleaning requirements in the hospital environment can be handled with one or more of the products described previously.

7-1-5   Detergent Evaluation

Evaluation is an extremely important part of detergent research and formulation because, obviously, if you cannot measure what the product is doing, then it is not possible to know whether or not you have made an improvement. Unfortunately, evaluation is extremely difficult and reliable reproducible standard methods are usually lacking. Thus, the careful researcher must use a variety of evaluation methods in the laboratory in order to "zero in" on the performance of a particular product for a specific purpose.

It is not feasible to go into much detail here on the subject of detergent evaluation—it is one on which entire books have been written. One of the biggest problems of course is determining the correlation between detergency performance in the laboratory and in actual practice. Unfortunately, it is also very difficult to compare products in the in-use situation. Extensive in-use trial may be the only practical means of product selection.

To give the environmentalist an idea of some of the tests and their inherent problems, two different laboratory tests will be described at this point: the Gardner Straight Line Washability Test, and the Detergent Capacity Test. These two tests have been selected because they are in common use and because in many respects they best describe the major factors involved in defining cleaning ability.

Basically, detergency might be described as a combination of two factors. One is the ability to remove hardened inorganic soil mixtures; the other is its ability to suspend, emulsify and disperse oily or fatty soils. The first type of soil is representative of common street and floor soil, such as would be normally found in a hospital corridor floor in quantities varying according to the weather and distance from the entrances. Fatty or oily soils are perhaps less common and generally found on kitchen floors, around heavy machinery, and where hands touch and rub frequently, as around door knobs.

The Gardner Straight Line Washability Test is the test most commonly used to measure the ability of a detergent to remove soil from a resilient tile floor. The product to be tested is diluted to its recommended use dilution and a measured quantity poured on to a weighted sponge. The sponge is then drawn repeatedly over a white vinyl tile which has been previously coated with a tenacious soil mixture of kerosene, stoddard solvent, petrolatum, lubricating oil, shortening and brown pigment.

After coating, the tiles are dried for 30 minutes and baked at 176°F for 15 minutes. Three tiles per product are used and four photometric reflectance readings are taken on each tile both before soiling and after cleaning to determine percent soil removal. The final data reported is an average with variability of individual readings shown in confidence intervals at the 95% probability level. In laymen's language, this means that if the test is repeated over and over again, 95% of the results would fall within a certain range. Such statistical analysis is vital for this test because it is notoriously unreliable. The same product can be tested repeatedly with widely differing results. Unfortunately, it is not well known that this test is so unreliable and product specifications built around this test are highly suspect.

The Detergent Capacity Test measures the ability of a product to suspend, disperse and emulsify fatty soils. Performance in this test gives an indication relative to other products of how much soil can be handled—practically speaking, how often a mop pail will have to be changed or how many dirty dishes can be washed before the detergent solution will have to be changed.

This test uses standard china dinner plates, soiled with a fixed amount of a mixture of tallow, corn oil, and a trace of an ultraviolet sensitive fluorescent dye. An in-use solution of the test product at controlled water hardness and temperature is put into a dish pan via a funnel held at a fixed height.

The measure of results on the test consists of both the number of plates washed until the suds disappear, and the number of plates washed until fatty soil becomes plainly visible on the plate not only under ultraviolet light, but to an experienced observer in daylight.

The suds end point is considered only for those products that normally have sudsing properties. In such cases, when a slight excess of unemulsified fatty soil begins to appear in the wash solution, the sudsing will disappear.

Results must be interpreted carefully and relative to detergents of known ability. Full consideration must be given to the actual intended applications of the product tested. If the product is to be used, for example, to clean operating room floors, heavy fatty soils would rarely be encountered and high performance on the Detergent Capacity Test would not be necessary.

The reader is cautioned against attempting to devise detergency tests of his own or to perform the two tests mentioned above without referring to the original references describing them in detail.

7-1-6   Optimization of Cleaning Procedures

All detergents must be used properly to be fully effective, but it is not the intent of this chapter to go into detailed cleaning procedures. This will be handled elsewhere in this book. However, there are some basic application principles which can be utilized in designing specific procedures which will go far to optimize results with minimum labor. The most important are the following:

Temperature

In general the hotter the temperature, the more effective the cleaning results. However, there are a few exceptions to this, such as with heavy blood soils, or other soils with a high percentage of proteins. Temperatures above 160°F may "set" or coagulate blood to a degree where cleaning is more difficult than at somewhat cooler temperatures.

The proper temperature, of course, is also determined by the way in which the product is to be used. Obviously, if hands are to be immersed, the temperature cannot exceed 120°F.

Time

The exposure time of the soiled surface to the detergent solution is very important. The longer the soiled surface can be exposed via soaking, the less agitation and friction will be required to remove the soil. With some tenacious soils, soaking may be absolutely necessary to clean the surface at all, with any reasonable amount of applied friction. Allow detergent solutions to remain on the surface as long as possible, before agitation and removal.

Concentration

The amount of detergent used varies considerably from product to product and soil to soil, but in general, manufacturer's directions should be followed explicitly. Beyond the manufacturer's recommended amounts, detergent is wasted and cleaning results are improved little, if any. Besides the expense involved, excess detergent may create problems of its own.

Friction

Friction or "elbow grease" is usually one of the major factors in any cleaning operation and despite claims to the contrary, detergents do not eliminate the need for such friction and agitation.

7-1-7 Disinfectants in Hospital Practice

The subject of disinfectants as they apply to hospital practice is a very complex and confusing matter. A great deal of misinformation has been written, much of it based on old data or ill-advised research techniques. Many manufacturers of disinfectant products contribute to the confusion with exorbitant claims and inconsistent documentation of their products.

One of the major causes of controversy and confusion has in the past been the lack of reliable standardized laboratory and in-use evaluation methods for disinfectants. In recent years, however, the U.S.D.A.* (United States Department of Agriculture), and the A.O.A.C. (Association of Official Analytical Chemists) have come up with standard test methods which are reasonably reliable and are being enforced through regulation by the U.S.D.A. to the point where it is possible to take supporting documentation for various competitive products and compare them side by side. A major portion of this chapter will be devoted to the description and discussion of the more important evaluation tests, so that the reader may form his own conclusions through careful study of the supporting literature offered by reliable manufacturers.

Definitions

Detergent-Disinfectants. A detergent-disinfectant is a disinfectant with cleaning ability. There are several other similar phrases used to describe such a product and they are all equivalent: germicidal-detergent, detergent-germicide, disinfectant-detergent, germicidal-cleaner. On occasion, a germicide with very high cleaning ability may be called a germicidal-detergent, and conversely, one with poor cleaning ability but high germicidal ability may be called a detergent-germicide. However, in practice, all of these terms are synonymous.

There are, of course, also products which have no cleaning ability and these would be known as straight disinfectants or germicides. However, in virtually all cases, the addition of detergency to a good disinfectant very much enhances the antibacterial performance of the product.

Disinfectant. The term disinfectant itself refers to a product which kills all vegetative bacteria with the exception of spores. A germicide and bactericide are just synonyms for disinfectant.

Sanitizer. A sanitizer is a product which has some bacteria killing ability but which is not as strong as a disinfectant. A generally acceptable definition is that a sanitizer is a product which reduces bacteria counts to a level generally acceptable by Public Health Standards. A product can be both a disinfectant and a sanitizer with the product functioning as

*The disinfectant regulation functions of the U.S.D.A. were transferred in 1971 to the E.P.A. (Environmental Protection Agency).

a sanitizer at one concentration and as a disinfectant at the stronger concentration.

Sterilize. The terms sterilize (verb) and sterilizer (noun) cannot be applied to disinfectants. Sterilization is a process which kills all living organisms including spores. Sterilization normally can be obtained only in a steam or gas autoclave. Chemical sterilization may, under certain controlled circumstances, be achieved via ethylene oxide gas or certain other exotic chemicals, such as beta-propiolactone, but these do not constitute circumstances of frequent practical use to the hospital environmental health specialist.

Bacteriostat. A bacteriostat is a product which prevents bacteria from multiplying without actually killing the bacteria. A bacteriostat has no practical value on hard surfaces because if the surface is dry the bacteria will not multiply anyway.

Antiseptic. An antiseptic is an antibacterial agent for use on the skin. An antiseptic may kill bacteria on the skin, or it may function only as a bacteriostat. Hexachlorophene is a common bacteriostat for skin use.

7-1-8 Disinfectant Evaluation Methods

It is widely known that no single germicide is ideal for all applications and the ability of a germicide to kill each representative bacteria should be known. Unfortunately, the bacteria themselves have their own individual resistance to germicides, which makes it difficult to know with any degree of certainty whether or not a particular germicide kills a particular bacteria unless actual tests have been carried out via reliable methods.

There are many test methods available. Some favor particular germicides against particular bacteria; other methods favor other germicides against other bacteria. The solution to this problem is always to conduct laboratory testing via the U.S.D.A. recommended A.O.A C. Test Method. If a hospital laboratory is unwilling or unable to carry out such A.O.A.C. Test Methods, then they should not be involved in the evaluation of a disinfectant. No other test methods are acceptable.

Unfortunately, some germicides on the market today have been largely documented by an old A.O.A.C. Test Method which by itself is not currently approved by the U.S.D.A. for the support of germicidal claims. This is the venerable Phenol Coefficient Method.

The Phenol Coefficient Method is the oldest and historically the most commonly used laboratory measurement technique. However, the results can be very misleading. It was developed originally to compare the highest killing dilutions of a given test germicide with the highest dilution of a 5% phenol solution on the same microorganism.

Basically, the method involves taking tubes of broth cultures of the particular test bacteria and adding the germicide to the tube in varying concentrations and allowing the germicide to act for five, ten and fifteen minutes. At the end of the specified time period a small sample of the germicide-bacteria broth culture mixture is transferred to a tube of sterile media and allowed to incubate 48 hours. If any bacteria are left alive, they will multiply and cloud up the tube of media indicating that, that particular dilution of the germicide was not completely effective.

The same thing is done with the standard 5% phenol solution.

The phenol coefficient number itself is simply the ratio of the killing dilution in ten minutes of the test germicide, to the killing dilution of the phenol solution. For example, a particular germicide might kill the organism *Salmonella typhosa* at a dilution of one part germicide to 900 parts water. The phenol standard typically kills *Salmonella typhosa* at a 1:90 dilution. Nine hundred divided by 90 equals 10 so the phenol coefficient of this particular germicide against *Salmonella typhosa* is 10.

Unfortunately, there are many ways in which the phenol coefficient number can be very misleading and all of the data leading up to it also. First of all, the most significant failing of the phenol coefficient method is its unreliability. You can repeat the test ten different times on the same bacteria with the same germicide and come up with ten different phenol coefficient numbers. Thus, it is very difficult to know with any degree of reliability what the true phenol coefficient is.

The purpose of the phenol coefficient number, of course, is to determine what dilution might be considered effective when used on hard surfaces. The conventional rule of thumb is the multiplication of the phenol coefficient by 20, and this is the number of parts water to which one part of the germicide can be added to come up with an efficient use dilution.

It is known today that this rule of thumb is largely invalid, and that in fact there is no reliable rule of thumb multiple. Some germicide manufacturers, however, use the phenol coefficient method to come up with a great deal of impressive documentation; but it is documentation which can be very misleading. Such manufacturers carry out the phenol coefficient method but report only the killing dilutions i.e., the dilution of the germicide in the tube of broth culture of the test bacteria that kills in a specified period of time. The implication is that, using the example above, we have a germicide which is effective in the test tube at a 1:900 dilution. Then if the manufacturer reports a 1:100 use dilution in his directions, you have a substantial margin of safety. Nothing could be further from the truth because there is no relationship between what happens in the test tube under these circumstances and what happens when the germicide is used under practical conditions.

Even a commonsense analysis of the phenol coefficient method would indicate why this should be so. The bacteria are exposed to the germicide under completely liquid conditions. The cells are floating around in the germicide solution and thus are exposed to the germicide under the most optimum possible conditions—conditions which would rarely be duplicated in practice.

Of course, the phenol coefficient method was designed originally to compare phenolic type disinfectants back to straight phenol, and not to compare nonphenolic disinfectants with phenol. Thus, the problems described above regarding the use of the phenol coefficient method are multiplied severalfold when the test method is used on other chemical types of germicides such as quaternary ammonium compounds. Quaternary ammonium compounds have the ability to give false high phenol coefficients.

For example, a phenolic disinfectant and a quaternary disinfectant both with proven disinfectant ability at a 1:100 dilution might give a phenol coefficient of 10 for the phenolic and 30 for the quaternary. Thus, while the rule of thumb multiple of 20×10 giving a 1:200 dilution for the phenolic product is wrong by a factor of 2, the phenol coefficient derived dilution of 1:600 (20×30) is wrong by a factor of 6, for the quaternary compound.

A.O.A.C. Use Dilution Confirmation Test

The A.O.A.C. Use Dilution Confirmation Test is as reliable and useful as the Phenol Coefficient is not. The Use Dilution Test is now required by the U.S.D.A. for all specific claims of germicidal effectiveness against specific bacteria—Mycobacterium tuberculosis, fungi, and spores excepted. These three exceptions are handled by other specific A.O.A.C. Test Methods as required by the U.S.D.A.

The A.O.A.C. Use Dilution Confirmation Test is carried out as follows:

Sterile stainless steel ring carriers simulating a hard surface are dipped in a broth culture of the test organism and dried for at least 20 minutes and up to 60 minutes. The contaminated carriers are then immersed in a tube of in-use solution of the germicide, for 10 minutes at 20°C. The supposedly disinfected carriers are then immersed in tubes of appropriate nutrient media and incubated for 48 hours. If only a few organisms survive on a carrier they will multiply and show signs of growth in the tube.

In order to pass this test, it is necessary to show "no growth" from ten ring carriers in separate tubes of media. However, in practice, the U.S.D.A. often requires perfect results in 60 or more ring carriers instead of the conventional 10.

The Use Dilution Test is very strict and demanding. One reason for this is obvious — the bacteria are buried in a film of organic media, dried on to a hard surface. This is a realistic situation and one which demands the utmost of the germicide.

The A.O.A.C. Use Dilution Confirmation Test is now required by regulation for all germicides shipped in interstate commerce. However, for hospital use only three test organisms are commonly required, they are: *Staphylococcus aureus*, *Salmonella choleraesuis*, and *Pseudomonas aeruginosa*. To be further assured of a broad spectrum performance by a germicide, some hospitals may prefer use dilution test data carried out on a much wider variety of microorganisms.

Tuberculocidal Testing

As mentioned, a separate test method is now required for the measurement of a disinfectant's ability to kill *Mycobacterium tuberculosis*. This organism, while highly resistant to chemical agents, is difficult to grow under laboratory conditions. Furthermore, the organism is highly subject to bacteriostatic effects which prevent its multiplication without destroying it. Therefore, laboratory evaluation of tuberculocidal activity in a disinfectant must include subculturing in a variety of specific nutrient media and extensive incubation to insure reliable detection of surviving organisms.

The U.S.D.A has recently finalized on a modification of the A.O.A.C. Use Dilution Test which takes all of these factors into consideration. The test is known as the A.O.A.C. Tuberculocidal Test and involves subculturing in three different media and 90 days of incubation. This is a very demanding test method and one that showed many popular germicides thought to have been tuberculocidal for many years, not to be so in fact. Reformulation of these products was necessary.

Similar modifications of A.O.A.C. Test methods are now standard and required for proof of claims of fungicidal and sporicidal action, but these will not be described here.

In-Use Testing

In the last analysis, no laboratory test method can be relied upon completely to predict disinfectant results under all practical use conditions. Unfortunately, there are just as many problems in reliable in-use testing as in laboratory testing. Bacteria are not scattered evenly over surfaces, like "carrots in a field," they are scattered in highly random clumps and clusters and many areas of a floor may have very few bacteria while other areas may have a very dense population. There is no such thing as a uniformly contaminated surface in nature. Obvious as this is, it is usual for hospital technicians carrying out in-use testing to fail to take this into consideration.

The typical hospital in-use test involves the laboratory technician's taking one or two swab or Rodac plate counts from a floor, having the janitor mop the floor with the test germicide and then taking one or two counts afterwards to see what the difference in bacteria count is. It is just as likely that the technician will have swabbed a low-count area before and a high count area afterwards or vice versa and the results from such in-use tests are accurate only by accident.

Reliable in-use testing on surfaces such as floors requires sophisticated statistical design and analysis techniques in which not one or two, but dozens or even hundreds of samples are taken from a given floor area at mathematically random locations. Then the results must be statistically analysed.

A relatively simple but statistically valid means of comparing disinfection procedures has been described by Pryor (Reference #6, p. 253) and is strongly recommended.

Various Disinfectants Compared

The question of whether the hospital germicide shall be phenolic, quaternary, iodophor, or chlorine is highly controversial. The basis of such controversy has historically been due to the questioning of evaluation methods, and unfortunately, accurate, objective, up-to-date information on the subject has been lacking. The discussion that follows about each of the major germicide types represents a distillation of the most current information available. As a result, it will on occasion be directly contradictory to what has often been published and frequently reported in the past.

Phenolic Disinfectant

Phenolic compounds and their many chemical derivatives are very popular in hospital use today because many are good products, and because they are historically the oldest. Despite all claims to the contrary, however, they are not unique in their performance characteristics and they are most certainly not ideal. There is no ideal product, at this time.

First of all, a well formulated phenolic product is a good disinfectant with competent activity over a wide range of organisms. However, many have certain weaknesses against some highly resistant Gram negative organisms like *Pseudomonas* and some are reportedly slow in their action against *Staphylococcus*. There is a wide variation of performance among the phenolic germicides from different companies and few generalities are possible.

Phenolics can be formulated by skilled and experienced chemists into fairly good combination detergent-germicides and these products are widely used for general purpose hospital housekeeping.

Phenolics are often not too expensive. However, when evaluating products for cost, the reader is advised to evaluate use-cost rather than the actual cost-per-gallon of a disinfectant. It is the cost per gallon of use solution which is critical and some of the most expensive products on the market on a per gallon basis, are the least expensive when diluted and used at the recommended concentrations.

One particularly notable disadvantage among phenolic compounds is that they are all quite irritating to the skin. This is not generally considered a dangerous type of skin irritation, but it is most annoying and requires careful handling. Lost time among housekeeping employees especially, is quite common due to this cause. Rubber gloves or protective hand creams (industrial type) are strongly recommended wherever a person is likely to be exposed even to use solutions of phenolic disinfectants.

Some of the older formulations are also objectionable because of strong phenolic odors, but modern formulations have largely eliminated this problem. It should be noted, however, that some manufacturers incorporate strong, heavy fragrances into their products and these are considered by some hospitals to be as objectionable as the older phenolic odors.

Chemically, there is almost an infinite variety of formulations possible with the phenolic disinfectants. There are many phenolic derivatives used such as ortho phenylphenol, ortho benzyl parachlorophenol, para tertiary amylphenol, and many others. The most widely accepted chemical formulation practice is to use two or more phenolic derivatives because it is not currently possible to use a single phenolic derivative and obtain the wide spectrum antibacterial performance required, unless an excessively expensive amount of the single ingredient is used in the formulation.

Likewise, there are a variety of detergent ingredients possible to incorporate into phenolic disinfectants but these must be selected very carefully. All detergent ingredients are incompatible to at least some degree with the phenolic ingredients and a careful balance is required of the various types of detergents used. Some types are totally inactivating, such as the nonionic synthetic detergents, and these must never be used under any circumstances in the formulation of a phenolic detergent germicide. Even accidental trace contamination must be avoided such as might occur if a mixing tank, used to mix a product containing a non-ionic, were not completely rinsed prior to making the phenolic product. Or at the use level, a mop used with a general purpose cleaner (usually contain nonionics) must be laundered before being used with phenolics.

Among the older and less expensive phenolic germicidal cleaners are those based on soap rather than synthetic detergents. While these products are still available, as a general rule, they should not be used in the modern hospital. The soap ingredients, while fair cleaners, usually leave a visible film on most surfaces which is aesthetically unpleasing and which is a safety hazard on surgical conductive floors. The soap reacts with the minerals in water and the resulting soap curd forms an insulating film on conductive floors. The use of soap based cleaners and germicides is one of the more common causes of conductive floor failure.

Phenolics are frequently thought to be very effective as tuberculocidal agents and while this is true for a few of the better products, it is not a generality which can be applied to the phenolic class as a whole. At this time, it is likely that many of the phenolic products on the market are not tuberculocidal as defined by the A.O.A.C. Tuberculocidal Test. Proof should always be required.

One common misconception on tuberculocidal performance in general is that if a germicide has proven tuberculocidal performance, it is going to be extremely effective against all other common microorganisms, too. This is definitely not true. The correlation between positive tuberculocidal performance and performance against such organisms as *Staphylococcus aureus* and *Pseudomonas aeruginosa* is not high. It is quite common to find a product effective against tuberculosis to be ineffective against *Pseudomonas* and visa versa. Similarly for *Staphylococcus aureus*.

One other disadvantage of all phenolic products is that they damage floor finishes and waxes, thus shortening the time between stripping and refinishing. This problem is especially acute without strictly enforced use directions or some automatic control device to combat the normal human tendancy to overuse cleaning products.

Quaternary Ammonium Germicide

The quaternary ammonium compounds are another major class of germicides and are, perhaps, the most subject to misinformation and false criticism. Much of the misinformation about quaternary ammonium compounds has been developed because of poorly reported and analyzed negative incidences based on a single quaternary ammonium compound originally developed over 30 years ago. As a result, the whole class of quaternary ammonium compounds has suffered in reputation, often quite unfairly. There are literally hundreds of chemically different quaternary compounds which have been synthesized and formulated over the years, many with vastly different properties than the old original compound. No one attributes to phenolic compounds in use today the highly undesirable characteristics possessed by the original phenol in use a hundred years ago, yet it is common to ignore similar progress in quaternary compounds.

Each brand of quaternary detergent-germicide should be examined on its own individual merits as supported by U.S.D.A. accepted A.O.A.C. Use Test Method documentation As with the phenolic compounds, there is an extreme range of performance found among the various brands.

The quaternary ammonium compounds which are the most effective germicidally are those formulated as combination detergent-germicide. Such formulations are occasionally synergistic and may be responsible for greatly improved antibacterial performance. As is the case with the phenolic detergent-germicides, proof must be required of the broad spectrum performance of the particular quaternary ammonium compound under consideration. Such proof must be via the A.O.A.C. Use Dilution Confirmation Test. Nothing should be taken for granted in the absence of such test data.

A well formulated quaternary detergent-germicide is an excellent cleaner and generally, a far more pleasant product to use by housekeeping employees. There is a virtual absence of hand irritation, which is a distinct advantage in hospital housekeeping. One of the more common problems with the phenolic germicides, other than the hand irritation potential, is that if they are used at significantly stronger concentrations than that recommended by the manufacturer there is the potential of damage to synthetic floor finishes. There is also possible attack on certain rubber and plastic goods. The hospital is advised to run tests on the potential deleterious effects of phenolic compounds on such plastic and rubber goods. Quaternary compounds, on the other hand, are generally not harmful to most materials and surfaces regardless of misuse.

One of the most common misconceptions is that quaternary compounds are seriously weak on Gram negative organisms. While this is true for some products it is definitely not true today for many others. There are some quaternary formulations available which are extremely effective on Gram negative organisms including resistant strains of Pseudomonas. These newer formulations are no less effective on Gram positive organisms. Another common belief is that quaternary compounds are not tuberculocidal. This is certainly true, but then as stated previously, so are many of the most popular phenolic compounds. It is known that good quaternary germicides, when mixed with fairly weak alcohol or acetone solutions instead of plain water, are effective tuberculocidal products. Obviously, this feature is not practical for anything other than immersion disinfection of objects like instruments.

It is an increasingly widely held position among hospitals today that tuberculosis is not a significant hospital-wide infection problem if patients are screened by X-ray on admission. Therefore the whole issue of tuberculocidal performance among germicides is badly over-emphasized.

A widely accepted statistic is that only about three out of every thousand patients admitted to a general hospital, are diagnosed eventually to have tuberculosis and of course these patients are promptly transferred. Furthermore, of these patients so diagnosed only a very small percentage will have the disease in an active infectious form. Thus, the issue of tuberculocidal performance need not ordinarily be considered for a hospital germicide, especially for one used in hospital housekeeping.

Another commonly held belief about quaternary ammonium compounds is that they are extremely susceptible to soil loads. There is no question that quaternary compounds are subject to inactivation by organic matter but so are other germicides. Well formulated quaternary disinfectants easily pass the A.O.A.C. Use Dilution Test in the presence of 5% horse serum — a severe test of their ability to function under heavy soil load conditions. Furthermore, the soil loads which do have a serious effect on the well formulated products are well beyond the level of aesthetic tolerance in any cleaning or disinfecting situation. Should such heavy soil loads be encountered the obvious answer, regardless of the type of the germicide used, is to clean first and then disinfect as a separate step.

Chemically, the more common quaternary ammonium detergent-germicides use one or more of a wide variety of compounds known under the general classification of alkyl dimethylbenzyl ammonium chlorides. There are hundreds of different quaternary ammonium compounds possible under this general chemical name, though this is not widely known among hospital personnel. The most common chemical difference is in the length of the carbon chain radical, which can vary typically anywhere from 6 to 20 or more carbons. The most effective germicidal chain lengths are currently thought to be mixtures of 12, 14, and 16 length carbon chains.

The main detergent ingredients in the quaternary detergent-germicide are synthetic nonionic types. The anionic detergents and natural soap cannot be used under any circumstances because they are incompatible.

Quaternary ammonium compounds are cationic in electrochemical nature and thus have a positive charge. Soap and anionic detergents have a negative charge and thus neutralize like quantities of quaternary ammonium compounds. The nonionics with no charge whatever are compatible, provided certain quaternary to nonionic ratios are not exceeded.

Other inorganic detergent ingredients are sometimes used and there are a wide variety of additives available.

One interesting phenomena of the quaternary ammonium compounds is that another chemical branch of the family is among the more popular ingredients in fabric softeners. The cationic nature of the quaternary compound makes them tend to absorb into many common fabrics and fibers. This absorption is not a continuous one and the build-up tends to stabilize. However, this characteristic does point up one precaution to take with regard to the use of such compounds.

This precaution is illustrated by one of the more infamous historical incidences of a negative nature with regard to quaternaries—a case in which Pseudomonas was found actually growing in a solution of a common quaternary used for skin antisepsis. Upon careful examination, however, it was found that the solution was at least several weeks old and cotton balls were stored there. As a cotton ball saturated with the solution was removed for use it was replaced with fresh cotton and over a period of time the quaternary ingredient was gradually leached out of solution, thus, permitting the Pseudomonas contamination. This occurrence is often referred to by those strongly prejudiced against quaternary compounds.

The particular compound used was the old original type (benzalkonium chloride) which is not nearly as effective as the more modern formulations. Nevertheless, germicidal solutions used in this fashion should be changed on a daily basis regardless of chemical types, and gross misuse of the product itself was responsible for the Pseudomonas contamination. Little if any real blame could be put upon the product in this instance.

It may also be pointed out by those prejudiced against quaternary compounds that their cationic nature may work against them in other ways. For example, it is not uncommon to have surfaces cleaned by anionic detergents followed by disinfection with a quaternary compound (cationic). The presumption is that the residual anionic detergent will effectively neutralize the cationic disinfectant and the hoped-for bacteria kill will be drastically inhibited. In answer to this hypothetical situation it is pointed out that, first of all, it is *not* common to find cleaning with an anionic detergent followed by a separate disinfection step — at least in hospital practice. This is simply too much labor and the detergent-germicide combinations are popular because they do permit one-step procedures. In any case, the amount of residual anionic detergent left on a surface would rarely, if ever, be sufficient to neutralize the quaternary disinfectant that might follow.

Finally, if this is in fact a problem with quaternary compounds it is also a problem with phenolic disinfectants, because most of the common anionic general purpose cleaners in use today also contain some nonionic detergent. Phenolics are far more sensitive to inhibition by nonionic detergents than quaternaries are to anionic detergents.

In conclusion, with regard to the great majority of hospital applications, there is little to choose between the best products of the quaternary family and the best products of the phenolic family. Good use procedures with products of either type, well documented by U.S.D.A. accepted A.O.A.C. Test methods, provide equally good antibacterial results.

Halogen Disinfectants

There is little controversy about halogen disinfectants such as iodine, chlorine, and bromine. They are universally accepted as excellent disinfectants per se, and in fact, considered strictly from the laboratory point of view, are probably more effective than even the best phenolic or quaternary germicides. However, they do have a number of notable disadvantages unrelated to their germicidal ability which restricts their use in the hospital. They are ordinarily quite corrosive to metals and other materials and they can be quite irritating.

The most interesting member of the halogen family and the one with the widest applications is iodine. Iodine can be chemically complexed with certain nonionic synthetic detergents to form iodophors. When iodine is in an iodophor form, it loses many of its disagreeable characteristics. Iodophors are relatively nontoxic and their corrosive properties are largely dependent upon the type of other ingredients formulated with it. For example, in order to be active germicidally, an iodophor has to be kept on the acid side of the pH scale. In the most common iodophors, phosphoric acid or hydrochloric acid is used to achieve this acid pH. If hydrochloric acid is used, the corrosive problems are much more severe than with phosphoric acid.

Iodophors are very rapid in their disinfecting action, accomplishing in seconds what other types of disinfectants often take minutes to do. This can be an advantage under some circumstances.

Iodophors are fairly good detergents, but in this capacity do not measure up to the performance of the quaternary or phenolic detergent-disinfectants. This is primarily due to the acid pH. Phenolics and quaternaries are on the alkaline side, a characteristic which contributes significantly to their detergency.

The characteristic reddish brown iodine color of iodophors is both an advantage and a disadvantage. The advantage is that iodophors are substantially self-monitoring as far as concentration and germicidal activity are concerned. The amount of iodine left in solution available to kill bacteria is directly and proportionately reflected in the color of the solution. However, iodine does stain temporarily and sometimes certain surfaces permanently. Permanent staining may occur with certain plastics and a temporary yellow color may be imparted to some white paints. A washable dark blue stain will occur on starched fabrics.

Iodophors are very broad in their antibacterial spectrum and may in general be depended upon to kill even the most resistant microorganisms. Some at sufficient concentrations and time of exposure even have some sporicidal action. However, this sporicidal action is not particularly practical and would not occur under any practical housekeeping conditions.

The greatest use of iodophors will be in nursing service and the dietary department. Nursing will find frequent uses for immersing thermometers, instruments, utensils, laboratory glassware, etc., and the dietary department will find them especially useful for disinfecting food contact surfaces such as pots and pans, and food preparation equipment. In the latter application, the iodophor is used at a relatively low concentration and the objects to be disinfected are cleaned and rinsed with fresh water prior to application of the disinfectant solution.

Chlorine is another very popular member of the halogen family but its applications are more restricted than for iodophors. Chlorine is far more corrosive and its bleaching properties are well known. It is an excellent disinfectant for fabrics when used with care and in this respect is quite effective on mops. However, it is too corrosive for soaking instruments and utensils, though it is often used as a final rinse sanitizer for food contact surfaces. In this respect it duplicates the function of the iodophor and there are few if any circumstances in which the iodophors would not do as good or better a job with greater safety.

Miscellaneous Disinfectants

There are a number of other miscellaneous disinfectants but these have very limited uses and will only be mentioned here. Among the more useful of these are the formaldehyde and gluteraldehyde products which are used for cold sterilization of heat sensitive instruments. Formaldehyde solutions are commonly sold under the trade name of Bard-Parker Solution and this type is quite effective and fairly inexpensive. The gluteraldehyde formulations are also effective and have the advantage of not being as disagreeable to use as the formaldehyde preparations. However, they are extremely expensive and probably justified only in rare circumstances.

Other cold sterilization chemicals include Beta Propiolactone and peracetic acid, but these materials are so hazardous to use that at the current time they would have no hospital application.

Other products based on heavy metals, such as mercury, are not true disinfectants at all and have no place in the hospital environment with the possible exception of skin antisepsis. There are one or two products being sold making disinfectant claims with organic forms of tin incorporated, but the tin, while a strong bacteriostat, has no germicidal ability and such products are of doubtful value.

Antiseptic hand soaps, such as those based on hexachlorophene or other bacteriostats are also not germicides at all. They are useful only to reduce bacteria counts on skin through bacteriastasis and have no application on inanimate surfaces.

7-1-9 Disinfectant Types Compared by Quality Ranges

Properties Overall Quality Range	Phenolic			Quaternary			Iodophor
	Poor	Average	Best	Poor	Average	Best	
Effectiveness against:							
Staphylococcus aureus	poor	good	excellent	fair	excellent	excellent	excellent
Salmonella choleraesuis	good	good	excellent	fair	good	excellent	excellent
Pseudomonas aeruginosa	poor	fair	good	poor	fair	excellent	excellent
Mycobacterium tuberculosis	poor	fair	good	poor	poor	poor	excellent
Speed of kill	poor	fair	fair	poor	fair	good	excellent
Detergency	poor	fair	good	good	good	excellent	fair
Skin irritation	poor	poor	fair	fair	excellent	excellent	excellent
Corrosion to metals	fair	fair	good	poor	fair	good	fair
Damage to floor finishes with overuse	poor	poor	poor	good	fair	good	good
Staining	good	good	good	good	good	good	fair
Odor of solutions	poor	fair	good	good	good	excellent	good
Degree of inhibition by organic soil	moderate	moderate	moderate	severe	moderate	moderate	severe
pH of solution	8.5–11.5	8.5–10.5	8.5–10.5	7.0–10.0	8.5–10.0	8.5–10.0	2.0–6.0
Toxicity (Acute oral)	moderate*	moderate*	moderate*	moderate	moderate	moderate	moderate
Deodorizing ability	poor	fair	fair	good	excellent	excellent	fair

*Phenolic concentrates cause severe burns to mucous membranes upon swallowing.

7-1-10   Optimization of Disinfection Results

There are many factors that effect the results to be obtained when using disinfectants and some of these are under the control of the user and some are not. First of all we have chemical factors that effect germicidal action. Among these would be the pH or the acidity or alkalinity of the use solution. As mentioned, iodophors have to be used at a pH in the acid range to be effective. There are circumstances under which very alkaline water supplies might neutralize the acid in a weak disinfectant solution and under these circumstances, even though iodine was present, it would be completely inactive germicidally. This characteristic again favors the phosphoric acid type products over the hydrochloric acid type, because under most circumstances there is only approximately 0.1% hydrochloric acid in these products whereas when phosphoric acid is used there is at least 5% and as high as 20% acid. This provides a far greater margin of safety in alkaline water conditions.

Quaternary compounds on the other hand are most active at an alkaline pH. However, some products are far more sensitive to pH than others in this respect. There are available certain quaternary ammonium compounds which are very nearly as effective in their disinfectant ability in moderately acid conditions as they are under alkaline conditions. These types of quaternaries would have application for example in acid type toilet bowl cleaners.

Phenolics, on the other hand, are most active germicidally when they are neutral or slightly on the acid side. Paradoxically, all phenolic disinfectants currently being sold are alkaline. The reason is that, when a phenolic disinfectant is in the neutral or acid condition, it forms milky solutions in water because the phenolic ingredients are in the free acid, non-water soluble (but dispersable) form. This milkiness, while it does no harm and even helps, is not very pleasing aesthetically, and all manufacturers compromise germicidal performance slightly by having the solution sufficiently alkaline to form clear use solutions. They add a slightly greater quantity of the phenolic ingredients to make up the difference.

Temperature is a strong factor in germicidal action. The higher the temperature, the faster and surer the activity of a disinfectant. However, in the case of iodophors you must limit temperatures to about 110–120°F, because at higher temperatures, the iodine will evaporate.

The ratio of germicide to a contaminated surface is important. Obviously, the more germicidal solution on a contaminated area the more germicide there is to attack microorganisms.

Time is a factor; the longer the exposure of the bacteria to the germicide the surer the results. But for most practical purposes, 3–5 minutes exposure is sufficient — especially in housekeeping applications.

Concentration, of course, is another obvious factor but in this respect the manufacturer's use directions should always be followed. There is a point of diminishing return with regard to increasing the concentration of a germicide, and for that matter there is such a point with regard to time, temperature, and quantity of germicidal solution on the surface too. As an example, with a 1% solution of a germicide, one might kill 95% of the bacteria under the use conditions and with a 2% solution this might increase to 97% kill. Therefore, these and other use factors must be placed into practical context.

One of the most important factors determining the end result of the disinfection process is the type and quantity of soil on the surface to be disinfected. Soil can be an inhibitor of germicidal action for all disinfectants, and under more critical conditions soil removal is at least as important as the application of the disinfectant itself. Under ideal conditions disinfectants (even the detergent-disinfectants) would be applied to essentially clean surfaces.

In hospital practice, soil removal is often impractical from a labor point of view. Hospital housekeeping for the most part has to be done via a one-step procedure. However, many of the disinfectant functions carried out by nursing service can be so critical that the extra labor becomes insignificant. For example, in decontaminating thermometers it is absolutely essential that the thermometers be washed carefully and ample "elbow grease" applied to remove all soil before immersion in the disinfectant. A similar procedure is followed, with instruments and utensils. In the food service area, of course, such prewashing of utensils is accepted practice prior to the application of a disinfectant (or sanitizer).

In the housekeeping function, single step procedures are largely a must. These procedures are described in greater detail in other chapters of this book. Basically, they encompass the various double pail mopping techniques; mop sterilization; double basin wiping techniques; use of disposable sterile cloths; and most importantly, the use of the spraying and wet vacuuming technique to replace mopping entirely.

One specific application technique which should be shunned is germicidal fogging. Fogging has become quite popular among hospitals, though despite the fairly extensive publication on the subject there has yet to be published any study that proves fogging is effective. In fact, most authorities, including the National Center for Disease Control, experts within The American Hospital Association, and the U.S. Public

Health Service, have concluded that fogging is simply not effective. Certainly, if the reader will critically analyze the properties of disinfectants, regardless of type, in view of the previously described factors effecting results, fogging will be found to violate virtually all of these. The amount of disinfectant on a surface is extremely small, the surface is dirty, there is no friction or agitation, the product is at room temperature, and on and on. The popularity of fogging is perhaps due mostly to psychological factors, i.e., it reminds people of fumigation and poison gas. But quaternary and phenolic germicides are neither fumigants nor poison gas and they should not be expected to function as such.

It can be argued that fogging (with the machine wide open) is a good means of thoroughly saturating the surfaces in an isolation room. But such a procedure takes at least 45 minutes (15 minutes of fogging plus 30 minutes of ventilation) and the same surface wetting can be accomplished in five minutes with a pump-up hand sprayer.

7-1-11 Detergent and Disinfectant Recommendations by Department and Cleaning Function

Code	Product	Code	Product
APC	All-Purpose Cleaner (Liquid)	MWD	Machine Washing Detergent
SHDC	Stripper and Heavy Duty Cleaner (Liquid) (may contain solvents)	LSC	Low Sudsing Cleaner
CC	Concrete Cleaner (Powder)	CS	Carpet Shampoo
WC	Wall Cleaner (Powder)	QDD	Quaternary Detergent-Disinfectant
PIC	Powdered Immersion Cleaner	PDD	Phenolic Detergent-Disinfectant
LIC	Liquid Immersion Cleaner	IDD	Iodophor Detergent-Disinfectant
MAD	Mild Acid Detergent	CD	Chlorine Disinfectant
SAD	Strong Acid Detergent (Toilet Bowl Cleaner)		

NOTE

Beside each cleaning function a product will be recommended by a code symbol. Where more than one product is applicable, the order of preference will be indicated by numbering. Where two or more products are judged equal, they will receive an identical ranking number. Occasionally, sequential treatment with two products may be advised – this will be indicated by the word "and" and the products will be listed in the correct sequence. In every case it is assumed that each product is of the highest quality.

Department	Cleaning or Disinfecting Function	Recommended Detergent Types	Recommended Disinfectants	Comments
Housekeeping	Manual cleaning of floors, furniture, equipment	APC	(1) QDD (1) PDD	

Department	Cleaning or Disinfecting Function	Recommended Detergent Types	Recommended Disinfectants	Comments
	Floors with auto-scrubber	LSC	QDD	
	Bathroom floors	MAD and APC	(1) QDD (2) PDD	
	Bathroom walls	APC and MAD	(1) QDD (1) PDD	
	Bathroom fixtures	APC and MAD	(1) QDD (1) PDD	
	Washing painted walls	(1) WC (2) SHDC	(1) QDD (1) PDD	
	Toilet bowls and urinals	MAD or SAD	(1) QDD (2) PDD	
	Waste cans	APC	(1) QDD (2) PDD	
	Stainless steel	MAD and APC		
	Windows	Ammonia		
	Light duty wall washing	(1) APC (1) SHDC	(1) QDD (1) PDD	
	Isolation rooms		(1) QDD (1) PDD	
	Tuberculosis decontamination		APC and (1) IDD (2) PDD	
	Wax or floor finish stripping	SHDC and Vinegar		Vinegar solution is for final neutralizing rinse
	Carpet cleaning	CS	(1) PDD (2) QDD	
Surgery	Floors and walls		(1) QDD (1) PDD	
Obstetrics	Conductive floors		(1) QDD (1) QDD	
	Deep scrubbing of conductive floors	SHDC and Vinegar		Monthly — Use vinegar final rinse to neutralize
	Cast room soil	MAD		
	Tables, fixtures equipment, cabinets		(1) QDD (1) PDD (1) IDD	
	Rubber goods		(1) QDD (1) IDD	or ethylene oxide sterilization
	Surgical instruments	(1) LIC (1) PIC		followed by autoclaving

Department	Cleaning or Disinfecting Function	Recommended Detergent Types	Recommended Disinfectants	Comments
	Heat sensitive instruments	LIC	(1) QDD (1) IDD (2) PDD	or ethylene oxide sterilization
	Machine washing of instruments	MWD		
Nursery	Bassinettes, isolettes	APC	(1) QDD (2) IDD	Phenolics may damage plastic
	Incubators	APC	(1) QDD (2) IDD	
	Humidifiers	MAD	(1) QDD (1) IDD	
Infant Form- ula Room	Bottles, nipples, racks, preparation vessels	(1) PIC (1) LIC	(1) CD (1) IDD	
	Removing lime and milk film from bottles, nipples, racks	MAD		
Physical Therapy	Hubbard tanks and whirlpool baths	APC	(1) QDD (2) IDD (2) PDD	
	Removing water mineral stains and films	MAD		
	Treatment tables	APC	(1) QDD (1) PDD	
	Paraffin baths	SHDC		Use very hot water
Anesthesia	Y-tubes, airways, laryngiscope blades, endo-trachael tubes	(1) LIC (1) PIC	(1) QDD (1) IDD	
	Rubber parts	(1) LIC (1) PIC	(1) QDD (1) IDD	
	Removing lime and rubber deposits	MAD		
	Gas machine	APC	(1) QDD (1) IDD	
Central Supply and Nursing Utility	Manual cleaning of: Patient utensils, instruments, bottles, rubber goods	LIC PIC		

Department	Cleaning or Disinfecting Function	Recommended Detergent Types	Recommended Disinfectants	Comments
Rooms	By machine	MWD		
	Ultrasonically	(1) LIC		
		(1) PIC		
		(1) MWD		
	Hypodermic syringes and needles—			
	manually	LIC		
	by machine	MWD		
	Ultrasonically	LIC		
Central Supply	Removing films from urinals, medicine glasses	MAD		
	Rubber gloves	LIC	IDD	Use 1/10 normal detergent amount
	Thermometers	LIC	(1) IDD	
			(2) QDD	Always clean first
			(3) PDD	
	Humidifiers	LIC and MAD	(1) IDD	
			(2) QDD	
	Inhalation therapy equipment	APC and MAD	(1) QDD	or ethylene oxide
			(2) IDD	sterilization
Laboratory-Pathology	Lab glassware by hand	(1) LIC	(1) IDD	Use QDD at temperatures above 140°F for tuber-
		(1) PIC	(2) PDD	culocidal activity
	By machine	MWD		
	Removing mineral films and urine film	MAD		
	Bench tops		(1) QDD	
			(1) IDD	
			(1) PDD	
	Autopsy table	APC and MAD	(1) QDD	
			(1) IDD	
			(1) PDD	
	Autopsy instruments	(1) LIC	(1) QDD	
		(1) PIC	(1) IDD	
			(1) PDD	
Dietary	Tableware	MWD		
	Cookware by hand	(1) LIC	(1) IDD	Wash first, then
		(1) PIC	(2) CD	rinse in
			(3) QDD	disinfectant

Department	Cleaning or Disinfecting Function	Recommended Detergent Types	Recommended Disinfectants	Comments
	Cookware by machine	MWD		
	Quarrytile floors, concrete floors	(1) CC (2) SHDC (3) APC	QDD	
	Refrigerators, coolers, store- rooms	APC	QDD	
	Food contact surfaces	APC	(1) IDD (2) QDD (2) CD	
	Hoods, heavy grease	SHDC		
	Waste cans	APC	QDD	
Laundry	Carts	APC	QDD	
	Floors	(1) APC (1) SHDC	QDD	
	Soap and detergent deposits	MAD		
	Chutes	SHDC	QDD	
Engineering	Air filters	SHDC	QDD	
	Filter rooms	(1) APC (1) SHDC	QDD	
	Heavy fans, equip- ment with heavy grease	SHDC		

REFERENCES AND SELECTED READINGS

A cooperative microbiological evaluation of floor cleaning procedures in hospital patient rooms. (A report of the Committee on Microbiol Contamination of Surfaces of The Laboratory Section of The American Public Health Association.) *Health Laboratory Science*, October 1970.

A new approach to cleaning rubbish and linen chutes, *The Executive Housekeeper*, July 1969.

LaFave, Edna, Pryor, A. K., and McDuff, C. R. A new method for decontaminating mops, *Hospitals, J.A.H.A.*, Vol. 41, July 16, 1967.

Mizuno, W. G. and Pryor, A. K. Considerations in selecting hospital detergent germicides, *Maintenance Supplies*, Vol. X, No. 1, January 1965.

Mizuno, W. G. Ph.D., and Pryor, A. K. Evaluating detergent-germicides for hospital use, *Hospitals, J.A.H.A.*, Vol. 40, January 16, 1966.

Pryor, A. K. A practical microbiol surveillance program, *The Executive Housekeeper*, March 1969.

Pryor, A. K. Are pathogenic spores a hospital threat? *Hospital Management,* Vol. 101, pp. 74–78, May 1966.

Pryor, A. K. Cleaning procedures for the operating room, *The Executive Housekeeper,* February 1970.

Pryor, A. K. Design for cleanability, *Modern Hospital,* April 1969.

Pryor, A. K. Detergent systems for laboratory glasswashing, *Laboratory Management,* November–December 1964.

Pryor, A. K. Evaluating hospital disinfectants, *Journal of Environmental Health,* March–April 1968.

Pryor, A. K. In use comparison of disinfection procedures in hospitals, *Journal of Environmental Health,* Vol. 27, No. 5, March–April 1965.

Pryor, A. K. Latest USDA requirements for germicide testing, *The Executive Housekeeper,* November 1969.

Pryor, A. K., M.A., Vesley, D., M.S., Shaffer, J. G., Sc.D., F.A.P.H.A., and Walter, W. G., Ph.D., F.A.P.H.A. Cooperative microbiol surveys of surfaces in hospital patient rooms, *Health Laboratory Science Magazine,* Vol. 4, No. 3, July 1967.

Pryor, A. K. Terminal cleaning of isolation rooms, *The Executive Housekeeper,* July 1970.

Pryor, A. K. Understanding germicide labels and brochures, *The Executive Housekeeper,* February 1968.

Vesley, D., Pryor, A. K., and Battles, D. E. Implications of environmental contamination control in an experimental surgery, (originally titled: Minnesota test finds sterile O.R. cuts infection death rate in half), *Modern Hospital,* Vol. 107, No. 4, October 1966.

7-2 ISOLATION PROCEDURES

7-2-1 Introduction

The use or misuse of isolation technique directly effects the spread of infection. The advent of powerful antibiotics; the closing of communicable disease hospitals; the change in role of the professional nurse, from intensive bedside care to administration; and the performance of some medical services, has contributed to the increasing infection problem in hospitals today.

General Control Procedures

1. Rapid diagnosis and isolation of infected patients or suspected infected patients who are admitted to the hospital.
2. All hospital employees adhere to established techniques:
   a. Handwashing when entering and leaving the isolation area.
   b. Gowning when in intimate contact with the patient.
   c. Leaving contaminated articles in the isolation area.
   d. Masking and gloving as indicated.
3. Care of excreta and other wastes.
4. Knowledge of infectious diseases and their modes of transmission.
5. Care of linens.

6. Proper food preparation and serving.
7. Proper ventilation systems.
8. Detection of carriers among staff and patients.
9. Proper disinfection of rooms where infected patients have been: patient room, physical therapy, O.R., morgue.

Written procedures should be available to all personnel, who should be closely supervised in their performances.

7-2-2 Admissions

Newly admitted patients who are known or suspected to be infected should be placed immediately into individual isolation rooms, and not into hallways, open wards, semi-private rooms, and so on. All patients, if their conditions permit, should be X-rayed with 70 mm chest films to determine if they have tuberculosis.

Infected pregnant women upon admission to the labor area should be placed in individual isolation and delivered in a separate delivery room. The babies of the infected mothers must be considered to be contaminated and therefore placed in isolation.

Hospital Acquired Infections

Patients who acquire an infection should be moved into individual isolation. If laboratory tests have been conducted and phage types have been determined, individuals with the same organism and phage type may be placed in a single isolation unit. The patient, his equipment, and his neighbor must all be considered to be contaminated and should be isolated until the patient shows no sign of infection.

Isolation Areas

When a patient is put into isolation, all personnel must adhere to the regulations imposed. The patient care area must be defined; and floor-to-ceiling walls are essential.

Isolation technique is ineffective in open wards since:

1. Man is a social being, and patients will not stay away from each other.
2. Curtains pulled around a patient will not serve as an effective barrier.

3. Sinks usually are at a considerable distance from the patient's bed; therefore, basins are used for handwashing and disinfecting of hands. The disinfectant is rapidly used up and the basin literally becomes a mass of contamination.
4. Special housekeeping procedures are not followed.

7-2-3   The Isolation Room

The isolation room should have its own lavatory and toilet facilities, at the front of the room. All personnel should perform a medical scrub before leaving the contaminated area. The room should be properly placarded "ISOLATION."

Reverse Isolation

Patients, such as burn victims and those suffering from leukemia, who are extremely susceptible to infections, are placed in protective or "reverse" isolation. The patient is usually placed between sterile sheets. Personnel perform medical scrubs and don sterile gloves, masks, caps, and gowns before entering the room.

The most recent advance in reverse isolation technique is the RES-Care (Regulated Environment for Safety Care) unit, which protects the patient from airborne microbes as well as those in the external environment. The patient is placed within a plastic tent, much like an oxygen tent, that encompasses the entire bed. Everything that goes into the tent is sterile. The tent is kept at maximum positive pressure while the patient is being placed into the bubble, to prevent air contamination. A private room is desirable for this unit, but it is not essential. No more than two units, however, should be housed in the same room.

Emotional support for the isolated patient, be he infected or not, is paramount in combating feelings of rejection and self-degradation. The patient in the RES-Care unit needs special attention, since physical contact is prohibited. Nursing personnel are directly responsible for psychological well-being of patients, especially those in isolation. Too often personnel tend to shy away from the isolated patients because of fear and ignorance. Communication between patient and personnel is important in determining how the patient feels and how emotional support may best be provided. Explanations of procedures and care should be thorough and understood by the patient.

Equipment and Materials

Equipment must not be removed without adequate disinfection. All patient equipment, such as thermometers, basins, bedpans, blood pressure apparatus, otoscopes, and stethoscopes, should stay within the unit. Patient charts should not be brought into the unit.

Disposables

Disposables tend to reduce the potential spread of infection. In isolation all disposables, whether they be plates or syringes, should immediately be placed in plastic or waterproof bags and then incinerated. Disposable needles should be stored in a used I.V. bottle until incineration.

Linens

Linens from isolation units should be double bagged. The laundry inner bag should be kept near the door within the isolation unit. The clean outer bag should be just outside of the unit. The interior bag should be made of soluble plastic. The outer one, which should be clearly marked "contaminated linen," should be made with a six inch overlapping flap and should only be two-thirds full. It is essential that this linen be transported separately and washed before sorting. Clean linens being returned to nurseries or reverse isolation units should be sterilized before use.

Human Wastes

Disposing of wastes, especially excreta, poses a real problem, especially for the isolation room without an adjacent bathroom. If toilet facilities are available adjacent to the isolation room, excreta may be emptied there. If the patient is ambulatory, he may use the toilet facilities. In this case, the toilet and toilet seat should be disinfected three times daily. If a hopper in a utility room is the only available receptacle for disposing of excreta, special precautions should be taken, especially when disposing of feces containing viral hepatitis organisms, salmonella or shigella organisms, or other infectious organisms.

Quality toilet tissue should be provided.

7-2-4 Patient Personal Hygiene

Patient personal hygiene is essential in preventing cross-contamination. When organisms are discharged in the feces of a patient who can care for himself, he should be instructed and supervised in thorough hand and nail cleaning techniques to prevent reinfection, or cross-infection. Nursing personnel must wash the hands of the patient who cannot care for himself, or who is incontinent.

Employee Protective Measures

The degree of infectiousness of the patient and the causative organism will determine how much isolation is necessary. However, the general controls of handwashing, masking, gowning, and gloving are always added protection if not always entirely necessary.

Nursing personnel, and others coming into close intimate contact with the patient, should wear a gown when providing care. Intimate contact includes such procedures as bathing, changing linens, giving the bedpan, providing physical therapy, doing a portable X-ray, etc. If the patient is incontinent of bowel movements and the organism is discharged in the feces, personnel should wear gloves. Disposable gloves are desirable since they are used only once and discarded. The nurse or doctor doing venapunctures should also wear gloves to prevent contamination, especially if the patient has viral hepatitis. Wearing gloves does not negate the need for the medical scrub when leaving the isolation room.

The mask should be worn when personnel care for patients who discharge organisms into the air. The mask may be made of cloth, double thickness; paper or plastic. It is ineffective when it gets damp or after 15–20 minutes. Double masking does not appreciably prolong its effectiveness. Masks should not be allowed to dangle about the neck of the wearer to contaminate him and those with whom he comes into contact. When in use, it should cover the nose and mouth.

Ventilation and Air Conditioning

Air-conditioning units have been known to spread bacterial contamination of the air. While the air conditioning is running, slime collects on the cooling coils. Bacteria may also collect there, finding a growth medium. When the air conditioning is turned off, the coils become warm; and the slime and bacteria dry and crack off to be spread throughout the entire ventilation system. Operating rooms, delivery rooms, reverse isolation units, and nurseries should have ventilating systems apart from that supplying other patients and nonpatient areas. These rooms should be under positive pressure. Isolation rooms for the infected patients should be under negative pressure.

7-2-5   Transportation

Infected Patients

Sometimes isolated patients have to be transported to other service areas in the hospital, such as X-ray or physical therapy. The patient should be scheduled. Immediately upon arrival he should be serviced rather than be allowed to lie in the hallway where he could contaminate everyone and everything. Clean sheets should be placed on the vehicle and the patient wrapped snugly in them. If the organism is airborne, the patient should wear a mask. The vehicle is then considered contaminated and should be disinfected before reuse. The room in the service area, into which the patient is taken, is contaminated and should be thoroughly disinfected before another patient enters. The transport personnel, as well as the service personnel, should be properly gowned at all times

Noninfected Patient in Reverse Isolation

The patient who is in reverse isolation may need treatment in other hospital departments, such as physical therapy. The patient should be scheduled and immediately serviced to prevent the acquisition of a super-infection. The reverse isolation technique applies in all areas where the patient is transported or serviced. Personnel should be gowned, masked, and gloved properly. The treatment room should be separate from other patient areas and should be properly pre-disinfected. Speed and asepsis are paramount when transporting a patient who is in reverse isolation. He should be provided with protective covering for his nose and mouth.

7-2-6   Discharge of Previously Infected Patients

If the patient is no longer infectious, he is either discharged from the hospital or taken out of isolation. Too often "taking out of isolation" means removing the placard, handling the linens as any other linen, and proceeding with regular care. The patient is left in his contaminated room and bed. The patient should be bathed with a soap containing hexachlorophene, and his hair shampooed. He should then be placed in clean clothes and transferred to a clean room. The isolation room should then be terminally disinfected.

If an infected patient is discharged from the hospital or treated at home, the family may readily become contaminated and show various clinical symptoms related to that organism. To reduce contamination in the environment, the family should use soap containing hexachlorophene. If the acquisition of a soap dispenser is impossible, individual bar soap should be used and discarded after one use. The hands should be washed frequently. Intimate contact with food should be avoided. All family members should be instructed in handwashing methods. Small children should be supervised. Linens should be disinfected in a chlorine solution, such as clorox, before laundering. The infected individual should not wear an article of clothing twice before it is laundered. Hand towels should be used only once; paper towels should be used wherever possible. Plastic mattresses and pillow cases should be used on all beds. Each child, if infected, should have his own bed and not be allowed to go from bed to bed.

Showers should be used whenever possible, and disinfected after each use. Water should be left running in bath tubs instead of accumulating. The infected individual should shower last. Toilet seats and other fixtures should be disinfected after each use. Hot water and a detergent-disinfectent should be used.

Paper products should be used whenever possible. Dressings and disposables should be placed immediately into plastic or waterproof paper bags and sealed, instead of accumulating in waste baskets to be strewn around by pets or small children. The house should be aired regularly. Visitors should be kept to a minimum.

The public health nurse is the key figure in home counseling when infection invades a family. Her responsibility includes teaching hygienic household measures, supervising the family in carrying out such measures, and providing support and hope for the infected individuals.

7-2-7   The Deceased Infected Patient

If the patient dies while he is infected, the body should be wrapped snugly in a sheet for transportation to the morgue. While en route to the morgue, personnel should be properly gowned. The body should leave the unit via the nearest elevator and not be allowed to lie in the hallway. If an autopsy is performed, isolation techniques of gowning, masking, and gloving should be enforced. The body should be handled carefully and closed adequately, so that body fluids do not escape. The casket should be sealed. The morgue should then be disinfected as any other room to prevent the spread of organisms on clean bodies that are autopsied. If the patient was even suspected to be infectious, precautions should be taken.

7-2-8   Preventive Techniques

The Medical Scrub

1. Remove jewelry, rings, watches, etc.
2. Turn on faucet. (Running water is essential.)
3. Wet hands.

4. Soap hands and wash them. Use much friction. Begin with hands, move to wrists, then to elbows (be sure to clean well between fingers and around thumb).
5. Rinse. (Rinse hands, arms to elbow, letting water run off the elbow.)
6. Clean nails under running water. Use orange stick and discard.
7. Repeat steps 4, 5, 6.
8. Dry hands. Blot water from hands to elbow with one paper towel. Use second paper towel to finish drying.
9. Turn off faucet. Use second paper towel if knee-action control is absent.

Gowning: Discard Method

1. Don gown before entering isolation room. Overlap the back flaps and tie strings.
2. "Roll out" of gown just before leaving isolation room
   a. Untie the waist strings.
   b. Untie the neck strings (being careful to touch only the strings).
   c. Grasp the gown, cross-armed, at the shoulders.
   d. Roll out of the gown, turning the outside in.
   e. Roll the gown, holding it away from the uniform and discard it.
   f. Do a medical scrub.
   g. Remove mask (touching only the strings).

Changing the Mask While Contaminated

1. Push up gown sleeves, touching only the outside of the cuff.
2. Wash the hands and wrists (be thorough) using much friction.
3. Untie mask strings (be careful to touch only the strings, holding arms away from the face).
4. Discard mask into proper container. (Container lid should be operated by a foot pedal.)
5. Don clean mask.
6. Push sleeves of gown back into place.
7. Continue task.

Care of Excreta

If excreta must be carried to a hopper outside the isolation room, precautions must be taken:

1. Cover bedpan *completely* with disposable plastic cover or newspaper.
2. Open hopper door with foot pedal.
3. Uncover and place bedpan inside hopper.
4. Close hopper door.
5. Using paper towel to protect clean handles, flush the hopper 3–5 times.
6. Incinerate bedpan covering.
7 Using paper towel, remove bedpan from hopper. Be sure all fecal matter is removed!

8. Immerse bedpan in 200 parts per million chlorine solution for 15 minutes or steam clean in automatic unit for three minutes before returning it to the patient's room.
9. Return to isolation room to finish task.

7-2-9   Education and Training

There is a great need for continuous in-service training, which relates to the spread of disease, for all personnel in all areas of the hospital. Techniques of gowning, masking, handwashing, food handling, waste disposal, linen handling, and various nursing procedures have to be taught. These presentations should be followed by practical training in the hospital, close supervision, immediate retraining where necessary, and long range periodic scheduled review sessions.

7-2-10   Summary

Several problems in the care of isolation patients have been identified: the admission of infected patients; the definition of the isolation area; the care of contaminated equipment and wastes; personnel and patient hygiene; the transportation of isolated patients; and the discharge of infected or once infected patients. Protective techniques have been recommended for controlling cross-contamination. Regular in-service education programs for personnel have been strongly recommended. With newer strains of organisms causing infections, personnel must be kept abreast of new techniques for preventing cross-contamination. Isolation and reverse isolation techniques should be learned and carried out with comfort and skill. The control of hospital acquired infection is a direct function of the use of modern medical techniques and the cooperative efforts of an informed staff.

REFERENCES AND SELECTED READINGS

Brown, Regina, and Wapner, Myra, A family's battle with staphylococcus, *American Journal of Nursing*, 64: 136, September 1964.

Colbeck, J. C. *Control of Infections in Hospitals*. Chicago: American Hospital Association, 1962.

Foster, Marion, A positive approach to medical asepsis, *American Journal of Nursing*, 62: 76–77, April 1962.

Ginsberg, Miriam K. and LaConte, Marie L. Reverse isolation, *American Journal of Nursing*, 64: 88–90, September 1964.

Gordon, J. E. (Ed.), *Control of Communicable Diseases in Man*. 10th ed., New York: The American Public Health Association, 1965.

Henderson, J. *Emergency Medical Guide.* New York: McGraw-Hill Book Co., 1963.

Jones, Julia M. A new view on breaking the chain of TB infection, *Bulletin,* 2–5, November 1967.

Kline, Patricia A. Isolating patients with staphylococcal infections, *American Journal of Nursing,* 65: 102–104, January 1965.

LaBoccetta, A. C. Halting the spread of infectious disease, *Hospitals,* 30: 68–69, September 16, 1956.

McClain, M. Esther and Gragg, Shirley Hawke, *Scientific Principles in Nursing.* 5th ed., St. Louis: C. V. Mosby Co., 1962.

National League for Nursing, *Nursing the Patient in Isolation: Policies and Procedures.* N.L.N., 1963.

New York State Department of Health, *Guide for the Handling of Communicable Diseases in Hospitals.* Bureau of Epidemiology and Communicable Disease Control, 1950.

Nichols, Glennadee A. Environmental stress: the isolated patient, *ANA Clinical Sessions,* New York: Appleton-Century-Crofts, Inc., 1966.

Nichols, Leola, When Staph comes home to roost, *American Journal of Nursing,* 63: 75–78, April 1963.

Prevention of Hospital Infection. London: The Royal Society of Health, 1963.

Sinton, Eleanor, Hardy, R., McCormick, Nell Vane, and Sheldon, Elnor C. Fingertip culture tests and handwashing instructions lower infection rates, *Hospitals,* 38: 63–65, May 16, 1964.

Smith, Alice L. *Principles of Microbiology.* 5th ed., St. Louis: C.V. Mosby Co., 1965.

Top, F. H. *Communicable and Infectious Diseases,* 5th ed., St. Louis: C.V. Mosby Co., 1964.

Uyeda, C. T. Successful ways of controlling infections, *Hospitals,* 37: 79–82, 96, July 1, 1963.

7-3 MICROBIOLOGICAL TESTING, AIR AND SURFACE SAMPLING TECHNIQUES

7-3-1 Introduction

The hospital and related medical care facilities present an environmental complex with animate components—patients, medical staff, support personnel, and visitors—in close, interacting relationships with an inanimate environment. A prime concern in the management of this complex is the control of microbial components with efforts to restrict or eliminate the transmission of bacterial, viral, and fungal agents from person to person, from persons to the environment, and from the environment to persons. The major route of transmitting microbial agents is by direct personal contact, a route of transfer that is controllable to varying degrees by barrier techniques of various designs. Protection of food and water supplies likewise are controllable to a high degree both during their initial processing and storage as well as in their distribution under standard conditions. These conditions should permit no, or limited, contact with potential sources of contamination.

Air as an environmental element has dynamic and random contact with both animate and inanimate components of the environment. Contact comes through air masses moving in patterns of natural and directed ventilation with exposure to patients, staff, and areas of various levels of contamination. Even in select areas requiring high levels of environmental contamination control, e.g., surgery, newborn nursery, intensive care, burns treatment areas, staff personnel and patients are constant sources of contamination of the clean air deliverable to these areas by presently available air handling methods.

The quantitative and qualitative determination of airborne microbial contamination has not been correlated with the frequency of cross-infection in the hospital to the extent that provides a predictive basis for evaluation. There are varying opinions of the relative importance of the air in transmitting infection in the hospital. However, lack of agreement not withstanding, there would be few who would not include air in considering the total environmental complex and its possible role in nosocomial infections.

7-3-2   Review of Basic Aerobiology

Particle Size and Aerodynamics

Settling velocity of viable airborne particles is fundamental to understanding their behavior, and practical importance in air hygiene and in control methods. Velocity can be expressed by Stoke's Law which gives the rate of fall of a small sphere in a viscous fluid as a function of the radius and density of the particle and the density and viscosity of the fluid (air). Since the density and viscosity of room air at normal temperatures are nearly constant, the relationship between settling rate and diameter of particles of unit density can be expressed as: $V = 0.006d^2$; where V is in feet per minute, and d is in microns. For practical usage when applied to particles in the size range found in intramural air, this formula gives an easily applied estimation of the relationship between particle size and settling velocity.

Since the shape and composition of viable airborne particles recovered from intramural air are not known, their exact size cannot be determined by settling rate, but approximation can be made by expressing particle size in terms of equivalent spherical diameter, viz., the size of a naturally occurring viable particle equal to that of a sphere of unit density and having the same settling velocity in still air. In normal usage, reference to particle diameter has this definition. It should be remarked that still air conditions are unlikely in the intramural environment where particle size determinations based on settling rate of naturally occurring particles might be carried out.

Particles of interest in air hygiene can be sized in broad categories represented by dust, droplets, and droplet nuclei. Dust-borne bacteria are usually associated with particles greater than 10 microns in diameter and occur characteristically in the size range 12–18 microns (Hatch, 1961). Sizes of droplets vary from less than 10 microns in diameter to over 100 microns with a mean size between 10 and 20 microns (Duguid, 1946a). In the early years of interest in airborne contagion, it was assumed that the large droplets containing microorganisms expelled during a sneeze or cough settled rapidly to the floor in the immediate vicinity of their source. However, droplets evaporate rapidly, droplets smaller than *c*. 80 microns in diameter exposed to 90% relative humidity have been shown to evaporate before falling a distance of six feet, leaving a residual "droplet nucleus" a few microns in diameter (Wells, 1934). Particles of diameter less than 10 microns are within the size range normally classified as droplet nuclei.

Viable airborne particles occur in a range of sizes which are distributed about a median diameter size in a naturally occurring particle population. The count median diameter (CMD), and standard deviation about the CMD can be determined from a plot of the cumulated size distribution on probability graph scale, arithmetic or logarithmic, depending on the distribution (Wolf, *et al.*, 1959).

Survival of Airborne Microorganisms

Disappearance of airborne viable particles from the air is a function of size (settling rate), removal by ventilation (room air volume change rate), and biological decay (death). Experimental studies of airborne microorganisms, particularly bacteria, have shown that air temperature, relative humidity, physiological age of the bacterial cells, conditions of growth, storage effect on the airborne organism, gaseous composition of the supporting atmosphere, radiation, and kind of microorganism are important factors affecting survival. Methods of producing the microbial aerosol, suspending fluid for atomization, and methods of collection of the aerosol are additional variables that must be considered in working with bacterial aerosols under experimental as well as field conditions. Comparative evaluation of published results from studies of factors affecting survival is difficult because of differences in procedures and the recognized interaction of variables affecting survival.

Evaluation of most factors known to affect survival is not possible for those viable particles collected from intramural air. Such particles originate from various sources and present heterogenous but unknown biological and physical histories. However, intramural environmental parameters of temperature and relative humidity are usually controlled, and are measurable for inclusion as part of the environmental data obtainable during air sampling.

The influence of temperature on the viability of airborne microorganisms is small as compared to the effects of relative humidity (Hemmes, 1960). Limited data suggest, however, that biological die-away of microbial aerosols increases with temperature. Low relative humidities have been reported favorable for survival of airborne vaccinia (Harper, 1961), influenza (Harper, 1961; Hemmes, 1960; Loosli, 1943), measles (DeJong, 1964), Venezuelan equine encephalomyelitis virus (Harper, 1961), and unfavorable to the survival of poliomyelitis virus (Harper, 1961; Hemmes, 1960). However, relative optimal recovery at high and low relative humidities has been reported for influenza (Shechmeister, 1950) and Columbia SK viruses (Akers, 1966).

Intermediate range of relative humidity has been reported to be most harmful for pneumococci, hemolytic streptococci (Dunklin, *et al.*, 1948), and *Serratia marcescens* (Kethley, *et al.*, 1957). Optimal recovery of airborne *S. marcescens* has been reported for this organism exposed to conditions of high relative humidity (Kethley, *et al.*, 1957; Webb, *et al.*, 1964) while low relative humidity as an optimal condition has been reported for *Salmonella pullorum* (DeOrme, 1944) and *Klebsiella pneumoniae*, Type A (Goldberg, *et al.*, 1958). Goldberg (*ibid.*) found *Staphylococcus albus*, *Pseudomonas sp.*, *Pseudomallei sp.*, *Pasteurella pestis* to occupy this comparative order of decreasing stability in air at 68–72% relative humidity. Strasters, *et al.* (1966) found a threefold decrease in the biological decay rate of a hospital strain of staphylococcus at 75% relative humidity compared to the decay rate at 39% relative humidity. Wide variation in the effect of relative humidity depended on several conditions of experimental procedure, but there was no indication that "epidemic" strains survive better than other strains under these conditions.

Prediction of the response of a particular microorganism to the airborne state based upon a comparison with that of similar microorganism(s) studied under experimental conditions should be done with caution because of multiple factors influencing survival.

Diseases Naturally Transmitted by the Airborne Route

Pathogenic microorganisms are transmitted from a host by direct contact; indirect airborne transfer of viable dust particles dispersed into the air from reservoirs of contaminated surfaces, clothing, and bedding as a result of human activity; droplet-nuclei; and direct droplet infection.

Airborne droplets containing infectious microorganisms have been classed as one form of direct or contact transmission (Langmuir, 1965). The short projection distance of droplets expelled by sneezing or coughing and the requirement that a recipient host be in close vicinity for transfer of the droplets before they are removed from the air by gravitational settling, are considered part of the direct transmission pattern. This does not take into account, however, the demonstrated high rate of evaporation of droplets which produces droplet-nuclei from the majority of the particles formed in a sneeze before they have fallen two feet (Wells, 1934). This settling distance as a function of particle size and evaporation rates, seems little affected by the range of relative humidity usually encountered in occupied spaces (Riley, *et al.*, 1961).

The distinction of size among the several designations of airborne particles related to natural airborne infections, pertains to their responsiveness to ventilation effects and to their deposition in the respiratory tract of the host. Particles in the size range of 0.25 to 0.5 micron are poorly retained in the lung. Efficiency of retention increases for particles above and below this range. Below 0.25–0.5 micron retention approaches 100%; above 0.5 micron, highest deposition of inhaled particles occurs in the one to two micron size range, with gradual reduction in retention as the particle size increases to 10 microns (Hatch, 1961). Larger particles, which are often more common and often contain larger numbers of microorganisms, may be of more concern in contamination of skin surfaces or open wounds. Droplet-nuclei are less than 10 microns in diameter; dust 10–100 microns in diameter with perhaps a small percentage of overlap of particles slightly less than 10 microns; and droplet particles which are over 100 microns in diameter (Wells, 1955). With these distinctions to emphasize airborne infection carried by small particles, airborne infection in nature includes psittacosis, Q fever, pulmonary tuberculosis, brucellosis, anthrax, histoplasmosis, pneumonic forms of plague and tularemia (Langmuir, 1965). The airborne route is also considered as one means of transmitting the viruses of measles (DeJong, 1964) and smallpox (MacCallum, *et al.*, 1950; Downie, 1951).

7-3-3 Hospital Environment

Animate Environment

Air as a natural transmission route of certain infectious diseases occurring among susceptibles within a normal population operates also in the hospital environment. A significant distinction between the normal population at large and the hospital patient population is the elevated susceptibility to infection that frequently exists among this latter group. In this regard, the role of the air can be extended beyond the transmission of a relatively limited number of infectious diseases to include its potential as a significant transfer medium of potentially infectious microorganisms. Susceptibility to infection varies among individual patients and groups, some representing increased susceptibility to infection resulting from impairment by disease of normal body protective defenses. Certain chemical and radiological therapies reduce the effective level of the immune response; surgical procedures of increasing complexity in restorative repair—open heart, organ transplant—have affected the actual and potential capability of extending the duration of patients' lives but have also incurred an increased potential of infection.

The patient population as an aggregation of individuals of varying susceptibilities to infection as well as individuals who are sources of infectious microorganisms, comprise a major element of the animate environment. Staff and support personnel in contact with the patient population also represent potential or active infection sources and carrier state reservoirs of infectious microorganisms

Methods to control transmission of infectious contamination in the hospital environment for protection of patients should also include safeguards for protection of staff personnel. Hospital-acquired infection by hospital personnel is an occupational risk and its recognition is an important element in implementing policies of employee safety. Increasing participation in patient care functions by subprofessional and nonprofessional staff presents additional requirements for actively directed control methods to reduce exposure risk to staff and prevent transmission of contamination to patients and patient care areas of the hospital. The animate environment is central to the relation of air hygiene and other segments of the hospital environment to the definition and control of nosocomial infections.

Inanimate Environment

The random dynamics and rapid contamination transport capability of air are unique qualities of this environmental element. Observations on transport of microbial particles within multistoried buildings have shown that contamination released in the basement is detectable within minutes in air circulating along corridors of the floors above, being conveyed by ventilation drafts caused by open stairwells and vertical shafts (Walter, 1958; Wells, 1935). Comparable transport of contamination has been observed in laundry chutes (Hurst, *et al.*, 1958; Michaelsen, 1964). Riley, *et al.* (1959) demonstrated the effectiveness of airborne tuberculosis cross-infection in air, transported in a ventilation system connecting the cases of acquired infection with those of infection sources.

Horizontal surfaces such as floors have been considered inanimate reservoirs of infectious particulate contamination, shed from human sources and related to airborne microorganisms as a contamination source generated through personnel activity (Walter, *et al.*, 1960). Resuspension of particles into the air is produced by mechanical dislodgement and agitation as a result of personnel activities. The size of these particles, principally dust, cause their resettlement in the absence of air currents, a condition not usually found in occupied, ventilated rooms. However, particles of 30 microns diameter settling at approximately five feet per minute in still air, could be transported throughout an average size room or beyond by the combined effects of turbulence and ventilation air currents. Studies of particle transport in an experimental room under normal ventilation conditions, have demonstrated lateral transport of 50 microns diameter particles as much as eight feet in the room (Kethley, *et al.*, 1963). Theoretically, room air currents could keep particles of unit density and 90 microns diameter in the airborne state (Corn, *et al.*, 1967). Room air velocities under draft-free conditions are unlikely to produce air re-entrainment of viable particles on exposed surfaces. The most likely mechanism remains the mechanical translation of personnel activities to contaminated surfaces.

7-3-4 Sources of Microbial Air Contaminants

Personnel Activity

Room areas requiring a high level of environmental control such as surgery and the newborn nursery will show low levels of airborne contamination when these areas are closed and unoccupied by personnel. However, when the area is occupied, the principal source of airborne contamination is introduced and aided in dispersal by personnel activities.

It has not been possible thus far to establish a close correlation between numbers of airborne microbial particles, numbers of personnel, and measures of activity. This is particularly difficult in the general areas of the hospital because of the multiple sources and high levels of airborne contaminants. In areas of high environmental control where sources of contamination are principally personnel, there have been reports of a significant relationship between the traffic count in areas such as the surgical corridor and the numbers of airborne microbial particles (Nimeck, *et al.*, 1959). Air samples of the exhaust air from an operating room during an operation have shown that the bacterial count fluctuated with the degree of activity in the room and was from two to ten times as high as in the air delivered to the room (Warner, *et al.*, 1963).

The handling of contaminated textiles such as bed linens and blankets can be a prolific source of airborne contamination. Rubbo, *et al.* (1962) using a marker organism, *S. citreus*, in a surgical ward demonstrated wide dispersion of this organism as a contaminant on cotton and woolen blankets. Blankets artificially contaminated with staphylococci and manipulated in a clean room according to routine use, were shown to disperse airborne viable particles settling out at distances of from one to eight feet from the source blanket (Anderson, *et al.*, 1959). Rubbo, *et al.* (1960) found the staphylococcal count as well as the total bacterial count to be relatively constant up to the nine foot height above the floor. The measurable fiber constant of the air fell off markedly with increasing height, and approached a constant level between approximately four to nine feet above the floor. It appeared that airborne organisms were seldom carried on the large woolen fibers. The term "fibre nuclei" was introduced in the postulate that airborne transmission of organisms takes place through the movement of free organisms, or organisms attached to microscopic fibers, the fibre nuclei probably consisting of cellulose, a large component of hospital dust. The significance of textiles, especially blankets, as sources of infection has not been clearly established. Although disinfection of blankets has been shown to reduce considerably *S. aureus* contamination of the air in the hospital ward, it did not reduce nasal colonization of patients (Caplan, 1962), nor was there evidence that blankets contaminated with Group A streptococci from nasal carriers caused respiratory infection among a large group of healthy men (Perry, *et al.*, 1957).

Transport of contaminated textiles from a patient area for processing should be done in a manner to prevent further dissemination of contaminants into the air. The use of chute systems for transporting laundry and refuse can be a source of contamination if the system is improperly designed (Hurst, *et al.*, 1958).

Cleaning methods are not only important in maintaining high levels of environmental hygiene, but can be a source of airborne microbial contamination. Methods generating the suspension of dust in the air have no place in environmental maintenance procedures for the hospital and the use of machine aids in cleaning, such as vacuum devices should be designed with adequate filtration for removal of small viable particles from the exhaust air stream (Wheeler, *et al.*, 1962; Allen, 1959).

Human Sources

Staff personnel and patients are highly significant sources of microbial contamination shed into the environment. Pathogenic organisms can be expelled from the nasopharynx by coughing and sneezing (Duguid, 1946b). The skin and clothing are also sources of large numbers of air-borne bacteria, slight to vigorous activity liberating 1000–10,000 bacteria-carrying dust particles per minute (Duguid, *et al.*, 1948).

It has been found that some carriers of *Staphylococcus aureus* contaminate the air with much larger numbers of these organisms than the majority of carriers, even when wearing sterile protective clothing. These individuals are "dispersers" (Hare, *et al.*, 1956). A higher frequency of "dispersers" and a greater profusion of shed bacteria in men than in women, has been reported (Bethune, *et al.*, 1965). The skin is the direct source of most of the bacterial particles arising from noninfected human sources, and in the absence of a sneeze or cough, the naso-pharynx contributes a minor fraction of the total shed into the environment. Although bathing appears to increase the numbers of viable particles shed, protective clothing of tight weave and applications to the skin are effective controls (Bernard, *et al.*, 1965a, 1965b; Speers, *et al.*, 1965). Increase in shedding rates continues five to six hours after washing, and tends to increase with increasing bacterial skin surface population. The rate of shedding varies with the individual and from day-to-day with the same individual (Heldman, *et al.*, 1967).

Air contamination with *S. aureus* has been traced to single patients ("dispersers") on wards where "broadcasts" of this organisms occurred (Noble, 1962). Perineal carriers of *S. aureus* (Ridley, 1959; Hare, *et al.*, 1958) and of streptococci (McKee, 1966) have been reported to be significant sources of airborne contamination by these organisms and to disperse greater numbers of staphylococci into the air than nasal carriers, although the majority of *S. aureus* on the skin of nasal carriers are derived from the nasal vestibule (Solberg, 1965). Frequency of skin contamination and air contamination during activities, appears correlated in those patients who are nasal carriers of larger numbers of staphylococci (White, 1961).

Further examples are found among patients with skin diseases who have been shown to be "dispersers" of streptococci (Loosli, *et al.*, 1950) and staphylococci (Cooke, *et al.*, 1963; Thomas, *et al.*, 1961), even from patients with significant but clinically inapparent infections of dermatological lesions (Selwyn, *et al.*, 1965). Infected lesions are sources of airborne microbial contamination if not covered, and during removal of the dressing cover the potential for aerial dissemination of dried infectious discharges is considerable (Thom, *et al.*, 1962; Hare, *et al.*, 1961; Shooter, *et al.*, 1958).

Air-Handling Systems

Cooling coils and other parts of the air-conditioning and ventilation system where moisture and dissolved nutrients present potential growth conditions are sources of contaminating microorganisms (Solberg, *et al.*, 1956). The significance of microbial contaminants from humidifier water as an infection source is not known, but efforts should be made to remove this potential source of risk (Blowers, *et al.*, 1962). Cole, *et al.* (1964) found a decrease in numbers of *E. coli*, *S. aureus*, beta-streptococci, *Bacillus sp.* under conditions simulating those found on direct expansion air-conditioning coils at 14°C and in coil condensate warmed intermittently to room temperature. Direct contamination of the cooling fins and coils and *S. aureus* resulted in the rapid disappearance of these bacteria, and the conclusion was made that the direct expansion air-conditioning coils of the window type unit are an unlikely source of airborne contamination. Many organisms isolated from the condensate of cooling coils or humidification units have not been associated with infection. *Pseudomonas aeruginosa* is a notable exception. This microorganism has adaptability to wide conditions of growth, and has been reported as a heavy contaminant of water associated with the cooling system and recovered from the air passing through the system (Anderson, 1959).

One survey of hospital air conditioning units showed that approximately 24% of the units contained *S. aureus* and approximately 63% of the units located in the nurseries contained *S. aureus* (Shaffer, *et al.*, 1962). Adequate maintenance should insure that such equipment does not become a source of gross contamination that might be transported to areas containing patients of high infection susceptibility.

Patient Equipment

Equipment for assisted breathing, maintaining high humidity breathing air, and administration of medication through the formation of fine particle aerosols can be a potential source of infectious contaminated liquid aerosols. However, inhalation equipment not incorporating aerosolization units have been considered to present no greater risk of infection than room air (Reinarz, *et al.*, 1965). Rubbo, *et al.* (1966) found heavy contamination of a suction apparatus and tubing by *Pseudomonas aeruginosa* in the course of a serious outbreak of infection in a premature nursery and demonstrated that this apparatus could also disseminate the organism as an aerosol.

Neonatal infections with *Pseudomonas aeruginosa* have been reported associated with contaminated resuscitation equipment (Bassett, *et al.*, 1965); others have reported dissemination of airborne microorganisms by a surgical pump (Ranger, *et al.*, 1958). Humidification components of inhalation equipment are the principal sites of gross contamination which in addition to *Pseudomonas aeruginosa* have been reported to include *Escherichia, Achromobacter, Alcaligenes faecalis, Staphylococcus aureus, S. viridans, enterococci*, yeasts and fungi (Sever, 1959); *Flavobacterium* sp., *Herellea* sp., *Alcaligenes* sp., *Achromobacter* sp., *Pseudomonas* (Reinarz, *et al.*, 1965); and *Klebsiella pneumoniae*, Type II, presumably having occurred in the nebulizer solution contaminated by an inhalation therapist who was a carrier of this organism (Mertz, *et al.*, 1967). Inhalation therapy equipment has been reported by others to be a source of cross-infection (Phillips, *et al.*, 1965) and a potential source of infection in Gram-negative pneumonias (Edmundson, *et al.*, 1966; Linton, *et al.*, 1965; Pierce, *et al.*, 1966).

7-3-5   Nature and Size of Airborne Microbial Contaminants

Microscopic examinations have shown flake-like particles recovered from the air which morphologically resemble skin scales but include also a number of fiber-like particles. These fibers consist essentially of cellulose (Pressley, 1958) and have been found to contain coagulase positive *Staphylococcus aureus* (Pressley, 1958; Gardner, *et al.*, 1960). The size distribution of bacterial particles dispersion by textiles is the same as that of the particles which contaminate the textiles (Rubbo, *et al.*, 1963). Small particles which do not settle do not contribute to residual contamination of the environment and are subject to the removal from the room by ventilation.

Particles of desquamated skin with a mean equivalent diameter of *c*. 8 microns have been reported from ward air; however, no estimate was made of the diameter of skin particles carrying bacteria (Davies, *et al.*, 1962). Airborne viable particles obtained from a dermatological ward have been reported to be in the range of 4 to more than 50 microns in diameter (Selwyn, 1965).

The size distribution of airborne particles carrying *S. aureus* has been reported to be relatable to the diagnosed disease of the skin producing these particles. In psoriasis 78% of the viable staphylococcal particles were greater than 8 microns; in eczema the majority (39%) were found in the range 10–18 microns. In other diagnosed skin diseases, 53% of the particle size distribution was found to be larger than 18 microns (Selwyn, *et al.*, 1965).

A difference in particle size associated with different types of bacteria has been reported from the measurement of airborne bacterial particles in a nursery for the newborn. The mean equivalent diameter of viable particles carrying *S. aureus* were found to be 16, 18.5 and 24 microns; viable airborne particles carrying group G streptococci were 5, 7, and 7.5 microns in diameter (Hughes, 1963). The number of staphylococci per particle in hospital ward air during quiet periods and during periods of activity have indicated on the average about 4 cocci per particle; over the particle size range of less than 4 microns to more than 18, the number of cocci increased from 1 to 6 with increasing particle size (Lidwell, *et al.*, 1959).

The "cloud-baby" reported by Eichenwald, *et al.* (1960) contaminated the air from the respiratory tract as a result of a bacterial-viral inter-action, the skin and clothing presenting a minor source of contamina-tion. Determination of sizes of particles dispersed by these babies under conditions of minimum personnel activity indicated that the airborne particles were almost entirely less than 5 microns in diameter. The majority of babies studied possessed low indices of infectivity or con-tagiousness while a small minority were highly infectious to others.

The size of airborne staphylococcal particles disseminated by a carrier, who was the source of airborne wound infections incurred during surgery, was made by Walter, *et al.* (1963). The carrier dressed and undressed under controlled conditions in a cubicle from which air samples were taken with the Anderson sampler. The count median diameter (CMD) of the particles was 5.3 microns. Shaking the carrier's woolen suit jacket, trousers, and laboratory coat under the same con-ditions produced airborne viable particles having a count median diameter (CMD) of 8.2 microns. The particle diameter indicated by these studies may be related to the time sequence of taking air samples during the last five minutes of a fifteen minute period during which the larger particles might have been removed by gravitational settling. The possible role of airborne staphylococci in surgical wound infections has emphasized the presence or absence of large staphylococcal-bearing particles, and it is of especial interest that this well documented case study implicated particles of diameters within the range of droplet-nuclei.

Noble, *et al.* (1963) reported diameters of airborne bacterial particles on hospital wards in the range of 13.3–15.7 microns with 25% of the particles of the cloud being less than 8 microns, and 25% greater than 20 microns in equivalent diameter. These authors also reported equivalent diameters of airborne fungi in the range 3–13 microns with 25% smaller than 2 microns, and 25% larger than 15 microns. Many fungi appear to be present in the air as single spores. These results indicate that organisms associated with human disease or carriage are usually found on particles in the range of 4–20 microns in equivalent spherical diameter.

7-3-6 Analytical Methods

Aerobiology

Sampling systems designed to determine the viable particulate contamination in the air are based upon two broad requirements: (1) the physical recovery of the particle from air, and (2) the culture system required to demonstrate the viability of the microorganisms associated with the particle. A number of sampling devices have been developed to meet these requirements, but many have been restricted mostly to the experimental laboratory and have not found wide application in intramural field studies. Review of air samplers, necessary auxiliary equipment, and operational methods have been published (Wolf, *et al.*, 1959; Batchelor, 1960).

There are several air sampling devices available from commercial sources that are very useful in determining the counts of airborne particulate contamination in intramural air. These samplers take in a measured volume of room air and remove the suspended microbial particles by filtration, impingement or impaction — mechanisms of collection that permit categorizing the various samplers under the following headings:

Impaction-Type Samplers. The slit-type sampler design is incorporated in three commercially available samplers that provide the most useful instruments for most requirements in intramural air sampling. The principle of operation of these samplers is the drawing of a measured volume of air through a slit positioned at a fixed distance above an impaction or collection surface. As a particle in the incoming air stream is accelerated by passage through the restricting slit, it impacts on the receiving surface as a result of inertial force. This impaction surface, in samplers used to collect viable airborne particles, is usually an agar medium containing necessary growth supporting nutrients. Coincident impaction of particles onto the same area is prevented by rotating the impaction surface at a constant rate beneath the slit so that the deposited material will be spread out over a continuous track. This sampler design permits the determination of airborne contamination with time, and permits a correlation of contamination levels and personnel activity. The Reyniers, Casella, and TDL air samplers are representative of the slit-type sampler.

Another impaction-type sampler that is very useful for the determination of particle size is the Andersen sampler (Andersen, 1958). This sampler consists of a cascaded arrangement of six stages, each stage consisting of a sieve plate of several hundred holes of the same diameter through which the air sample is drawn, accelerating the airborne particle for impaction on an agar surface beneath each sieve plate. Succeeding stages of the sampler contain progressively smaller hole diameters and as the air sample passes from one stage to another, the velocity of the air jet is increased with the result of collecting progressively smaller particles. Each stage is calibrated in terms of sizes of particles collected which enables a particle size distribution to be made from the microbial colony count occurring on each stage (Wolf, *et al.*, 1959). This sampler has been proposed as a reference standard sampler for viable particles in low airborne concentration, and when sizes of particles are being determined (Brachman, *et al.*, 1964).

Microbial colonies growing on the agar surface represent particles containing one or more viable microorganisms and can be reported in terms of colony forming units per cubic foot of air (cfu/ft^3). The Reyniers, TDL, Andersen, and Casella impaction samplers operate at one cubic foot per minute (28.3 lpm); also available is a model of the Casella sampler that has a sampling flow rate of *c.* 25 cubic feet per minute (700 lpm).

Impinger-Type Sampler. The high velocity liquid impinger has high efficiency and effectiveness in collection and demonstration of viable airborne microbial particles. An example is the All Glass Impinger (AGI), particularly the AGI-30 which operates at 12.5 liters of air per minute. This sampler has been proposed as a reference standard sampler (Brachman, *et al.*, 1964). It is commercially available, as part of a hospital contamination analysis kit, from the Millipore Filter Corporation.*

A disadvantage of this sampler is the low rate of air sampling—an important limitation under conditions of low concentrations of airborne

*Millipore Filter Corporation, Bedford, Massachusetts.

contaminants. This limitation can be removed, in part, by increasing the number of sampler units operating simultaneously to obtain a representative sample of the room air. Some loss of viability may occur among collected bacterial cells because of the high velocity of the impinging air jet and because of extended continuous operation.

During the collection process, the microbial particles will tend to be disrupted by the force of impingement. A single particle containing multiple cells may produce more than one bacterial colony when the collection medium is cultured. The results, therefore, are more indicative of the number of viable cells in contrast to the number of colony-forming units (cfu) reported from the solid surface, impaction-type sampler.

Filtration-Type Sampler. Various applications of the filtration principle have been made, and one of the most useful for intramural surveillance is the membrane filter. This is a very efficient collector of airborne particles, but its effectiveness of demonstrating viable microorganisms is restricted by the desiccation effect on the organisms collected on the filter surface. It can be useful for sampling in situations where a small device is required to avoid interference with a procedure being carried out on a patient, and when a limited volume air sample is adequate.

A vacuum source is required to operate volumetric samplers and should provide volume and vacuum capacity meeting requirements of the particular type sampler. During operation, the sampler should be connected to flowrator, critical-orifice, or manometer for measurement and regulation of the volume, and rate of air sampling. Periodic calibration of sampler systems should be done for accuracy and to insure a leak-free system. Detailed guidance in instrument calibration can be found in *Sampling Microbiological Aerosols* (Wolf, *et al.*, 1959).

Sedimentation. The standard Petri dish containing a suitable nutrient medium in an agar base has been widely used as a semiquantitative air sampler because of its availability, cheapness, and simplicity of use. Collection of viable airborne particles by the open Petri dish depends upon the gravitational settling of the particle and because of this, when used under normal intramural conditions will discriminate against the small particles that remain airborne and transported about by air currents. Theoretically, if the settling plate is exposed to airborne contaminants in still air with only the effect of gravity acting on the suspended particles and zero biological decay, the settling plate would eventually collect all particles in a closed column of air above the exposed surface. However, for many applications the settling plate can be used to advantage and has been suggested as the sampler of choice when employed under certain conditions and recognized restrictions on the evaluation of the air counts obtained (Kethley, *et al.*, 1967). Settling plates were reported by Wellman, *et al.* (1965) as a practical method for establishing the baseline of bacterial contamination in two nonsurgical patient areas of a hospital.

Routine monitoring of microbial contamination of the air should include basic data of: the location of the sampler; the time of day the sample was taken; the volume of air sampled; the nature of the collection medium; temperature and relative humidity of the air; record of number and activity of personnel; particle size distribution; and the air count reported as the number of colony-forming units per cubic foot of air (cfu/ft^3). Detailed information has been published on various air samplers and their use in air monitoring for viable contaminants in the hospital (Fincher, 1966).

Air sampling equipment used for the recovery of airborne bacterial particles has also been employed in the recovery of viral particles from the air. Liquid impinger samplers (Artenstein, *et al.*, 1964; Thorne, *et al.*, 1960; Douglas, *et al.*, 1966); slit sampler (Dahlgren, *et al.*, 1961), and Andersen sampler (Guerin, *et al.*, 1964; Jensen, 1964), and filtration techniques (Meiklejohn, *et al.*, 1961) have been employed to recover different types of viruses and bacteriophages from the air. Requirements for physical collection of airborne viruses are not basically different from those for airborne bacteria. Although a great deal is unknown about the distribution of naturally-occurring airborne viral particles, it is reasonable to assume, on the basis of what is known of bacteria-containing particles, that the viruses also occur in a complex of carrier material that contributes to the mass and size of the particle. Technical difficulties, of recovering viruses from intramural air, are associated more with processing the collected sample, and removal of the viruses from associated debris and bacteria than to special growth systems required for their cultivation.

A problem occasionally encountered is the requirement to recover a specific bacterial or viral agent when it occurs in very low concentration in the air; or, when the total numbers of viable airborne particles are very low, such as in ultra-clean rooms or in evaluation of high-efficiency air filters.

The need for high volume rate sampling in the range of 1000–15,000 liters of air per minute (35–525 cfm) can be met by two commercially available devices—the Large Volume Air Sampler,* and the Lundgren

*Applied Science Division, Litton Systems, Inc., 2003 East Hennepin Avenue, Minneapolis, Minnesota 55413.

Air Sampler.* These devices utilize inertial and electrostatic forces for efficiently and continuously collecting airborne particles and concentrating them into a small volume flow of liquid. Use of the Large Volume Air Sampler (LVAS) has been used in the assessment of viral aerosols (Gerone, *et al.*, 1966).

A summary of selected samplers for airborne microorganisms that are commonly used for intramural sampling requirements are presented in the following table.

Summary of Selected Samplers for Airborne Microorganisms

Type of Sampler Impaction	Collection Medium	Sampling Rate	Comments
Slit Type			Provides data of airborne concentrations with sequential timing. No dilution or plating of sample required after collection. High particle concentration may over-load collecting surface. Viable particles collected and cultured *in situ*. Counts expressed as colony-forming units per cubic foot of air (cfu/ft[3]).
Reyniers[1]	Agar surface	1 CFM (28.3 lpm)	
Casella[2]	Agar surface	1 CFM (28.3 lpm);	
TDL[3]	Agar surface	1 CFM	
Cascade-Sieve Type			Separates and collects particles into six size ranges. Viable particles collected and cultured *in situ*. High concentration of airborne particles limits sample size. Results expressed as colony-forming units per cubic foot of air (cfu/ft[3]).
Andersen[4]	Agar surface	1 CFM (28.3 lpm)	
Impingement			Low sampling rate limitation with low airborne particle concentration. Disruption of collected particles. Results expressed as viable cell count per unit volume of air sampled. Vacuum source must be sufficient for operating sampler at critical flow velocity.
All Glass Impinger[5,6] (AGI)	Liquid	0.44 CFM (12.5 lpm)	

*Environmental Research Corporation, 3760 North Dunlap Street, St. Paul, Minnesota 55112.

Type of Sampler Impaction	Collection Medium	Sampling Rate	Comments
Filtration			
Membrane filter[6]	Membrane	Var: function of flow resistance, area of filter, and vacuum	High efficiency of collection. Some viability loss among sensitive cells — bacterial resistance to desiccation during continuous sampling a factor in effective collection of viable cells. Counts reported as colony-forming units per volume of air sampled.
Sedimentation			
Petri Dish	Agar surface	Nonvolumetric	Simple to use; inexpensive. Semiquantitative. Collected particles cultured *in situ*. Counts reported as number of colony-forming units per unit area per unit time.

[1]Reyniers & Son, 3806 North Ashland Avenue, Chicago 13, Illinois.

[2]C. F. Casella & Co., Ltd., Regent House, Britannia Walk, London, N. 1, England.

[3]Scientific Products, Division of American Hospital Supply Corp., 1210 Leon Place, Evanston, Illinois.

[4]Andersen Samplers & Consulting Service, 1074 Ash Avenue, Provo, Utah.

[5]Ace Glass, Inc., Vineland, New Jersey 08360; Millipore Filter Corporation, Bedford, Massachusetts.

[6]Millipore Filter Corporation, Bedford, Massachusetts; Gelman Instrument Co., P.O. 1448, Ann Arbor, Michigan 48106.

Temperature and Relative Humidity

Fundamental data in air hygiene measurements should always include measurements of ambient air temperature and relative humidity. Instrumental methods for making these determinations range from a simple wall-mounted wet and dry bulb hygrometer to precision instruments such as the Electric Hygrometer Sensing Unit*. A standard instrument for accurate determination of water concentration in air and relative humidity by means of wet and dry bulb temperature difference is the sling psychrometer. Two thermometers are attached to a folding swiveled handle in such a way as to provide ventilation for the wet bulb. Temperature readings—dry bulb and wet bulb—are used with an

*Hygrodynamics, Inc., 949 Selin Road, Silver Spring, Maryland.

accompanying psychometric chart for determining relative humidity, viz., the ratio of the quantity of water vapor present in the atmosphere to the quantity which would saturate at the existing temperature.

For most purposes in areas under controlled air conditioning, periodic direct readings in the room are sufficient. However, for continuous air monitoring and for conditions where temperature and relative humidity fluctuate, it may be necessary to use a continuous recording system in order to obtain a mean and range of atmosphere values.

Ventilation Measurements

Ventilation is displacement of air from a space by the introduction and removal of air from and to a source external to that space. In contamination control, ventilation removes gaseous (odor) contaminants and airborne small particles from the space by dilution ventilation. This refers to the gradual removal of contamination and, when the contamination concentration is constant (not being added to at the start of ventilation), the speed of contaminant reduction is a function of room volume and total air flow through it.

The expression of a room volume air-change does not mean, however, that the airborne contamination has been completely removed. Silver (1946) verified experimentally, that within a chamber with perfect mixing of a gaseous contaminant and air, the number of chamber volume air changes (K), is related to the removal, in percent, of the gaseous contaminant with time. This can be expressed at $t\% = K(a/b)$, where $t\%$ is the percent contaminant removed in time t. K is a constant, a is chamber size, and b is the rate of air flow. The values of K were shown to be:

% Removal of Contaminant $(1-e^{-k})$	K
99	4.605
95	2.996
90	2.303
85	1.897
80	1.609
63	1.000

It should be noted that the ratio a/b is the time required for one air change and from the above values of K it can be seen that one volume air change will remove only 63% of the contaminant; succeeding contaminant removal occurs at progressively decreasing rates. For example, a chamber of 3000 cubic feet volume, ventilated at 300 cubic feet per minute (18,000 ft^3/hr = 6 air changes/hr) has $a/b = 0.166$ and would require c. 45 minutes for 99% removal of the contaminant ($t^{99} = 45$ min). This example is valid for a gaseous contaminant in a chamber where perfect mixing of the contaminant occurs.

In normal room ventilation this theoretical dilution ventilation does not hold because of (1) perfect mixing does not occur, and (2) airborne particles, except very small particles, do not behave as a gas. Small particles are liable to removal by dilution ventilation, larger particles being removed primarily by sedimentation. The above example is presented as the principle of dilution ventilation and under theoretical chamber conditions indicates the minimum time required for contamination removal. Actual performance of room ventilation is considerably more complex and requires the use of tracers for empirical determination of ventilation rates (Lidwell, 1960).

Practical estimates can be made of ventilation performance by determination of input and exhaust air volumes together with room dimensions. The most readily made measurements are taken as air velocity readings at the air inlet and air exhaust grill faces in the room. For such measurements the Biram Type Anemometer or the Model MRF FloRite Air Velocity Indicator* are applicable. The Alnor^R Velometer^R† is a versatile, simple direct-reading instrument with suitable attachments that enable direct measurements to be made also in supply and return air ducts.

Air velocity readings at grill faces of inlet and exhaust openings into the room and in air ducts are in velocity units of feet per minute. The volume air flow rate, in cubic feet per minute, is a product of the average velocity of the air stream multiplied by the area of that air stream. Measurements taken across grill or diffuser facings usually require a correction factor in the calculation; this factor should be obtained from the equipment manufacturer.

Determination of air currents and patterns of turbulence can be estimated by the use of test smoke such as stannic chloride or titanium tetrachloride. Available*‡ in tubes for ease and convenience of use, the

---

*E. Vernon Hill & Co., P.O. Box 189, Lake Geneva, Wisconsin 53147.

†Alnor Instrument Co., Div. of Illinois Testing Laboratories, Inc., 420 North LaSalle Street, Chicago, Illinois 60610.

‡Controlled Environment Equipment Co., 344 South Avenue, Whitman, Massachusetts 02382.

smoke test is a quick method in determining directional flow of air in critical areas such as surgeries, nurseries, and delivery rooms, where the air is under positive pressure in relationship to adjacent areas.

For detailed technical direction in measurement of temperature, pressure, fluid velocity and volume, and humidity of air, reference should be made to *ASHRAE Guide and Data Book* (1965), Chapter 16.

Temperature and relative humidity requirements for selected areas in the hospital are shown below.

Temperature and Relative Humidity Requirements in Selected Areas*

Area Designation	Temp. °F	RH%
Operating	70–76†	50–60
Delivery	70–76†	50–60
Recovery	75	50–60
Nursery (observation)	75	50
Nursery (full-term)	75	50
Nursery (premature)	75–80†	50–60†
Intensive care	70–80†	30–60

*PHS Publication No. 930-A-7, December 1967, U.S. Dept HEW, Div. Hospital and Medical Facilities.

†Variable range required.

A minimum temperature of 75°F should be provided in all other occupied areas (PHS Publ. No. 930-A-7, 1967). Air pressure relationships and ventilation of certain hospital areas contained in the regulations of the Hill-Burton Program Under General Standards of Construction and Equipment for Hospital and Medical Facilities are shown in the table on pages 284–285.

For a more detailed analysis of mechanical design and performance of hospital ventilation and air-conditioning, reference should be made to the writing by Gaulin (1966).

Surface Sampling

Surface sampling techniques are usually carried out by using swabs or Rodac Contact plates. As explained in the section on Disinfectant Evaluation Methods (*see* p. 233), bacteria are scattered in highly random clumps and clusters on surfaces and therefore dozens or hundreds of samples would have to be taken to achieve accurate results. These techniques are recommended only for special studies and not for routine evaluation.

General Pressure Relationships and Ventilation of Certain Hospital Areas*

Area Designation	Pressure Relationship to Adjacent Areas	Minimum Air Changes of Outdoor Air per Hour	Minimum Total Air Changes per Hour	All Air Exhausted Directly to Outdoors	Recirculated Within Room Units
Operating room	P	5	25	Optional	No[5]
Emergency operating room	P	5	25	Optional	No[5]
Emergency exam. and treatment	E	2	6	Optional	Optional
Delivery room	P	5	12	Optional	No[5]
Nursery, all	P	5	12	Optional	No[5]
Recovery room	P	2	6	Optional	No[5]
Intensive care	P	2	6	Optional	No[5]
Patient room	E	2	2	Optional	Optional
Patient room corridor	E	2	4	Optional	Optional
Isolation room	E	2	6	Yes	No
Isolation room-alcove or anteroom	E	2	10	Yes	No
Examination room	E	2	6	Optional	Optional
Medication room	P	2	4	Optional	Optional
Pharmacy	P	2	4	Optional	Optional
Treatment room	E	2	6	Optional	No[5]
X-ray, fluoroscopy room	N	2	6	Yes	No
X-ray treatment room	E	2	6	Optional	Optional
Physical therapy and hydrotherapy	N	2	6	Optional	Optional
Soiled workroom or soiled holding	N	2	10	Yes	No
Clean workroom or clean holding	P	2	4	Optional	Optional
Autopsy	N	2	12	Yes	No
Darkroom	N	2	10	Yes	No
Non-refrigerated body holding room	N	Optional	10	Yes	No
Toilet room	N	Optional	10	Yes	No
Bedpan room	N	Optional	10	Yes	No
Bathroom	N	Optional	10	Yes	No
Janitor's closet	N	Optional	10	Yes	No

Sterilizer equipment room	N	Optional	10	Yes	No
Linen and trash chute rooms	N	Optional	10	Yes	No
Laboratory, general[1]	N	2	6	Optional	Optional
Laboratory, media transfer[2]	P	2	4	Optional	No[5]
Food preparation centers[3]	E	2	10	Yes	No
Ware washing area	N	Optional	10	Yes	No
Dietary day storage	E	Optional	2	Optional	No
Laundry, general	E	2	10	Yes	No
Soiled linen sorting and storage	N	Optional	10	Yes	No
Clean linen storage	P	2	2	Optional	Optional
Anesthesia storage[4]	E	Optional	8	Yes	No
Central medical and surgical supply					
Soiled or decontamination room	N	2	4	Yes	No
Clean workroom	P	2	4	Optional	Optional
Unsterile supply storage	E	2	2	Optional	Optional

P = Positive; N = Negative; E = Equal.

*This table, provided by the Health Care Facilities Service, Health Services and Mental Health Administration, U.S. Dept. HEW, has been proposed for inclusion in the 1973 edition of *Minimum (cq) Standards of Construction and Equipment for Hospital and Medical Facilities.*

[1]*See* Sec. 7-29D2j and Sec. 7-29Dk for additional requirements.

[2]*See* Sec. 7-29D2j for additional requirements.

[3]*See* Sec. 7-29D2f for exceptions.

[4]*See* Sec. 7-29D2n for additional requirements.

[5]Recirculating room units meeting the filtering requirement for sensitive areas in paragraph 7-29D2f may be used.

7-3-7   Evaluation of Airborne Contamination

The significance of airborne contamination, within the total complex of microbial contamination present in the environment, is difficult to assess. Excluding those diseases listed above, principally respiratory, that are naturally transmitted by the airborne route, airborne microbial contaminants occupy an equivocal position in the ranking of environmental sources of infection. The recovery of microbial contaminants from these sources, air or surfaces, cannot be interpreted as direct evidence of infection sources. However, such findings are important as presumptive evidence of infection source and must be included in the total evaluation of the multifactorial system that is usually operative.

As part of a fundamental approach to environmental control in critical areas such as surgery, newborn nursery, and other areas where individuals of high susceptibility to infection are housed, provision for maintenance of high levels of air contamination control should be included as standard practice. Ventilation design and air-cleaning practices are well-developed and provide practical implementation of minimum measures to improve significantly the quality of air hygiene in these areas.

Sources of microbial contaminants in the hospital environment, uniqueness of patient population susceptibility to infection, and selected episodes where microbial air-contaminants can be directly implicated in cross-infection emphasize the potential circumstance and opportunities for infection that are peculiar to the hospital environment. Assumption of the premise of significance of air hygiene requires a broad interpretation of the role of airborne microbial contamination in critical patient areas.

Air, as one source of microbial contamination, has been included among other factors in studies on origins and control of wound (surgical) infection. Major prevention of surgical infection has been most singularly effective through the development of barrier techniques that control the most frequent and efficient mechanisms of contamination transmission—direct contact. The contaminant-laden air remains an indirect route of transmission.

Reduction or removal of airborne contaminants should be followed by a reduction in rates of infection if infections acquired during wound exposure are caused by microorganisms from this source. The absence of a measurable reduction in infections in other wound classes indicates that contamination sources, other than air, are largely responsible for infections in these wounds (NAS-NRC, 1964).

Air control in surgery, by changes in ventilation and directional flow of air by pressurizing the room, has been reported to reduce the average counts of bacterial particles in the room air and to have been accompanied by a significant reduction in surgical wound infection rate (Shooter, *et al.*, 1956). Ventilation as well as the activity of personnel and the use of blankets have been considered important contributors to high counts of airborne *Staphylococcus aureus*. Most infections were considered to have occurred from airborne sources during the time of operation. Control measures applied to these factors were followed by a reduction in infection rate from 10.9% to 3.9% (Blowers, *et al.*, 1955).

Changes in ventilation control and personnel practices resulting in a decrease in airborne bacterial particle counts, have not always been followed by a reduction in infection rates. Kinmouth, *et al.* (1958) reported that during a brief time when the positive pressure ventilating system was inoperative, there occurred an accompanying increase in infection rate. Reversal of the positive pressure ventilation system of an operating room, with reversion to high airborne bacterial air counts and implicated airborne route of infection, has been reported by Shooter, *et al.* (1956).

The role of host susceptibility factors and virulence of the airborne staphylococci contaminating a surgical wound and with resulting infection is indicated from the studies by Burke (1963). Sixty-eight percent of the wounds studied showed the same strain of staphylococcus in the wound as in the air in contact with it. Staphylococci were found in the air and in the wounds in all 50 operations studied. Two infections occurred, one of which was caused by a strain of staphylococcus recovered only from the air.

Walter, *et al.* (1963) demonstrated airborne surgical infection due to *S. aureus* that was traced to a single individual present in the operating room. This person was a "disperser" or "shedder" who disseminated particles of less than 10 microns in diameter (count median diameter); the total count of bacterial particles recovered from the air was a mean of 3.7 ± 2.7 per cubic foot, *S. aureus* being present in 11.2% of the 169 operations studied. Two patients were infected by staphylococci from this "disperser." An individual "disperser" who was found to have been a perineal carrier of Group A beta-hemolytic streptococci has also been reported as the source of a probable airborne transmission resulting in eight cases of streptococcal puerperal endometritis and three cases of streptococcal postoperative wound infection (McKee, *et al.*, 1966).

The significance of airborne transmission of bacterial contaminants is also suggested where clinical infection is not a direct result but where a potentially infectious microorganism is transmitted from patient to patient. An example of this is in the results reported by Mortimer, *et al.* (1966) that infants acquired an index staphylococci in the anterior nares and umbilicus by the airborne route (10%) compared to a 14% transmission rate via physical contact by carefully washed hands of attending nurses.

The frequency of cross-infection due to airborne transmission of microorganisms in areas of high environmental control is believed to be low. Average counts of airborne contamination in such areas can be maintained at levels as low as two bacterial particles per cubic foot of air (Baldwin, *et al.*, 1965) or less with specially designed systems (McDade, *et al.*, 1968). In circumstances where low frequency of occurrence of an event (infection) and low levels of agents causing that event are present, the statistical requirements to demonstrate a reduction in a low infection rate by a further improvement in the air component of control is considerable, as has been indicated by Lidwell (1963).

While recent experience in hospital air hygiene has emphasized studies on airborne staphylococci, one application of monitoring levels of airborne microbial contamination is the use of such information as part of an environmental hygiene index. Sampling procedures may have utility in comparing maintenance methods in environmental protection programs, particularly in restricted areas requiring high levels of control. Such sampling is easily employed while the area is in use and thereby giving an actual assessment of activity and procedures as they are sources *per se* and/or generators of environmental contaminants liable to airborne transport.

In conclusion, airborne microbial contaminants are an important concern in environmental protection. Assessment of that importance must be done with a full appreciation of the total factors — animate and inanimate — operating in a given situation.

REFERENCES AND SELECTED READINGS

Akers, T. G., Bond, Sheila, and Goldberg, L. J. Effect of temperature and relative humidity on survival of airborne Columbia SK group viruses, *Appl. Microbiol.*, 14: 361–364, 1966.

Allen, H. F. Air hygiene for hospitals. I. Arrestment of airborne and dustborne staphylococci by a hospital vacuum cleaner, *J. Am. Med. Assn.*, 169: 533–559, 1959.

Andersen, Ariel A. New sampler for the collection, sizing, and enumeration of viable airborne particles, *J. Bact.*, 76: 471–484, 1958.

Anderson, A. F. and Sheppard, R. A. W. Dissemination of *Staphylococcus aureus* from woolen blankets, *Lancet*, 1: 514–515, 1959.

Andersen, K. *Pseudomonas pyocyanea* disseminated from an air-cooling apparatus, *Med. J. Aust.*, 1: 529, 1959.

Artenstein, M. S. and Cardigan, Frances C. J. Air sampling in viral respiratory disease, *Arch. Environ. Hlth.*, 9: 58–60, 1964.

ASHRAE Guide and Data Book (1965–6) Fundamentals and Equipment. Publisher: Amer. Soc. Heat., Refrig., and Air-Cond. Engineer., Inc., 345 East 47th Street, New York, N.Y. 10017.

Baldwin, M., Weatherby, R. J., and MacDonald, F. D. S. Microbiological characteristics in a neurosurgical environment, *Hospitals*, 39: 71–78, 1965.

Bassett, D. C. J., Thompson, S. A. S., and Page, B. Neonatal infections with *Pseudomonas aeruginosa* associated with contaminated resuscitation equipment, *Lancet*, 1: 781–784, 1965.

Batchelor, H. W. Aerosol samplers. *In: Advances in Applied Microbiology*. New York: Academic Press, Vol. 2, pp. 31–64, 1960.

Bernard, H. R., Speers, R. Jr., O'Grady, F., and Shooter, R. A. Reduction of dissemination of skin bacteria by modification of operating-room clothing and by ultraviolet irradiation, *Lancet*, 2: 458–461, 1965a.

Bernard, H. R., Speers, R. Jr., O'Grady, F. W., and Shooter, R. A. Airborne bacterial contamination. Investigation of human sources, *Arch. Surg.* (Chicago) 91: 530–533, 1965b.

Bethune, D. W., Blowers, R., Parker, M., and Pask, E. A. Dispersal of *Staphylococcus aureus* by patients and staff, *Lancet*, 1: 480: 483, 1965.

Blowers, R., Mason, G. A., Wallace, K. R., and Walton, M. Control of wound infection in a thoracic surgery unit, *Lancet*, 2, 786–794, 1955.

Blowers, R., Lidwell, O. M., and Williams, R. E. O. Infection in operating theatres in relation to air conditioning equipment, *J. Inst. Heat, & Vent. Engineers* (London), pp. 244–245, October 1962.

Brachman, P. S., Ehrlich, R., Eichenwald, H. F., Gabelli, V. J., Keithley, T. W., Madin, S. H., Maltman, J. R., Middlebrook, G., Morton, J. D., Silver, I. H., and Wolfe, E. K. Standard sampler for assay of airborne microorganisms, *Science*, 144: 1295, 1964.

Burke, J. F. Identification of the sources of staphylococci contaminating the surgical wound during operations, *Ann. Surg.*, 158: 898–904, 1963.

Caplan, H. Observations on the role of hospital blankets as reservoirs of infection, *J. Hyg.* (London), 60: 401–410, 1962.

Cole, W. R., Bernard, H. R., and Dunn, B. Growth of bacteria on direct expansion air-conditioning coils, *Surgery*, 55: 436–439, 1964.

Cooke, E. Mary and Buck, H. W. Self-contamination of dermatological patients with *Staphylococcus aureus*, *Brit. J. Derm.*, 75: 21–25, 1963.

Corn, M. and Stein, F. Mechanisms of dust redispersion. *In: Surface Contamination*, New York: Pergamon Press, Ltd., 1967.

Dahlgren, C. M., Decker, Herbert M., and Harstad, J. B. A slit sampler for collecting T-3 bacteriophage and Venezuelan equine encephalomyelitis virus, *Appl. Microbiol.*, 9: 103–107, 1961.

Davies, R. R. and Noble, W. C. Dispersal of bacteria on desquamated skin, *Lancet*, 2: 1295–1297, 1962.

DeJong, J. G. and Winkler, K. C. Survival of measles virus in air, *Nature* (London) 201: 1054–1055, 1964.

DeOrme, K. B. The effect of temperature, humidity and glycol vapour on the viability of airborne bacteria, *Am. J. Hyg.*, 40: 239–250, 1944.

Douglas, R. G. Jr., Cate, T. R., Gerone, P. J., and Couch, R. B. Quantitative rhinovirus shedding patterns in volunteers, *Am. Rev. Resp. Dis.*, 94: 159–167, 1966.

Downie, A. W. Infection and immunity in smallpox, *Lancet*, 1: 419–422, 1951.

Duguid, J. P. The size and the duration of air-carriage of respiratory droplets and droplet-nuclei, *J. Hyg.*, (Camb.), 44: 471–479, 1946a.

Duguid, J. P. Expulsion of pathogenic organisms from respiratory tract, *Brit. Med. J.*, 1: 265–268, 1946b.

Duguid, J. P. and Wallace, A. T. Air infection with dust liberated from clothing, *Lancet*, 2: 845–849, 1948.

Dunklin, E. W. and Puck, T. T. The lethal effect of relative humidity on airborne bacteria, *J. Exp. Med.*, 87: 87–101, 1948.

Edmundson, E. B., Reinarz, J. A., Pierce, A. K., and Sanford, J. P. Nebulization equipment. A potential source of infection in Gram-negative pneumonias, *Amer. J. Dis. Child.*, 111: 357–360, 1966.

Eichenwald, H. F., Kotsevalov, Olga, and Fasso, Lois A. The "Cloud-baby": an example of bacterial viral interaction, *Amer. J. Dis. Child.*, 100: 161–173, 1960.

Fincher, E. L. Air sampling, applications, methods, recommendations. *In: Control of Infections in Hospitals.* Continuing Education Series No. 138. The University of Michigan, School of Public Health, Ann Arbor, Michigan. Pp. 200–209, 1966.

Gardner, A. W. and Pape, K. G. *Staphylococcus aureus* from airborne fibers in a hospital ward, *Med. J. Aust.*, 47: 127–129, 1960.

Gaulin, R. P. Hospitals. *In: ASHRAE Guide and Data Book—Applications for 1966 and 1967.* Publisher: Amer. Soc. Heat., Refrig. & Air-Cond. Engineers, Inc., 345 East 47th Street, New York, N.Y. 10017, Chap. 29, 1966.

General Standards of Construction and Equipment for Hospitals and Medical Facilities, U.S. Dept. of Health, Education and Welfare, USPHS, Division of Hospital and Medical Facilities. Public Health Service Publication No. 930-A-7, December 1967.

Gerone, P. J., Couch, R. B., Keefer, G. V., Douglas R. G., Derrenbacher, E. B., and Knight, V. Assessment of experimental and natural viral aerosols, *Bact. Rev.*, 30: 576–584, 1966.

Goldberg, L. J., Watkins, H. M. S., Boerke, E. E., and Chatigny, M. A. The use of a rotating drum for the study of aerosols over extended periods of time, *Am. J. Hyg.*, 68: 85–93, 1958.

Guerin, L. F. and Mitchell, C. A. A method for determining the concentration of airborne virus and sizing droplet nuclei containing the agent, *Canad. J. Comp. Med. and Vet. Sci.*, 28: 283–287, 1964.

Hare, R. and Thomas, C. G. A. Transmission of *Staphylococcus aureus*, *Brit. Med. J.*, 2: 840–844, 1956.

Hare, R. and Ridley, M. Further studies on transmission of *Staphylococcus aureus*, *Brit. Med. J.*, 1: 69–73, 1958.

Hare, R. and Cooke, E. M. Self-contamination of patients with staphylococcal infections, *Brit. Med. J.*, 2: 333–336, 1961.

Harper, G. J. Airborne microorganisms: Survival tests with four viruses, *J. Hyg.*, (Camb.), 59: 479–486, 1961.

Hart, Deryl, Bactericidal ultraviolet radiation in the operating room. Twenty-nine year study for control of infection. *J. Amer. Med. Assn.*, 172: 1019–1027, 1960.

Hatch, T. F. Distribution and deposition of inhaled particles in respiratory tract, *Bact. Rev.*, 25: 237–240, 1961.

Heldman, D. R., Sunga, Fe C. A., and Hedrick, T. I. Microorganism shedding by human beings, *Contam. Control*, 6: 28–31, 1967.

Hemmes, J. H., Winkler, K. C., and Kool, S. M. Virus survival as a seasonal factor in influenza and poliomyelitis, *Nature*, 188: 430–431, 1960.

Hughes, M. H. Dispersal of bacteria on desquamated skin, *Lancet*, 1: 109, 1963.

Hurst, Valerie, Grossman, M., and Ingram, F. R. Hospital laundry and refuse chutes as source of staphylococci cross-infection, *J. Amer. Med. Assn.*, 167: 1223–1229, 1958.

Jensen, M. M. Inactivation of airborne viruses by ultraviolet irradiation, *Appl. Microbiol.*, 12: 418–420, 1964.

Kethley, T. W., Fincher, E. L., and Cown, W. B. The effect of sampling method upon the apparent response of airborne bacteria to temperature and relative humidity, *J. Inf. Dis.*, 100: 97–102, 1957.

Kethley, T. W., Cown, W. B., and Fincher, E. L. Mock-up surgery tests air flow patterns, *Mod. Hosp.*, 100 (3): 99–102, 1963.

Kethley, T. W. and Cown, W. B. In defense of settling plates, *Hosp. Management*, 103: 84, 87, 1967.

Kinmouth, J. B., Hare, R., Tracy, G. D., Thomas, C. G. A., Marsh, J. D., and Jantet, G. J. Studies of theatre ventilation and surgical wound infection, *Brit. Med. J.*, 2: 407–411, 1958.

Langmuir, A. D. Airborne infection. *In: Preventive Medicine and Public Health*. 9th ed. Philip E. Sartwell (Ed.), Appleton-Century-Crofts, Chap. 10, 1965.

Lidwell, O. M., Noble, W. C., and Dolphin, G. W. The use of radiation to estimate the numbers of micro-organisms in air-borne particles, *J. Hyg.*, 57: 299–308, 1959.

Lidwell, O. M. The evaluation of ventilation, *J. Hyg.* (Camb.), 58: 297–305, 1960.

Lidwell, O. M. Methods of investigation and analysis of results. *In: Infection in Hospitals*. R. E. O. Williams and R. A. Shooter, (Eds), Philadelphia, Pa.: F. A. Davis Co., pp. 43–46, 1963.

Linton, R. C., Walker, F. W., and Spoerel, W. E. Respirator care in a general hospital: a five-year survey. *Canad. Anaesth. Soc. J.*, 12: 450–457, 1965.

Loosli, C. G., Lemon, H. M., Robertson, O. H., and Appel, E. Experimental airborne influenza infection. Influence of humidity on survival of virus in air, *Proc. Soc. Exp. Biol.*, N.Y., 53: 205–206, 1943.

Loosli, C. G., Smith, M. H. D., Cline, J., and Nelson, L. The transmission of hemolytic streptococcal infections in infants' wards, with special reference to "skin dispersers," *J. Lab. & Clin. Med.*, 36: 342–359, 1950.

MacCallum, F. O., McPherson, C. A., and Johnstone, D. J. Laboratory investigation of smallpox patients with particular reference to infectivity in the early stages, *Lancet*, 2: 514–517, 1950.

McDade, J. J., Whitcomb, J. G., Rypka, E. W., Whitfield, W. J., and Franklin, Carol M. Microbiological studies conducted in a vertical lammar airflow surgery, *J. Amer. Med. Assn.*, 203: 125–130, 1968.

McKee, W. M., DiCaprio, J. M., Roberts, C., Evans, Jr., and Sherris, J. C. Anal carriage as the probable source of a streptococcal epidemic, *Lancet*, 2: 1007–1009, 1966.

Meiklejohn, G., Kempe, C. H., Downie, A. W., Berge, T. O., Vincent, St. L., and Rao, A. R. Air sampling to recover variola virus in the environment of a smallpox hospital, *Bull. Wld. Hlth. Org.*, 25: 63–67, 1961.

Mertz, J. J., Scharer, L., and McClemment, J. H. A hospital outbreak of Klebsiella pneumonia from inhalation therapy with contaminated aerosol solutions, *Amer. Rev. Resp. Dis.*, 95: 454–460, 1967.

Michaelsen, G. S. Waste Handling. *In: Proceedings of the National Conference on Institutionally Acquired Infections*. USPHS Publication No. 1188, U.S. Govt. Printing Office, Washington, D. C. Pp. 65–69, 1964.

Mortimer, E. A., Wolinsky, E., Gonzaga, Antonia J., and Rammelkamp, C. H. Role of airborne transmission in staphylococcal infections, *Brit. Med. J.*, 1: 319–322, 1966.

National Academy of Science—National Research Council, Report of an *Ad Hoc* Committee. Postoperative Wound Infections: The Influence of ultraviolet irradiation of the operating rooms and of various other factors. *Ann. Surg.*, 160 (2): 1–192 (Suppl.), 1964.

Nimeck, M. W., Myers, G. E., and MacKenzie, W. C. An evaluation of aseptic and antiseptic techniques as practised in a modern hospital. I. Operating theatres. *Canad. J. Surg.*, 2: 233–241, 1959.

Noble, W. C. The dispersal of staphylococci in hospital wards, *J. Clin. Path.*, 15: 552–558, 1962.

Noble, W. C., Lidwell, O. M., and Kinston, D. The size distribution of airborne particles carrying micro-organisms, *J. Hyg.* (Camb.), 61: 385–391, 1963.

Pierce, A. K. and Sanford, Jay P. Treatment and prevention of infections associated with inhalation therapy, *Mod. Treat.*, 3: 1171–1174, 1966.

Perry, W. B., Siegel, A. C., Rammelkamp, C. H., Wannamaker, L. W., and Marple, E. C. Transmission of Group A streptococci. I. The role of contaminated bedding, *Am. J. Hyg.*, 66: 85–95, 1957.

Phillips, I. and Spencer, G. *Pseudomonas aeruginosa* cross-infection due to contaminated respiratory apparatus, *Lancet*, 2: 1325–1327, 1965.

Pressley, T. A. The fibre composition of hospital dust, *Lancet*, 2: 712–713, 1958.

Ranger, I. and O'Grady, F. Dissemination of microorganisms by a surgical pump, *Lancet*, 2: 299–300, 1958.

Reinarz, J. A., Pierce, A. K., Mays, Benita B., and Sanford, Jay P. The potential role of inhalation therapy equipment in nosocomial pulmonary infection, *J. Clin. Invest.*, 44: 831–839, 1965.

Ridley, M. Perineal carriage of *Staphylococcus aureus*, *Brit. Med. J.*, 1: 270–273, 1959.

Riley, R. L., Mills, C. C., Myka, W., Weinstock, N., Storey, P. B., Sultan, L. U., Riley, M. C., and Wells, W. F. Aerial dissemination of pulmonary tuberculosis. A two-year study of contagion in a tuberculosis ward. *Am. J. Hyg.*, 70: 185–196, 1959.

Riley, R. L. and O'Grady, F. Airborne Infection—Transmission and Control. New York: MacMillan, 1961.

Rubbo, S. D., Pressley, T. A., Stratford, B. C., and Dixson, Shirley. Vehicles of transmission of airborne bacteria in hospital wards, *Lancet*, 2: 397–400, 1960.

Rubbo, S. D., Stratford, B. C., and Dixson, S. Spread of a marker organism in a hospital ward, *Brit. Med. J.*, 2: 282–287, 1962.

Rubbo, S. D. and Saunders, J. Liberation of organisms from contaminated textiles, *J. Hyg.* (Lond.), 61: 507–513, 1963.

Rubbo, S. D., Gardner, Joan F., and Franklin, J. Clare. Source of Pseudomonas aeruginosa infection in premature infants, *J. Hyg.*, (Camb.), 64: 121–128, 1966.

Selwyn, S. The mechanism and prevention of cross-infection in dermatological wards, *J. Hyg.*, 63: 59–71, 1965.

Selwyn, S. and Chambers, D. Dispersal of bacteria from skin lesions: a hospital hazard, *Brit. J. Derm.*, 77: 349–356, 1965.

Sever, J. L. Possible role of humidifying equipment in spread of infections from the newborn nursery, *Pediatrics*, 24: 50–53, 1959.

Shaffer, J. G., and McDade, J. J. Air-borne *Staphylococcus aureus*, *Arch. Envr. Hlth.*, 5: 547–551, 1962.

Shechmeister, I. L. Studies on the experimental epidemiology of respiratory infections. III. Certain aspects of the behavior of Type A influenza virus as an airborne cloud. *J. Inf. Dis.*, 87: 128–132, 1950.

Shooter, R. A., Taylor, G. W., Ellis, G., and Ross, J. P. Postoperative wound infection, *Surg. Gyn. & Obst.*, 103: 257–263, 1956.

Shooter, R. A., Smith, M. A., Griffiths, J. D., Brown, M. E. A., Williams, R. E. O., Rippon, J. E., and Jevons, M. P. Spread of staphylococci in a surgical ward, *Brit. Med. J.*, 1: 607–613, 1958.

Silver, S. D. Constant flow gassing chambers: principles influencing design and operation, *J. Lab. & Clin. Med.*, 31: 1153–1161, 1946.

Solberg, A. N., Shaffer, H., and Kelley, G. A. The collecting of air-borne microorganisms, *Ohio J. Science*, 56: 305–313, 1956.

Solberg, Claus Ola. A study of carriers of *Staphylococcus aureus* with special regard to quantitative bacterial estimations, *Acta Med. Scand.* 178: Suppl. 436: 1–96, 1965.

Speers, R., Bernard, H. R., O'Grady, F., and Shooter, R. A. Increased dispersal of skin bacteria into the air after shower-bath, *Lancet*, 2: 478–480, 1965.

Strasters, K. C. and Winkler, K. C. Viability of hospital staphylococci in air, *Bact. Rev.*, 30 (3): 674–677, 1966.

Thom., B. T. and White, R. G. The dispersal of organisms from minor septic lesions, *J. Clin. Path.*, 15: 559–562, 1962.

Thomas, C. G. A. and Griffiths, P. D. Air-borne staphylococci and the control of hospital cross-infection, *Guy's Hosp. Rept.*, 110(1): 76–86, 1961.

Thorne, H. V. and Burrows, T. M. Aerosol sampling methods for the virus of foot-and-mouth disease and the measurement of virus penetration through aerosol filters, *J. Hyg.*, 58: 409–417, 1960.

Walter, C. W. Environmental sepsis, *Mod. Hosp.*, 91: 69–78, 1958.

Walter, C. W. and Knudsin, R. B. The floor as a reservoir of hospital infections, *Surg., Gyn. & Obst.*, 111. 412–422, 1960.

Walter, C. W., Knudsin, Ruth B., and Brubaker, Mary M. The incidence of airborne wound infection during operation, *J. Amer. Med. Assn.*, 186: 908–913, 1963.

Warner, P. and Doherty, Jane, Bacteriology of air-conditioning ducts with special reference to operating rooms, *Canad. Med. Assn. J.*, 88: 416–419, 1963.

Webb, S. J., Cormack, D. V., and Morrison, H. G. Relative humidity, inositol and the effect of radiation on air-dried microorganisms, *Nature* (London), 201: 1103–1105, 1964.

Wellman, W. E. and Ulrich, J. A. A bacterial survey of two areas in one hospital by the settling plate method, *Mayo Clin. Proc.*, 40: 708–713, 1965.

Wells, W. F. On air-borne infection. II. Droplets and droplet nuclei. *Am. J. Hyg.*, 20: 611–618, 1934.

Wells, W. F. Air-borne infection and sanitary air control, *J. Indust. Hyg. & Toxicol.*, 17: 253–257, 1935.

Wells, W. F. Ray length in sanitary ventilation by bactericidal irradiation of air, *J. Franklin Institute.* 238: 185–193, 1944.

Wells, W. F. Circulation in sanitary ventilation by bactericidal irradiation of air, *J. Franklin Institute*, 240: 379–396, 1945.

Wells, W. F. Airborne Contagion and Air Hygiene. Cambridge, Mass.: Harvard University Press, 1955.

Wheeler, W. E. and Milaras, M. S. Testing a vacuum cleaner for hospital use, *Hospitals*, 36: 92–94, 1962.

White, A. Relation between quantitative nasal cultures and dissemination of staphylococci, *J. Lab & Clin. Med.*, 58(2): 273–277, 1961.

Wolf, H. W., Skaliy, P., Hall, L. B., Harris, M. M., Decker, H. M., Buchanan, L. M., and Dahlgren, C. M. *In: Sampling Microbial Aerosols.* Public Health Monography No. 60. U.S. Government Printing Office, Washington, D.C., 1959.

7-4 STERILIZATION

7-4-1 Introduction

In the institutional environment such as hospitals, clinics, laboratories, and particularly nursing homes, the need for practical information on the methods of sterilization is acute, particularly where numerous non-professional workers are employed. The professional and nonprofessional worker depends upon the science of sterilization and surgical asepsis as the chief means of protecting the patient against infectious disease and to combat cross-infections in hospitals and institutions.

The importance of sterilization of materials cannot be underestimated where the patient's welfare is concerned. When a patient is subjected to improperly sterilized material, there is a possibility of cross-infection. This possibility must be eliminated. Hospitals and hospital personnel, as well as institutional personnel, have a moral obligation to the patient to provide the best services possible so the hospital stay or convalescence will not be prolonged by a nosocomial infection. Therefore, anyone who accepts the responsibility for providing properly sterilized material for patient care should thoroughly understand the underlying principles upon which aseptic procedures and techniques are based.

In order to be responsible and understand the principles and methods of sterilization, there are commonly used terms which should be reviewed and understood. These are sterilization, disinfection, and sanitization.

The first term, *Sterilization*, means the complete destruction of all forms of microbial life. *Disinfection* is the destruction of pathogenic organisms, including the tubercle bacillus, but does not guarantee destruction of all spore forms of bacteria by chemical means. The third term, *Sanitization*, is the reduction in the total number of microorganisms, but does not necessarily imply that any particular organism is affected to a greater degree than others which might be present. In essence, a sanitizing process may be nothing more than a thorough cleaning procedure, since this in itself, if conducted properly, would remove or reduce microorganisms from a given surface. The United States Public Health Service recognizes or defines sanitization as a surface containing less than 100 microorganisms per a four inch square of surface.

From the definition of these three terms it is obvious that only one carries a definition of exactness, sterilization.

There is another term that will be seen and heard more in relation to care of materials after use before further handling by personnel. The term, *Decontamination*, is the equivalent of sterilization in that all agents of infection must be destroyed or permanently inactivated.

7-4-2   Microbiological Background

In considering the death of microorganisms during a sterilizing procedure, the question may be raised, how does this phenomenon take place. Investigations have shown that when a population of bacteria is exposed to a sterilizing influence, the rate by which the individual organisms die (are killed) is governed by definite laws. The order of death adheres to a definite uniform and consistent course and is described as being logarithmic. This means that in a given population of bacteria exposed to a sterilizing medium, death occurs in such a manner that the logarithm of the numbers of living cells at any particular time when plotted against that time will fall in a descending straight line. This is illustrated in Figure 7-1.

Thermal Death Time and Point

The slope of the line depends upon the rate of death. The logarithmic order of death implies that the same percentage of living bacteria die in

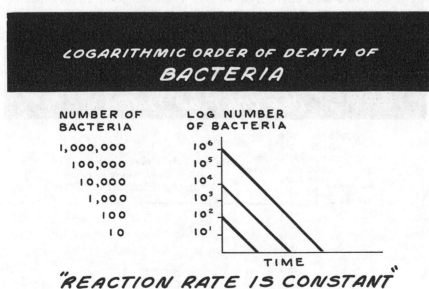

Figure 7-1   (Reprinted with permission from Amsco Equipment Co., Erie, Pa.).

a given unit of time. As a theoretical example, we can assume that a suspension of 1,000,000 bacteria/milliliter is exposed to a sterilizing agent and that 90% of the bacteria are killed each minute of exposure. At the end of the seventh and eighth minutes of exposure, the number of survivors would be 0.1 and 0.01 bacteria/milliliter, respectively, as shown in Figure 7-2. This, of course, appears ridiculous on the basis of a one milliliter sample, but it does mean that there would be one bacterium remaining alive in 10 ml and in 100 ml of suspension at the end of these respective exposure times. Theoretically, one bacterium would still survive in 1000 liters of suspension after 12 minutes exposure. This example, as illustrated in Figure 7-3, shows that in practical application of sterilizing procedures, a proportionally greater time period of exposure to a sterilizing influence is required for increasingly higher contamination levels of microorganisms.

This principle, definitely must be considered when establishing minimum exposure periods for sterilization of items. However, it is all too often neglected when exposure cycles are established for sterilization procedures.

Factors Which Influence the Ability to Kill Microorganisms

The destruction of microorganisms is usually dependent on a number of factors which are directly related to the killing or sterilizing agent,

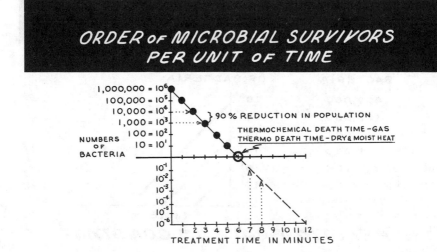

Figure 7-2   (Reprinted with permission from Amsco Equipment Co., Erie, Pa.).

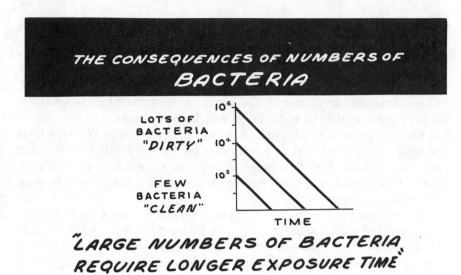

Figure 7-3   (Reprinted with permission from Amsco Equipment Co., Erie, Pa.).

and to the organisms directly involved. Briefly, the main factors influencing the killing powers of a microbicidal agent include: the intensity of the agent if physical, or the concentration if a chemical agent; the time in which the agent is allowed to act on the organisms; and the temperature occurring at the time of reaction. Factors which influence the susceptability of organisms to sterilizing agents include: the kind or type of organisms; the resistance of the organisms to a particular sterilizing agent; the numbers or population of organisms to be killed; the conditions or the type of environment in which the killing process is to take place; and the previous history of the organism. Awareness of these factors when attempting to sterilize a given material is important in achieving sterility.

Microbial Resistance

Microorganisms exhibit varying degrees of resistance to physical and chemical sterilizing agents or processes. Spores of microorganisms are generally more resistant to sterilizing agents than vegetative cells, although slight variations in resistance of different groups of vegetative cells may be found. Mold spores are usually only slightly more resistant than their vegetative forms whereas bacterial spores may be many times more resistant than their vegetative parents. Data has been compiled showing the relative resistances of bacterial spores, mold spores, and viruses to various sterilizing agents when the resistance of *Escherichia coli* is taken as unity.* This data indicates that viruses and mold spores are somewhat more resistant than the vegetative *E. coli* and that the bacterial spores are many times more resistant than the vegetative cell. For example, the death rate of *E. coli* in the case of moist heat is 3,000,000 times as great as that of bacterial spores, but only two to ten and one to five times as great as mold spores and viruses, respectively. With dry heat conditions *E. coli* is killed at a rate only 1000 times as great as that for spores of bacteria. This data indicates resistance not only varies with the type of biological condition of the organism but also varies with the type of sterilizing agent.

The resistance of viruses to sterilizing agents has come into prominence during the past several years and this subject must be given due consideration since many of our serious diseases are caused by a viral agent. In general, most viruses may be considered similar to vegetative bacterial cells in relation to their resistance to heat inactivation. One notable example of the exception of this rule is the virus of serum hepatitis. This virus appears to exhibit a high thermal resistance. Because of this potential resistance, it is important that materials such as hypodermic syringes and needles and other similar instruments are decontaminated or treated by a recognized sterilizing process.

7-4-3 Sterilizing Processes

There are three practical and effective methods of sterilization used in present-day hospitals. These are (1) saturated steam under pressure, (2) dry heat, and (3) ethylene oxide gas. The mechanisms by which microorganisms are killed or inactivated by the above mentioned processes are (1) saturated steam under pressure-coagulation, (2) dry heat-oxidation, and (3) ethylene oxide-alkylation as shown in Figure 7-4.

Saturated steam

Sterilization by moist heat or steam is probably the most commonly used method in all modern hospitals today. It is the most dependable process known for the destruction of all forms of microbial life. Even the most resistant bacterial spores are susceptible to these conditions and can be destroyed within a period of 15 minutes. The reaction of moist heat or steam at these relatively high temperatures on microorganisms

*Rahn, O. Physical methods sterilization of microorganisms, *Bact. Rev.*, 9: 1–47, 1945.

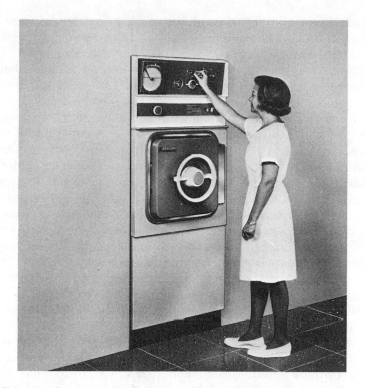

Figure 7-4 A modern autoclave. (Reprinted with permission from Amsco Equipment Co., Erie, Pa.)

closely parallels that of heat coagulation on proteins, i.e., bacteria are destroyed as a result of the denaturation by heat of protein materials that make up the bacterial cell.

Steam is used for sterilizing for several reasons:

It has a high heat content for its weight.
It gives up heat at constant temperature readily.
It is cheap, clean, odorless and tasteless.
It is readily distributed.
It heats rapidly but can behave as a gas and penetrate capillaries readily.
Its temperature and condition may be readily controlled.
Bacteria are best killed by heat in moist conditions; steam supplies both.

The achievement of sterility by steam under pressure is based on the fact that pressurized steam produces moist heat temperatures much higher than those obtainable by boiling water, and it is these high moist temperatures and not pressure which destroy microorganisms. Under these conditions, steam has a relatively rapid heating and penetrating effect on porous materials such as fabrics. It is known that steam heats largely through the transfer of its heat of vaporization as it condenses upon the surface of materials. This can be illustrated by describing the reaction of steam on porous materials. When in contact with porous surfaces, steam leaves a film of moisture on the outer surface. The next film of steam passes through to the second surface layer and during condensation on this layer releases heat to the material. This process continues until the material or fabric equilibrates to and remains constant at the temperature of the surrounding steam. For solid surfaces, there is, of course, no penetration of steam, and sterilization is effected only by the continual condensation of steam on the surface until the article is heated to the steam temperature. Because of the rapid heating effect and the abundance of moisture, however, it is possible to use shorter exposure periods for sterilizing metallic or other solid surface materials, as compared to porous materials which require time for steam to permeate to the inner surfaces.

The worst enemy of proper steam sterilization is air which may be trapped in the load of materials being processed or within the chamber itself. Mixtures of air and steam do not produce the proper temperature for sterilization. The greater the proportion of air in the air-steam mixture, the lower the ultimate temperature will be. For example, when only one-third of the air within the chamber has been discharged, a high temperature of 228–230°F is obtained, considerably below what is needed for sterilization. Since air under pressure has no germicidal effects, a small amount of air entrapped in a sterilizer can lead to serious sterilization failures.

Sterilization, by steam or moist heat under pressure, is normally conducted in a specially designed metal chamber surrounded by a steam jacket and sealed by a specially constructed door. Nonjacketed chambers and such equipment as pressure cookers can be employed as steam sterilizers; however, for accuracy in temperature, pressure and timing controls, it is much more desirable to employ a standard, commercially available, jacketed, steam sterilizer designed and constructed for reliable, dependable, and reproducible sterilization.

In most hospitals, steam is generated in a boiler and is conveyed through steam lines to the sterilizers. Usually, the pressure of the steam in such lines is about 60–80 pounds per square inch gauge. This pressure, however, is too high for the sterilizing cycles routinely conducted. Therefore, the pressure must be reduced to a working level suitable to the design strength of the sterilizer. This is done by passing the steam through a pressure regulating valve which reduces the steam pressure to about 16–18 pounds pressure per square inch (250–254°F) or 27–28 pounds pressure per square inch (270°F).

After it has passed through the pressure regulator, the steam enters the jacket which completely surrounds the sterilizer with the exception of the door, and in most cases, the rear wall of the sterilizer chamber.

The conventional type steam sterilizer is usually referred to as the gravity discharge type, in that steam is forced under pressure into the rear of the chamber where it displaces and forces the air out through a port in the lower front of the chamber known as the chamber drain line. On entering the chamber, the steam rises to the top and compresses the air at the bottom of the chamber. As indicated above, the cooler air must be removed from the chamber through the drain line; otherwise, air pockets within the chamber and the load of materials being sterilized can easily develop. In such cases, the presence of air greatly reduces the ultimate temperature of the steam below that of pure saturated steam, and the temperatures in the lower areas of the chamber and load will be substantially lower than in the upper areas due to differences in specific gravities and a reluctance of the steam and air to mix.

It is extremely important, therefore, that the opening to the chamber discharge line and the discharge line itself are free from any obstructive substances which might impede the discharge of air from the sterilizing chamber.

Steam sterilizers which are currently manufactured, are equipped with an automatic and manual control operational system. Accurate thermometers, pressure gauges, electrically operated timing mechanisms, and reliable and dependable thermostatic valves for air elimination and condensate removal are installed on each sterilizer. A recording chart is also provided on each unit for purposes of recording chamber drain-line temperatures as well as for maintaining a record of each conducted cycle. Some of the more modern sterilizers contain pilot lights in the control panel which indicate each phase of the sterilizing cycle. For convenience, and to free the operator for other duties, current sterilizers are constructed on a push-button basis which requires only the push of a button to start the sterilizing cycle after the load has been placed in the chamber and the door closed.

Representative of the gravity feed-type sterilizer commercially available are the general-purpose types, which are used for the sterilization of dressings, surgical packs, trays of instruments, and other similar materials, and the more specialized laboratory types which are designed for the sterilization of bacteriological culture media, either under steam pressure or at low temperatures, and for infant formulas.

In a properly designed steam sterilizer, effective sterilization of materials can be attained very shortly after the materials reach a temperature of 250–254°F (121–123°C). No possible benefit can result from exposing materials to heat above that necessary for the destruction of all microorganisms. To ensure that sterilization will be attained, all articles placed in the chamber should be positioned so as to allow the least possible interference to passage of air from within the article to the chamber discharge line. For example, a pack containing several layers of muslin should be placed in the chamber in such a way that the layers are vertical to the base of the sterilizing chamber. This allows free flow of air from material. Utensils such as pans, basins, or any other solid bottom container should not be placed in an upright position in the chamber since this results in air being trapped within the utensils, resulting in temperatures lower than 250°F. Items such as these should be placed on their sides, or, if possible, inverted, so that the air will be eliminated and steam will take its place.

Rubber goods present special problems in steam sterilization, particularly gloves and rubber tubing. All surfaces must be exposed to the steam. In the case of gloves, air can be trapped in the fingers. This air must be removed. In order to promote the egress of air and the intake of steam, a "wick" of steam permeable paper, muslin, or gauze must be placed in the palm of the glove, as far as the fingers. Opposing rubber surfaces of the formed cuff should be separated. In the case of rubber tubing, leave the lumen (interior) distinctly moist. This residual moisture plus the heat of the steam sterilizes the interior.

Sterilization of instruments, in steam, can be readily accomplished if the following conditions are met:

1. All instruments must be clean.
   a. All surfaces free from soil, oil, grease, or any anhydrous substance.
2. All surfaces must be exposed to permit direct contact with steam.
3. Instruments must be arranged in a tray and/or wrapped which permits free circulation of steam.

Saturated steam at 250–254°F (121–123°C) will destroy the most resistant forms of microbial life in a brief interval of exposure, and is not deleterious to most materials and supplies. Exposure periods for attaining sterility under these conditions are well within practical limits and allow ample time for heat penetration into loads of porous materials. Any given exposure period is measured from the instant the chamber drain line thermometer registers a temperature of 250°F, which is the minimum range considered safe for sterilization.

Many materials are normally sterilized by steam under pressure; however, there are some materials which should be sterilized by dry heat. These include such items as oils, greases, powders, and similar materials. Minimum exposure periods have been established for sterilizing many materials compatible with steam. These exposure times are based on the proper methods of material packaging, proper loading of the sterilizer chamber, and temperatures of 250–254°F (121–123°C). The table on page 304 lists some of the standardized exposure periods which provide minimum time for heat penetration and sterilization.

During the past decade, developments in steam sterilization have resulted in relatively short time cycles through the use of a vacuum pump for mechanical removal of air from the chamber and load, plus a higher sterilizing temperature (270–285°F). It has been determined that by drawing a vacuum on the chamber to an absolute pressure of 25 mm of mercury, almost all of the air removal under proper vacuum conditions is accomplished in a short period of time and this, plus a temperature of 270–285°F, will result in a considerable shortening of the penetration time or load lag, the minimum time-temperature ratio, and the safety factor. Utilization of equipment such as this increases productivity and prolongs the life of materials.

Failure to attain sterility in a properly designed steam sterilizer can easily occur if one is not cognizant of the principles of steam sterilization.

The following items are probably the most common factors causing sterility failures:

1. Failure to obtain the proper temperature in the sterilizer and load of materials.
2. Reliance on an incorrect or malfunctioning pressure gauge as an indicator of temperature in the chamber.
3. Entrapped air in the chamber or the load of materials.
4. Improper packaging of materials.
5. Use of steam-impermeable wrapping materials.
6. Improper loading of items within the sterilizer resulting in the formation of air pockets or protection of contaminated articles from contact with the steam.
7. Exposing materials which are incompatible with steam.

Minimum Exposure Periods for Sterilization of Supplies, Using Steam Under Pressure in Gravity Discharge Type Hospital Sterilizers

	250–254°F (121–123°C) Minutes	270°F (132°C) Minutes
Brushes, in dispensers, in cans or individually wrapped	30	15
Dressings, wrapped in paper or muslin	30	15
Dressings, in canisters (on sides)	30	15
Square-Pak Flasked solutions		
75 ml	20	
250–500 ml	25	
1000 ml	30	
1500 ml	35	
2000 ml	40	
Glassware, empty, inverted	15	3
Instruments, metal only, any number (unwrapped)	15	3
Instruments, metal, combined with suture, tubing or other porous materials (unwrapped)	20	10
Instruments, metal only, covered and/or padded tray	20	10
Instruments, metal, combined with other materials (in covered and/or padded tray)	30	15
Instruments, wrapped in double thickness muslin	30	15
Linen, packs (maximal size: 12 inches × 12 inches × 12 inches; maximal weight: 12 pounds)	30	
Needles, unwrapped (lumen moist)	15	3
Needles, individually packaged in glass tubes or paper (lumen moist)	30	15
Rubber gloves, wrapped in muslin or paper	20	
Rubber catheters, drains, tubing etc. (lumen moist), unwrapped	20	10
Rubber catheters, drains, tubing, etc. individually packaged in muslin or paper (lumen moist)	30	15
Treatment trays, wrapped in muslin or paper	30	
Utensils, unwrapped	15	3
Utensils, wrapped in muslin or paper	20	10
Syringes, unassembled, individually packaged in muslin or paper	30	15
Syringes, unassembled, unwrapped	15	3
Sutures, silk, cotton or nylon, wrapped in paper or muslin	30	15

To obtain satisfactory sterilization routinely, it is much more desirable that the sterilizer is properly operated, as much air as possible is removed from the chamber, the temperature of the discharge line is taken as a guide for the degree of heat attained in the chamber rather than a steam pressure gauge, and that all materials to be sterilized are properly wrapped or packaged and loaded into the chamber.

Dry Heat

Sterilization of materials by dry heat is a method commonly employed in many hospitals and laboratories. It is a restrictive method, however, as it is recommended only where the direct contact of materials or items to saturated steam is impractical or unattainable. The method also requires the use of specially designed equipment as the temperatures required to achieve sterilization are otherwise difficult to control within narrow limits. The slow and uneven penetrating powers of dry heat, plus the relatively long exposure periods required for effective sterilization, further limit this method as an ideal process.

Generally, dry heat sterilization, which is essentially an oxidation process, is conducted at a temperature of 320°F (160°C) for a minimum period of two hours, although two and one-half hours are preferred. This condition refers to the actual temperature of the materials being exposed, and does not allow for the time required for the materials to reach this temperature. Other dry heat temperatures can be effectively employed in achieving sterility and minimum standards have been suggested, e.g.,

340°F (171°C) for one hour
320°F (160°C) for two hours
300°F (179°C) for two and one-half hours
285°F (140°C) for three hours
250°F (121°C) for six hours or longer.

The ability of dry heat to sterilize is influenced by a number of factors. For example, microorganisms show a relatively wide variation in their resistance to dry heat, with bacterial spores showing much higher resistances than bacterial vegetative cells. Mold spores, although showing a certain resistance to dry heat, appear to fall in between the vegetative and sporulating bacteria. Another factor is the presence of organic matter, such as a film of grease or oil surrounding the organism and forming a protective or insulating carrier to heat.

Hot air or dry heat sterilizers are basically of two types, i.e., the gravity convection unit, and the mechanical convection or forced air circulation type. When electrically operated, sterilization temperatures can be accurately and dependably controlled. The gravity type sterilizer is much slower in heating, as it depends entirely upon the natural rise of warm air currents to the top of the sterilizer and the downward movement and heating of the cooler air. The speed of circulation is dependent upon the ventilation mechanism on the top of the sterilizer and its adjustment, and the temperature differential between the area over the heaters and the exhaust port.

Longer exposure periods are required for this type of sterilizer, as there is less uniform temperature throughout the chamber. It should be used only for applications where rapid and precisely controlled heating and accelerated air circulation are not required. For maximum functional efficiency at a minimum cost, the mechanical convection or forced air circulating sterilizer is preferred. A rapid movement of large volumes of hot air to convey heat directly to the load under controlled temperature is provided in this sterilizer by a motor-driven, turbo-blower. Uniform controlled temperatures can be maintained as well as air velocity, direction of circulation, and heat intensity within the chamber regardless of the type of load. On some units of this type, an exposure timer which does not actuate until the desired chamber temperature is reached, and an alarm system signaling the end of a desired exposure time are provided.

As indicated above, dry heat sterilization is applicable to only certain materials. For example, certain instruments have component parts that must be sterilized. If, in the steam sterilization of these instruments, moisture cannot directly contact all parts, then sterility of the instrument cannot be guaranteed. The method of choice of these cases is dry heat. The action of dry heat on objects such as these is that of conduction. Heat is absorbed by the exterior surface and eventually it heats the interior. Other items which can be sterilized by dry heat include anhydrous oils, fats, petrolatum, and other petroleum products and powders. Surgical items such as instruments, suture needles, and glass syringes are often sterilized by dry heat as well as scalpel blades and other instruments with sharp cutting edges. Medicants, including several of the sulfonamide powders, talcum, zinc oxide, and zinc peroxide, can also be sterilized by hot air provided they are properly prepared in recommended quantities and containers.

Materials which cannot be sterilized by dry heat include fabrics, rubber goods, and a number of plastic items, as they will rapidly deteriorate when exposed to the high temperatures. The proper loading of a hot air sterilizer is as equally important as the loading of a steam sterilizer. When loading for example: never load the chamber to the limit; allow space between packaged items; and keep all articles away from the chamber sidewalls, so that the hot air may freely circulate. It is also important to keep in mind that all materials, when placed in a hot air sterilizer, do not reach the desired sterilization temperature at the same time. This fact places an additional responsibility on the operator of the hot air sterilizer in terms of knowing or determining the time required for a given load of materials to come up to the desired sterilization temperature before the actual exposure or sterilizing time is started.

Ethylene Oxide

Sterilization by ethylene oxide gas is rapidly gaining in popularity throughout the medical and industrial fields. Sterilizing equipment is commercially available for the processing of materials in relatively any volume or load size. The main advantage of gaseous sterilization is that it enables one to sterilize any item which is heat-labile or moisture-sensitive.

Ethylene oxide is highly toxic, flammable, and explosive in its pure state; however, by diluting the gas with such inert gases as nitrogen, carbon dioxide, or some of the halogenated hydrocarbons (Freon or Ganetrol 11 and/or 12), ethylene oxide can be made quite safe for normal usage. Some of the mixtures in current use are: Carboxide* (10% EtO–90% Co_2), Benvicide† (11% EtO–54% Freon 12 and 35% Freon 11), Oxyfume Sterilant 12* (12% EtO–88% Freon 11) or Pennoxide‡ (12% EtO–88% Freon-12).

Ethylene oxide sterilization is a somewhat more complex process when compared to steam or dry heat sterilization, as there are several factors which should be understood by the individual contemplating gaseous sterilization. To illustrate, the effectiveness of ethylene oxide is dependent upon its concentration; the time in which it is allowed to remain in contact with materials; the temperature of the materials and the atmosphere surrounding the materials, and the moisture content (humidity) of the materials to be sterilized. The importance of these factors is briefly described below.

Concentration. To achieve sterilization, a suitable concentration of ethylene oxide gas must be introduced into the sterilizing chamber. For practical applications, a minimum concentration of 450 milligrams per liter of chamber space is required in order to achieve sterilization in a reasonable period of time (6–16 hours). Higher concentrations are desirable as exposure periods can be considerably reduced.

Exposure Time. The destructive effect of ethylene oxide on micro-organisms is not a rapid process. However, in normal practice where

*Linde Products, Union Carbide Corp., New York.
†Matheson Co., East Rutherford, New Jersey.
‡Pennsylvania Engineering Co., North Howard Street, Philadelphia, Pa.

articles to be sterilized have been properly cleaned and suitably packaged in recommended packaging materials, exposure times of approximately two hours can be employed using proper gas concentration and temperature.

Temperature. Temperature has a significant effect on ethylene oxide as it enhances the penetration properties of the gas and affords a reduction in the exposure time. In normal practice, temperatures of 49–60°C (120–140°F) are employed; however, there are some instances, such as the sterilization of heat-labile plastic materials, where lower temperatures are required.

Humidity. Humidity or moisture has been established as necessary in ethylene oxide sterilization, and in some cases, it is desirable to have it present on, or in the materials to be sterilized. Sterilization of porous materials can be achieved at relatively low humidities of 20–30% RH, whereas, hard or solid-surface items require humidities of 50–60% RH because of moisture absorption characteristics. Normally, humidities of 50–60% RH are recommended for gaseous sterilization because of the possibilities of loads containing both porous and nonporous articles or materials.

There are two other important factors which have a significant influence on the sterilizing efficiency of ethylene oxide. These are the resistance and protection of microorganisms by extraneous materials and packaging materials. It has been established through research that microorganisms vary greatly in their resistance to ethylene oxide.

Vegetative cells are much less resistant than spores, and spores can vary in resistance, depending upon their state of hydration. Resistance of microorganisms is also found when they are protected by extraneous materials. For example, organisms suspended in salt solutions and dried on materials are often very difficult to kill because they become embedded in dried crystals which are impervious to the ethylene oxide. Heavily contaminated areas on materials are also difficult to sterilize, as organisms can be protected by other surrounding organisms.

Although ethylene oxide has unusual penetrative properties, it cannot permeate through impervious packaging materials, such as aluminum foil or certain plastic films commonly used for wrapping purposes. It is important, therefore, that only those materials which are permeable to moisture and ethylene oxide be used in this type of process. Further information on packaging materials will be presented later in this chapter.

Sterilization of materials by ethylene oxide is usually conducted in specially designed gas sterilizing chambers. These units are operated on either an automatic or manual basis according to a predetermined plan or cycle. A typical cycle comprises the following steps:

1. The materials to be sterilized are placed in the chamber which has been preheated to $54 \pm 3°C$ ($130 \pm 5°F$) and the door is closed.
2. The operator sets the desired exposure time on the timing mechanism and pushes the starting button. At this point, the operator usually leaves the sterilizer, to perform other duties, as the sterilizer is normally operated on an automatic basis.
3. When the starter button is pushed, the gas cycle is initiated and undergoes the following phases:
   a. The chamber is evacuated to approximately 27 inches mercury to remove the greater portion of air within the chamber and packaged materials.
   b. The materials are heated and moisturized.
   c. The ethylene oxide gas mixture is introduced into the chamber to a preselected pressure and is automatically shut off when the pressure is reached.
   d. The exposure time is started as soon as the desired chamber pressure level has been attained and the gas flow has been stopped.
   e. Following the exposure time, the chamber is again automatically evacuated to approximately 27 inches mercury.
   f. Freshly filtered air is admitted into the chamber to release the vacuum to atmospheric pressure.
   g. The materials are then removed from the chamber in a sterile condition.

Figure 7-5 illustrates a schematic diagram of a typical gas cycle employing an ethylene oxide-halogenated hydrocarbon mixture.

To maintain exposed materials in a sterile condition, it is customary to wrap the items in a suitable packaging material. Certain criteria have been established in the selection of proper wrapping materials which should be compatible with the gas sterilizing cycle, as well as affording the maintenance of sterility in the exposed articles. These criteria include:

1. The wrapping material must be permeable to the ethylene oxide— the sterilizing agent—and to moisture.
2. The wrapping material must act as a dust filter in preventing the free passage of air through the package after sterilization. This includes the ability to properly seal the wrapping material after enclosing the articles to be sterilized.

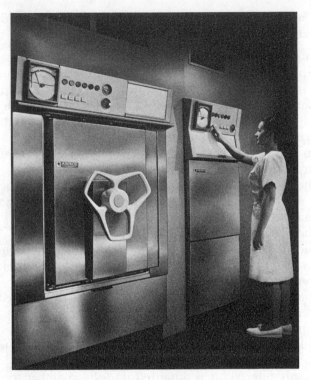

Figure 7-5 A modern combination steam and gas sterilizer with an ethylene oxide gas console. (Reprinted with permission from Amsco Equipment Co., Erie, Pa.)

3. The wrapping material must be durable in order to withstand necessary handling.
4. The wrapping material must be pliable and flexible so that the package can be easily opened and the contents removed without becoming contaminated.
5. The wrapping material should provide a certain amount of protection to delicate or breakable items.
6. The wrapping material should be relatively inexpensive and commercially available.

In current practices of gaseous sterilization, packaging materials such as paper, muslin (cloth), and certain plastic films are commonly employed because of their relatively high permeable properties to moisture and ethylene oxide. Plastic films are quite popular in that they are pliable and flexible and enable the operator to identify the articles enclosed in the film because of their transparency. Polyethylene film (low density — 3.0–4.0 mil) is highly recommended for gaseous sterilization based on experimental evidence and actual use in the field. There are many other plastic films which are used for packaging purposes; however, their compatibility to a gas sterilizing process has not been fully determined at this time. Therefore, care must be taken in selecting a wrapping material for this purpose.

A final factor concerning ethylene oxide sterilization pertains to the necessity of adequately aerating exposed materials or articles prior to use. This is predicated on the established fact that most, if not all, materials other than metal, absorb ethylene oxide during exposure and that this residual gas must be removed from the exposed items before use, to prevent toxic effects on human tissues. The removal of residual ethylene oxide from exposed items is normally accomplished by holding or quarantining the items for a period of time at room temperature in a well ventilated area. Under these conditions, aeration periods of not less than 24 hours are recommended as the dissipation of the ethylene oxide from materials at room temperatures is relatively slow. In some instances, aeration times have been extended up to seven days, particularly in relation to plastic tubing which is to be used on heart-lung machines and four to five days for certain human implants such as heart pacemakers. Because of the wide variety of materials which are gas sterilized and the broad variations in their ability to absorb and retain ethylene oxide, it is extremely difficult to determine precise aeration periods for each individual item processed by this method; consequently, it is recommended that all exposed articles be aerated for at least 24 hours or longer at room temperature in a well ventilated area. Aeration periods for some materials can be reduced, however, if facilities are available for subjecting the exposed articles to elevated temperatures of 49°C (120°F).

Methods of aeration, other than allowing exposed materials to stand at room temperature, have been explored. These include the subjection of gas-sterilized articles to multiple vacuum in a chamber and allowing bacterial free air to enter the chamber after each vacuum, or exposing the sterilized materials to forced air circulation in a ventilated area or chamber. None of which were useful in desorbing gas from the materials at an accelerated rate. Tests in the authors' laboratories indicate that the removal of total residual gases from certain exposed items can be accelerated by holding them at 120°F (49°C) for a period of five to eight hours. A series of tests were conducted in a recently developed gas aeration unit. This unit is shown in Figure 7-6.

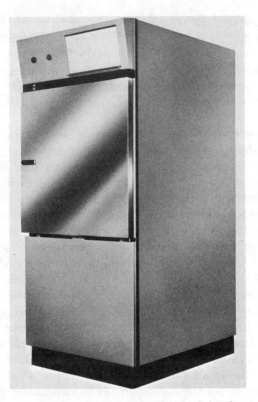

Figure 7-6   Ethylene oxide aerator. (Reprinted with permission from Amsco Equipment Co., Erie, Pa.)

These tests comprised the exposure of weighed (2.0 gram) samples of Tygon, gum rubber, vinyl tubing and polyethylene film to various gas mixtures. Immediately following exposure, all exposed samples were weighed to determine the quantity of total gas absorbed. The materials were then aerated at room temperature and in the Gas Aerator (120°F–49°C) and reweighed at periodic intervals to determine the dissipation rate of the absorbed gas. The aeration of the exposed materials at an elevated temperature enhanced the dissipation rate of absorbed gases, resulting in a faster removal. The general observation was that most gas-sterilized items could be aerated in one third the time in a Gas Aerator, than it takes to aerate at ambient temperatures.

It is impossible, unfortunately, to establish a single criterion or aeration period required for the removal of ethylene oxide and/or its diluent gases from every article or commodity which can be gas sterilized as this depends on: the nature of the article; the materials in which it is packaged; the intended use of the article; and the lack of definite information on the levels of ethylene oxide which can be demonstrated to be nontoxic to all human tissues and blood.

It is felt by the authors that the extent and judgment to which gas-sterilized articles are treated to remove residual gases following exposure, should rest with those personnel who are responsible for patient care in the medical and surgical fields. In view of this opinion, it is imperative that all personnel who use and/or operate gas sterilizing equipment be properly and thoroughly instructed on the need for proper aeration of gas-sterilized materials and the consequences which may arise from the use of such materials immediately after exposure to ethylene oxide. The final judgment on required aeration times of ethylene oxide sterilized articles is the responsibility of those concerned with the medical and/or surgical application of these articles and materials, and the circumstances under which these are to be employed.*

As previously indicated, ethylene oxide sterilization is a relatively complex process and the failure to achieve sterility by this method is as easy as it is with steam or dry heat. It is, therefore, the responsibility of the sterilizer operators to:

1. Prepare, assemble, and package or wrap materials to be gas sterilized in a proper manner.
2. Use only recommended packaging materials.
3. Use care in loading the sterilizer, ensuring that the packaged items are properly spaced for gas circulation.
4. Use only recommended exposure times.
5. Understand thoroughly the principles of gaseous sterilization and the relationship of each of the four factors (time, temperature, concentration and humidity) involved in this process.
6. Regard the sterilizer as a relatively sensitive instrument in that it requires proper care and maintenance for continued performance and reproducible sterilization cycles.
7. Avoid all tendencies to find or employ short-cuts in the sterilization of materials.

7-4-4   Sterilization Controls

The attainment of sterility in a load of exposed materials can be determined only by a suitable control system. The use of such a system is

*For further information and additional reading: Ethylene oxide sterilization, *The Journal of Hospital Research*, Vol. 7, No. 1, February 1969, is available.

essential in that, it is almost invariably impossible to test each exposed item for sterility because it may be too large for convenient testing, or it may constitute only one of its kind available, etc.

Sterilization controls are divided into three groups: (1) mechanical, (2) chemical, and (3) biological. The mechanical controls comprise certain instruments or devices installed on, or in the sterilizing chambers. These include such items as pressure regulating valves, indicating and/or recording thermometers, and pressure gauges for showing chamber and/or chamber jacket pressures. These controls are essential and should be used in the operation of all sterilizers as they provide a means of showing whether sterilizing conditions are occurring or being reached within the sterilizer. They will not, however, definitely show that materials exposed to sterilizing conditions are actually sterile.

Chemical sterility controls are also mechanisms which indicate only that materials have been exposed to sterilizing conditions. Examples of these controls include: chemical tapes which change color when subjected to specific temperatures, or ethylene oxide concentrations; and certain chemical solids, enclosed in sealed glass tubes, which melt when exposed to certain temperatures for a period of time.

Biological controls are recommended as the preferred sterility control system, as the ultimate purpose of a sterilizer is the destruction of microorganisms. On this basis, biological controls comprise a number of different, specially prepared, and packaged items or substances which are contaminated with or contain known, populations of spores from known species of bacteria. The selected spores* also have a known resistance to moist heat, dry heat, or ethylene oxide. In use, the biological controls are placed in a test pack to be exposed and subjected to the same sterilizing condition as the load. Following the removal of the load from the sterilizer, the sterility controls are aseptically removed from their respective enclosures and cultured in tube of suitable bacteriological culture media. The tubes are incubated at the optimum temperatures of the test organisms for a minimum period of seven days.† If, at the end of this incubation period, all the tubes are free of bacterial growth, the exposed materials are regarded as sterile. Controls of this type should be used in every load of materials processed until the operator is satisfied that the sterilizer is operating correctly. From this point, biological controls should be used at regular, periodical periods as a constant check on the exposure time of the sterilizer.

Bacillus subtilis var *globigii* for gas sterilization and dry heat, *Bacillus stearothermophilus* for moist heat under pressure.

†The United States Pharmacopeia, (USP), Eighteenth Revision, Sept. 1, 1970, page 855.

Sterilization is an essential requirement of many materials in many fields and is of special importance in the medical field where the life or death of a patient depends on the use of sterile materials. Because of this importance, it is mandatory that personnel operating sterilizing equipment must be properly trained in all phases of sterilizer operation as well as in the principles of sterilization.

REFERENCES AND SELECTED READINGS

Ethylene oxide sterilization, *Journal of Hospital Research*, Vol. 7, No. 1, February 1969.

McCulloch, E. C. *Disinfection and Sterilization*. Philadelphia: Lea & Febiger, 2nd ed., 1945.

Perkins, J. J. *Principles and Methods of Sterilization*, Springfield, Ill.: Charles C Thomas, 1956.

Pre-vacuum, high temperature steam sterilization, *Journal of Hospital Research*, Vol. 1, No. 3, July 1963.

Reddish, G. F. *Antiseptics, Disinfectants, Fungicides, and Chemical and Physical Sterilization*. Philadelphia: Lea & Febiger, 2nd ed., 1957.

Rubbo, S. D. and Gardner, J. F. *A Review of Sterilization and Disinfection*, London: Lloyd Luke, 1965.

Stumbo, C. R. *Thermobacteriology in Food Processing*. New York: Academic Press, 1965.

Sykes, G. *Disinfection and Sterilization*, Princeton: D. Van Nostrand, Inc.

51